Therapy, Spirituality, and East Asian Imaginaries

Therapy, Spirituality, and East Asian Imaginaries

Edited by
Ioannis Gaitanidis,
Luis Fernando Bernardi Junqueira,
Avery Morrow, and
Sangyun Han

Routledge
Taylor & Francis Group
LONDON AND NEW YORK

First published in 2025 by Amsterdam University Press Ltd.

Published 2025 by Routledge
4 Park Square, Milton Park, Abingdon, Oxon OX14 4RN
605 Third Avenue, New York, NY 10158

Routledge is an imprint of the Taylor & Francis Group, an informa business

ISBN: 9789048559015 (hbk)
ISBN: 9781041189534 (pbk)
ISBN: 9781003708261 (ebk)
NUR 728

Cover image: Cançado, Juracy Campos. *Do-In: Livro dos primeiros socorros* [Do-In: The Book of First Aid]

Cover design: Coördesign, Leiden

DOI: 10.5117/9789048559015

This work was supported by the Wellcome Trust [Reference: 217661/Z/19/Z].

Funded by

wellcome

For Product Safety Concerns and Information please contact our EU representative:
GPSR@taylorandfrancis.com
Taylor & Francis Verlag GmbH, Kaufingerstraße 24, 80331 München, Germany.

Table of Contents

Part 3 Alternative Therapies Across Epistemic Fields and Professions

Part 4 Alternative Therapies and National Identities

Figures and Tables

Acknowledgements

The topic of this volume and several of the chapters composing it are based on the first international conference of the East Asian Network for the Academic Study of Esotericism (EANASE), held entirely online over four weekends in November 2021. The conference's theme was *Spirituality, Healthcare and Social Movements in East Asia: A Transnational Perspective*. It gathered 25 presentations, and its recordings were later made available for seven days on EANASE's YouTube channel and were viewed nearly 200 times. EANASE is the brainchild of Professor Yoshinaga Shin'ichi 吉永進一 (1957–2022), the foremost scholar of the academic study of esotericism in Japan, who was also famous for his unrelenting efforts to encourage connections among researchers around the globe. As the first academic publication coming out of EANASE's activities, we dedicate this volume to Professor Yoshinaga and hope that he would have been proud of what we have been able to achieve thanks to the fruits of his labour.

A volume such as this one cannot be anything else than the result of collaboration. We, the co-editors, would like to thank all the chapter authors for their impeccable cooperation, the two anonymous reviewers for their insightful and extensive comments, the series editor and the editorial committee of the Health, Medicine, and Science in Asia series, as well as Amsterdam University Press for their support. All remaining shortcomings are our responsibility.

Note on Naming, Use of Italics, and Other Conventions

All Japanese, Chinese, and Korean names are given in the order of surname first, followed by forename(s), with a few exceptions where a scholar's primary language of publication is English and they have adopted the Anglophone naming convention of forename(s) first, followed by surname. Except for therapies, such as yoga, which have entered English vocabulary, all names of therapies (such as *shiatsu*) and concepts (such as *ki* or *chi*) originally written in Chinese, Japanese, and Korean are italicised. These conventions are followed throughout the main text, notes, and references sections of this book.

Therapy, Spirituality, and East Asian Imaginaries: An Introduction

Ioannis Gaitanidis, Luis Fernando Bernardi Junqueira, Avery Morrow, and Sangyun Han

Abstract: This volume is a transnational, transcultural, and transepistemic study of post-1970s alternative therapies and spiritualities associated with East Asia. Although the East and the West remain formative in discourses of authenticity surrounding spirituality and therapy, they have led to problematic usages of *-isation* (Easternisation, Westernisation) arguments to describe the changes such practices undergo in transnational settings. We argue that these descriptions ignore that the therapeutic cultures associated with East Asia blossomed in an already intertwined world. Instead of assuming a common 'East Asia-ness', we propose, therefore, to pay attention to how forms of knowledge identified as 'East Asian' came to be adopted, adapted, and disseminated by individuals and groups across the globe in order to achieve specific therapeutic and spiritual agendas.

Keywords: post-1970s, alternative medicine, New Age, transnational movement, spirituality

In this volume, we will discuss a range of ideas and techniques that tend to fall loosely under the umbrella of 'complementary and alternative medicine' and that have, since the 1970s, been increasingly associated with concepts, ideologies, and practices considered to be stemming from East Asia – namely China, Japan, and South Korea. However, as some of the authors will demonstrate, the alternativity of these therapies is often a subject of contestation and dispute. Their knowledge may be perceived as 'marginal', 'fringe', or 'heterodox' vis-à-vis biomedicine (Bivins 2008; Bernard 2018; Bynum and Porter 2018), but it is often not 'rejected' – at least not amongst the population at large. Indeed, the mainstream to which these ideas are

Gaitanidis, Ioannis, Luis Fernando Bernardi Junqueira, Avery Morrow, and Sangyun Han (eds), *Therapy, Spirituality, and East Asian Imaginaries*. Taylor & Francis Group 2025
DOI: 10.5117/9789048559015_INTRO

compared is already entangled with them conceptually and, even more often, politically, through the opening of spaces of collective processes of sense-making, therapeutic experience, and national imagination.

More recently, the growing global concern with mental health and the perceived limitations of biomedicine in addressing psychological and spiritual needs has sparked the publication of a series of outstanding works dedicated to the interdisciplinary study of spirituality and healthcare, combining insights from varied fields such as anthropology, history, religious studies, psychology, and the medical humanities (e.g., Harrington 2008; Zhan 2009; Moreira-Almeida et al. 2021; Hickey 2019; Lüddeckens et al. 2022). With a few exceptions, the majority of these works focus on the modern Euro-American world. While some authors have acknowledged East Asia as a fertile ground for research, only a handful of studies written in English have examined the intersection between spirituality and healthcare from a broader transnational perspective centred around modern East Asia (e.g., Gaitanidis 2022; Stein 2023). The present volume's main objective is to ask how localised movements have been initially inspired by and have continuously taken shape in relation to global concerns. The period starting in the 1970s is particularly relevant as it marks the heyday of the counterculture and the New Age, a wave of transnational movements that have consciously – and sometimes stereotypically – drawn on East Asia to challenge conventional Euro-American conceptions of healing, health, and well-being.

Consider the following vignette, extracted from Ioannis Gaitanidis' fieldwork in contemporary Japan.

Satoko, a Japanese therapist, has been practising reiki and other 'spiritual therapies' in the western outskirts of Tokyo for the last 20 years. She has turned a small study room of her apartment into a salon, where she receives clients, primarily through word of mouth, but also thanks to a very simple internet blog updated regularly with photos of day trips that she takes with her pet or of desserts that she enjoys with friends. Scholars of Japan may associate Satoko with a 'spiritual-but-not-religious' mood that has been discursively linked to the popular criticism against religion after the 1995 attack on the Tokyo subway by the religious organisation Aum Shinrikyō. Yet, she confesses to having been interested in collecting fortune-telling cards and in the aesthetics of esoteric imagery she found in Japanese translations of New Age books since the 1980s. When sociologists started talking of a shift of consciousness from 'religion' to 'spirituality' in the late 1990s, Satoko was already learning about clairvoyant healing from an American Wiccan who had relocated to Tokyo and who ended up establishing a school in

Japan for the next two decades. Today, Satoko sounds nostalgic about that period when 'Western teachers embraced the East, bringing in all these new therapies one after the other. [...] But, you know, they were more influenced by Asian ideas than we were buying into their theories'.

The confluence of 'spirituality' and 'therapy' with representations and imaginations about 'East Asian wisdom' is not uncommon or novel within practices that are explained as alternatives to, or as overcoming the limitations of, each of these two terms. As an alternative to religion, the 'rise of spirituality' has often been linked to the absorption by countercultural writers of East Asian philosophies, whereas much of complementary and alternative medicine shares structural arguments about illness aetiology and symptomatology with new, old, and most often reinvented healing traditions originating within the Asian continent. These contacts and exchanges with especially East Asia are commonly expressed using *-isation* concepts that end up dichotomising the world: the more than 100-year-old idea of the 'westernisation of the East' (see Holcombe 2017, 259–87; also Davidann 2018 for a critique) was later accompanied by the 'eastern*isation* of the West' (Campbell 2008). This conceptualisation attempts to capture the changes that are associated with the global flows of knowledge, while unavoidably assuming that sometime, somewhere there have always been homogenous or authentic 'East(s)' and 'West(s)' ready to be transformed, improved, or corrupted by their opposite 'Other'. What further prevents scrutiny is the identification of key historical moments – such as the Aum attack in Japan in 1995 or China's systematic crackdown on *qigong* in the late 1990s – that are employed by scholars as harbingers of radical social change, eternal points of reference between a before and an after that undercut any possibility of slow, gradual, and emergent shifts to which such events could be mere outliers.

Personal narratives such as those of Satoko make clear that even though the 'East' and the 'West' remain critical formative elements in discourses of authenticity surrounding spirituality and therapy, the game of verifying who influenced who, when, and how is fraught with essentialist traps. To put it more simply, is there a point in arguing that Satoko has become a practitioner of Westernised spiritual therapies learned from Eastern-inspired or Western reinterpretations she found in books and seminars produced by American authors who had relocated to Japan? This sentence tells us little about how underlying stories of the evidently far more complex origins of Satoko's spiritual therapies have shaped her practice and worldview, impacting her clients and Japanese society more broadly. How are imaginations of 'East Asia' as an origin point, 'East Asia' as a label of authenticity, and 'East Asia' as an epistemic frame entangled, and what does this entanglement tell us about what these practices do? These are the two basic questions that inform this volume. Still, these same questions can also be used to problematise common uses of the concepts of 'spirituality' and 'therapy'.

Beyond East/West Reifications of Spirituality and Therapy

In religious studies literature, 'spirituality' is typically defined by its relationship – whether complementary or alternative – to 'religion' (Woodhead 2010, 38). As such, the term has been used to estimate the size and value of religion. It has, for example, been employed to indicate what lies beyond the purview of organised or institutionalised religion, namely 'the spiritual but not religious' (Fuller 2001). In this context, spirituality has been either a gauge of secularisation – following a hypothetical decline of institutional religion – or an indicator of religion's transformation in a secular environment. From a second, recently more familiar perspective, spirituality, especially in its casual appearance, has been associated with qualitative descriptions attached to religious vocabularies, such as the notion of 'fuzzy fidelity', described by David Voas (2009) as a 'casual loyalty to tradition'. Here, the use of spirituality as a category underscores existing methodological problems of naming and quantifying religious identities and works as a descriptor for the indescribable. De-traditionalised, de-institutionalised religion, detached from whatever we thought it had been previously anchored to, is now fluid, floating, implicit, generic, individual, or light. The past seems at least relatively coherent and straightforward, while the present is unstable, blurry, and relative.

As Gaitanidis has argued elsewhere (2022, 3–8), to make these ambiguous and novel phenomena more understandable within their contemporary context, scholars often employ one or more strategies to argue for their significant impact and organisation, akin to that of 'religion'. Replying to Matthew Wood's (2007) critique of the non-formativeness of the New Age movement, for example, Ann Taves and Michael Kinsella (2013) point to the existence of organisational forms, such as the Theosophical Society or Alcoholics Anonymous, that are distinct from conventional religious institutions and that have had a significant impact on the global religious landscape, without having been acknowledged for that role until very recently. The formativeness of 'spirituality' is sought in structures that are not 'religion' but 'religion-like', reinforcing thus the idea that spirituality – whatever it entails in practice – is the alternative and perhaps the religion appropriate to the modern global world. Interestingly, many of the descriptions of what spirituality means for those who espouse it across the globe tend to reflect the diffusion of an understanding of spirituality associated with no other than Daisetz T. Suzuki (1870–1966).

Suzuki is famous for his sustained efforts to popularise a specific version of Zen Buddhism in the so-called Western world, fashioned by Suzuki's own life story and varied interests within and particularly without contemporaneous Buddhist thought, including Swedenborgianism and Theosophy. Suzuki's participation in the production of the 20th century's orientalist idea of spirituality has been given ample attention, as has his influence on Japanese discussions of *reisei* 霊性, the two-character word he adopted to translate the English concept of 'spirituality' into Japanese. More specifically, in his most famous work, *Japanese Spirituality* (1972; originally published in Japanese as *Nihon-teki reisei* 日本的霊性 in 1944), Suzuki discusses *reisei* as something akin to a universal essence that transcends the duality of mind and body, and whose institutionalised form gives birth to religion. The often-heard idea that spirituality is a sort of primaeval, universal religion, which organised religions around the world have sought to canalise, control, and manipulate, is very much D.T. Suzuki's phrasing. But it is also an idea born out of what many contemporaneous scholars would not have associated with 'religion'.

Andō Reiji (2020, 67–68) notes, indeed, that Suzuki probably borrowed the compound *reisei* from the work of Guifeng Zongmi 圭峰宗密 (780–841), the fifth Chinese patriarch of the Huayan (Kegon) school of Buddhism. The first time Suzuki employed *reisei* to mean 'spirituality' was in his Japanese translations of Emanuel Swedenborg's (1688–1772) works, most notably *Heaven and Hell* (1785) (Yoshinaga 2005). Behind the choice of that word, however, Andō locates Suzuki's understanding of 'spirituality' as influenced by the work of the American zoologist Edward Drinker Cope (1840–1897), who had claimed that the force behind the evolution of species connects mind and matter and originates from a universal and transcendental consciousness. Cope's works about this idea, as well as Henri Bergson's texts on the *élan vital* (vital force), also inspired by Cope, were published by Open Court Press (La Salle, Illinois), where Suzuki worked for 11 years as a translator and interpreter, and where he published some of his own texts. The spirituality that Suzuki incorporated into his alleged self-orientalist, sometimes 'Westernised' extrapolations of Zen stemmed from the worldview of a 19th-century devout Quaker scientist!

Knowing the above, trying to explain the very usage of 'spirituality' using the epithets 'Eastern' and 'Western' may invite derision: a Japanese scholar uses an originally Chinese word to describe in his lectures on Zen Buddhism an idea that he adapted from a 19th-century American zoologist. Does that mean that 'spirituality' is the Westernisation of an Eastern concept? Or is it Suzuki who should be accused of Easternising a Western idea? Replying to these questions does not seem to be leading us anywhere, but knowing that Cope inspired Suzuki perhaps sheds new light on the reasons why D.T. Suzuki's English writings became so popular and influential worldwide. Indeed, as noted by Jørn Borup and Marianne Q. Fibiger, rather than merely focusing on one-way directions of influence, it is more fruitful to locate these entanglements 'into broader understandings of the dynamics of religion and spirituality including human circulation (through migration, mission and personal encounters) and circulation of ideas, practices, concepts, materiality and imaginaries' (2015, 2). Here, not only do we wish to stress the role of the 'East' and 'West' as social imaginaries rather than ontological or reified categories, but also, and in contrast to Borup and Fibiger (2015, 5–6), we contest the use of 'spirituality' as an analytical category that is fundamentally distinct from 'religion' and 'medicine'.

The same argument can be made in regard to normative understandings of the concept of 'therapy'. However one chooses to categorise them – alternative medicine, complementary medicine, natural medicine, fringe medicine, heterodox medicine – it is undeniable that therapies originated in or inspired by East Asian elements have by now become an integral part of the daily life of millions worldwide. Recent studies on global therapeutics (Sax and Lang 2021; Nehring et al. 2020) have critiqued past assumptions that the construction and globalisation of modern autonomous individuals have been driven exclusively by the psychological disciplines that arose out of specific Euro-American scientific theories and professional associations during the long 20th century. In reality, we know now that therapeutic cultures – in and outside the psychological disciplines – have constantly been formed in dialogue with several conceptual universes from across the globe, particularly from East Asia (Lüddeckens et al. 2021; Moreira-Almeida et al. 2021). But this dialogue should not be reduced to *-isation* arguments. As the case studies in this volume will illustrate, the therapeutic cultures associated with East Asia – from Traditional Chinese Medicine and mindfulness to *shiatsu* and GiCheon – blossomed in an *already* interconnected world. To understand their initial formation and enduring appeal to a wide range of practitioners and customers, it is thus paramount to move between transnational concerns (macro) and local appropriations (micro), an approach Jacques Revel (1996) has called *jeux d'échelles* (scale games). In other words, we should avoid polarising arguments that either appreciate the global as a mere backdrop to the local or overemphasise the global over local factors.

In this volume, we are more concerned with how the above entanglements actually work rather than with the description of these entanglements in terms of simple processes or flows. To what extent have, for example, transnational movements like the counterculture and the New Age facilitated, if not fostered, this interplay between the macro and the micro? And what kind of stories have been generated from such seamless therapeutic and spiritual networks?

From mesmerism, spiritualism, and Theosophy in the 19th century to the counterculture, the New Age, and mindfulness movements in the 20th and 21st centuries, multiple actors in and outside East Asia have invoked the therapeutic and spiritual cultures of China, Japan, and Korea as means to challenge the limitations of reductive materialism and thereby offer alternatives to biomedical views of the body and mind, health and illness, life and death (Caplan 1998; Harrington 2008; Vargas-O'Bryan and Xun 2015; Hickey 2019; Cohen 2021). Furthermore, the wave of new religious movements that have flourished across East Asia over the last two centuries has rarely sought to reject 'Western science' altogether; on the contrary, many of these groups have aimed to incorporate science into their belief systems, sometimes in provocative and creative ways (Yoshinaga 2004; Palmer 2007; Pokorny and Winter 2018; Clart, Ownby and Wang 2020; Ichiyanagi 2011; Junqueira 2023). Such entanglements have had long-lasting effects. For example, the formation of modern psychology and the mind-cure craze that swept across the world from the late 19th through the first half of the 20th century led to the emergence of 'mind' and 'mental health' as distinct frames of reference to understand health and sickness (Moreira-Almeida et al. 2021; Hickey 2019; Cohen 2021) – and these categories have played an equally fundamental role in new religious and esoteric movements, in both East Asia and beyond (Palmer 2007; Harding, Iwata and Yoshinaga 2016; Pokorny and Winter 2018; Zheng 2018; Chang 2020; Junqueira 2023).

Since the 1960s, following the rise of the counterculture and alongside a growing frustration with what people interpreted as the false promises of mainstream medicine, there has been an unprecedented surge in the variety, availability, and visibility of such complementary and alternative therapies in the public sphere – not only in Europe, North, and Latin America but also in China, Korea, and Japan. As a result, the New Age quest for 'alternative lifestyles' and 'personal wellbeing' has become a critical driving force behind the reinvention and popularisation of East Asian therapies worldwide, giving a new lease on life to healing practices and cosmologies once dismissed as incompatible with 'science' and 'modernity'. Despite being home to the world's largest Japanese community living outside Japan, for instance, it is hardly a coincidence that East Asian therapies – such as acupuncture, *shiatsu*, and macrobiotics – began to take roots in Brazil precisely from the 1970s, the same period when the counterculture and New Age were making their way into the country from Europe and the United States (Sigolo 2022; Sigolo and Junqueira 2021). As Rodrigo Toniol (2016) has pointed out, it is paramount to attend closely to the internal dynamics within each region, such as its state-driven policies and regulations for alternative therapies, which have often deliberately avoided any explicit religious connotations. And the same goes for the term 'East Asia'.

East Asian Imaginaries and the Study of Esotericism

The time when East Asia was perceived merely in geopolitical terms or as a homogeneous culture stuck in the past has long passed. In recent years, a series of groundbreaking studies have begun to approach East Asia primarily as a historical construction, an 'imagined community' so to speak, which has been reshaped and reinvoked for various reasons by a variety of actors, many of whom have come from outside the geopolitical frontiers of China, Japan, and Korea (Smith et al. 2019; Otmazgin 2016; Mori and Hirano 2007; Zhan 2009; Chen 2010). From a methodological perspective, whereas an East Asian-centred approach might initially be helpful to counterbalance white, Euro-American-centred views still dominant in academic settings, it is undeniable that East Asia as a concept has flourished in an always-changing, closely interconnected world. This volume does not aim to identify what kinds of knowledge are genuinely East Asian – or how that knowledge might have been 'misused' or 'distorted' by non-Chinese, non-Japanese or non-Korean communities worldwide. Instead, we are interested in issues of knowledge production, translation, circulation, and appropriation (Burke 2015). In this sense, we follow recent warnings that 'when disembodied ideas are seen to simply "mutate" in a different environment, no attention is given to the local minds and bodies in which such ideas existed, or the intentions and agendas through which they were adopted, adapted and eventually disseminated further' (Asprem and Strube 2021, 4).

These warnings around agency and appropriation come from scholars of esotericism, a field that has, in the last 25 years, established itself as an authoritative community of researchers dedicated to investigating the history of certain ideas and practices that had previously been rejected or overlooked within academia due to their divergence from normative interpretations of religion, science, or culture (Hanegraaff 2012). As the field grew in size and significance – landmarked by its own dictionary (Hanegraaff et al. 2006), specialised journals (e.g., *Aries*; *Melancolia*), book series (e.g., Oxford Studies in Western Esotericism), and the publication of several edited volumes (Bogdan and Djurdjevic 2013; Magee 2016; Rudbog and Sand 2020) that revealed overlaps with other histories, such as those of spiritualism, premodern medicine, or art – it became increasingly obvious that the adjective 'Western' could only refer to the location of the intellectuals, practitioners, and groups that these scholars studied, and not to any kind of 'Western essence'. This is particularly notable in studies of 'contemporary esotericism', which are more prone to problematise the concept of 'tradition' in order to avoid, among others, the tropes of 'colonialist discourse whereby the self is created by the construction of the Other (i.e., "modern" versus "traditional")' (Asprem and Granholm 2013, 27).

Of course, the problems of Orientalism (Said 1978) are not new, but they necessarily come back to the fore when we try to make sense of the histories of contemporary transnational phenomena characterised by claims of possession of knowledge framed as 'esoteric' or even 'occult' because that knowledge came from the Other – namely the Far East. The immediate post-WWII period, with the Beat generation and the ensuing countercultural movement, are famous for having continued the spiritualist and theosophical traditions' search for inspiration in the East (see, for example, the influence of Zen Buddhism on American literary authors in Fields 1992, or the rise of mindfulness in Harrington 2008 and Hickey 2019). Still, it is only from the 1970s onwards that these entanglements have taken truly global attention and significance. There are several reasons for this, some of which we summarise below.

From the New Age movement to the Iranian Revolution and the contemporaneous controversies around newly emerging religious groups, the 1970s announced the 'death' of the secularisation thesis. Sociologists started talking of the return of religion into the public sphere, while others pointed at methodological flaws that had led their predecessors to restrict religion to church-going and faith-claiming behaviours (Josephson-Storm 2017). While novel definitions of religion were thus being proposed, terms such as 'spirituality' took on new meanings that attempted to make sense of alleged new forms of religiosity (Platvoet and Molendjik 1999). At the same time, the golden age of scientific medicine, initiated around the turn of the 20th century, came to a halt in the 1970s when the concept of health was expanded and came to be associated with more than the mere absence of disease (Bivins 2008; Peng-Keller et al. 2022). Scholars talked of a 'turn inwards', a striving to look for more than what was on offer and the idea that 'being healthy' is a human right for which each individual is responsible. People criticised biomedicine's shortcomings in failing to take proper care of its patients' psychological and spiritual needs. New fields, such as transpersonal psychology, sought to answer these calls by offering solutions that purportedly combined or even went beyond the traditional confines of science and religion.

The argument that the 'spiritual East' could save the 'materialistic West' – typical of what Mark Jerng has called 'the Asiatic Modal Imagination' – namely, discourses that 'invoke "Asianness" in order to establish possibilities for and set limits on the imagination of the future' (2021, 173) – expanded to cover Western science too. Such ideas gained even more prominence as the second millennium approached its end and society became increasingly aware of ecological catastrophes linked to human activities. Everyone started to look for alternative ways of protecting the environment, and with 'mother Earth' now reimagined as a self-regulating and complex system named Gaia, the Asian East once again provided valuable mythological accounts of 'forgotten' ways of living harmoniously with nature.

All this was reflected in an increasingly interconnected world mediated through popular cultural narratives and products translated, reinterpreted, and popularised in all four corners of the globe. By the 1970s, television sets were a common commodity in many developed countries worldwide. Although the internet later surpassed the capacities of connectedness that television (and cinema) first established, the 1970s framed how scholars talked about the ways alternative, rejected, or minor ideas reached the masses. Colin Campbell imagined a 'cultic milieu' (Campbell 1972), a pool of fringe material that keeps replenishing our novels, films, and dramas. Christopher Partridge updated Campbell's term with his concept of 'occulture', in which he includes a profusion of ideas and practices that have gained unparalleled global popularity since the 1970s: 'magick, extreme rightwing religio-politics, radical environmentalism and deep ecology, angels, spirit guides and channelled messages, astral projection, crystals, dream therapy, human potential spiritualities, the spiritual significance of ancient and mythical civilisations, astrology, healing, earth mysteries, tarot, numerology, Kabbalah, feng shui, prophecies (e.g. Nostradamus), Arthurian legends, the Holy Grail, Druidry, Wicca, Heathenism, palmistry, shamanism, goddess spirituality, Gaia spirituality and eco-spirituality, alternative science, esoteric Christianity, UFOs, alien abduction and so on' (Partridge 2005, 70).

It might come as a surprise to see such a diverse collection of thoughts put together under a single label. However, we contend that this approach, which has been typical in the study of the Other/the Alternative, has similarly affected the examination of East Asia's impact on alternative spiritualities and therapies. For many years, scholars defined their subjects based on normative understandings of difference. For example, there are very few similarities between 'alien abduction' and 'palmistry' other than perhaps that some people would consider them 'strange', 'unscientific', or 'difficult-to-prove' matters. But this is precisely why they appear together in scholarly exegeses: they tend to fit normative ways of imagining the 'non-orthodox' or 'non-mainstream'. In short, they are things to be grouped together because of their alleged 'alternativity'.

The same can be said about how 'East Asia' has been discussed, in both academic and popular literature. Certain ideas or practices are often treated as East Asian or Far Eastern because of the assumed commonalities that they are assigned based on their alleged 'East Asia-ness'. In this volume, however, by 'East Asian imaginaries' we mean that we will pay attention to why and how forms of knowledge identified by their practitioners as 'East Asian' came to be adopted, adapted, and disseminated by individuals and groups across the globe in order to achieve specific therapeutic and spiritual agendas. More specifically, we are interested in the ways in which multiple actors worldwide have invoked an (re)imagined, mysterious, or exotic East Asia as a means to challenge prevailing biomedical views of health, illness, and well-being – views denounced as too materialistic and out of touch with people's current psychological and spiritual needs (Harrington 1997; Scheid and MacPherson 2011; Sax and Lang 2021).

As a result, by acknowledging that 'East Asia' is a sort of imaginary and that even practices with a long history in the region blossomed in an already intertwined world, we are not presuming that what we talk about is, in essence, 'East Asian'. Instead, we maintain that those who talk about what they are doing as 'East Asian' have unique insights to offer, and their perspectives should no longer be dismissed. In doing so, we follow Tina Chen's (2021) conceptual framework of 'imaginable ageography', examining China, Japan, and Korea not simply in terms of geopolitical boundaries but primarily as interpretative paradigms rooted in the imaginary of what East Asia signifies or represents to those who reference it. Our wish to consider the practitioners' discourse more seriously also extends to another one of our concerns. As the following outline of chapters will demonstrate, we sought to bring together scholars of spirituality, alternative medicine, and esotericism from regions still largely underrepresented in English-language scholarship, including Brazil, Russia, China, Japan, and Korea.

Outline of Chapters

The volume is structured into four sections and 11 chapters. Each chapter is a case study and does not purport to be an overview of any single topic. Case studies were selected based on three criteria: 1) they deal with some sort of therapeutic technique/ritual; 2) part of the knowledge necessary to fully understand that therapy is considered or framed as accessible only to certain people (may those be learners of the technique or initiates to a certain school of thought); 3) as case studies, they complicate simplistic and essentialist notions of East Asia by focussing on phenomena of cross-regional circulation, (re)interpretation, and innovation of ideas and practices imagined as, and/or claimed to be of East Asian origin.

The first three sections deal with the flow of East Asian concepts around the globe (Chapters 1, 2, and 3), the circulation of therapeutic narratives in which such concepts are integrated into larger meaning-making processes (Chapters 4, 5, and 6), and the professionalisation of therapy-based 'disciplines' influenced by East Asian concepts and locales (Chapters 7, 8, and 9). The last section, Section 4, considers one obvious effect of the phenomena discussed in Sections 1 to 3: how such movements of ideas and practices are used to legitimise and/or (re)invent national identities (Chapters 10 and 11).

More specifically, Section 1 deals with the elephant in the room, namely the concepts and elements considered prototypically 'East Asian' shared by most therapies examined in this volume. Our authors here are particularly interested in how such concepts and practices are re-imagined when flowing through different therapeutic contexts within and beyond East Asia. Chapter 1, written by Emily Baum, focuses on a group of parapsychologists from China, the United States, Japan, and Russia whose publications were instrumental in the post-1970s conceptual transformation and contemporary understanding of *qi*. Inspired by Chinese medicine, these parapsychologists began to posit that perhaps *qi* was no different than the 'energy fields', or coronal discharges, captured by Kirlian electrophotography. Their hypothesis ushered in a new paradigm for Western definitions of *qi* that tied it closely to the concept of 'energy'. Chapter 2 discusses the work of the innovative *shiatsu* therapist and Japanese author Masunaga Shizuto (1925–1981), considering the meaning of the term *kyo* (deficiency) as he deployed it in his writings. Peter Skrivanic examines how contemporary students, practitioners, and teachers of *shiatsu* in Canada and Japan variously enact this idea within their embodied practices of *shiatsu* training and treatment. The author argues that the cultural translation of *shiatsu* from Japan to Canada has both embodied and sensorial dimensions that are crucial to its localisation and transformation. Building on this emphasis on bodily experiences, Huang Xinzhe examines, in Chapter 3, the translation of *qigong* from China to Japan, using the case study of a school of *qigong* based in Kyoto. Through his participant observation of Amano-sensei's classes, Huang describes how the notion of *qi* (pronounced *ki* in Japanese) – typically seen as central to the practice of *qigong* – has been upstaged by Amano's conviction that *qigong* should lead its practitioners to a state of *kimochi-ii* (feeling good), a goal he believes is attainable through unity with Shinto and Japanese nature. Section 1 thus announces several important tropes that reappear throughout the rest of the sections of this volume: a context-dependent translation of East Asian concepts that often borrows from other-than-religion epistemic vocabularies; the inherent transformations of meaning as subsequent generations of practitioners enact such concepts across the globe; and the meaning-making processes that such therapies contribute to when they are implicitly or explicitly connected with a reiteration of national identities.

Concepts only make sense, of course, when they are embedded in therapeutic narratives. Section 2 moves, therefore, beyond specific ideas and into how narratives of therapy and healing, expressed in dedicated salons, printed matter, or digital texts, play a role in legitimising certain techniques by positively enacting their perceived alternativity to other epistemic fields. In Chapter 4, Yang Yi shows how Five-Element Acupuncture imbued Chinese medicine with the countercultural values of British alternative medicine from the 1960s through the 1980s. Using oral history interviews with pioneers of Five-Element Acupuncture (FEA), Yang demonstrates that acupuncture was reinvented as a superior healing system in opposition to the ontological limitations of materialistic biomedicine. In doing so, FEA practitioners negotiated the boundaries of science and culture on the one hand, and modernity and tradition on the other. In Chapter 5, Luis Fernando B. Junqueira and Renata Palandri Sigolo discuss the zenith of the counterculture and New Age movements in Brazil in the 1970s. Their exploration focuses on the translation and reception of *From Eden to Aquarius: The Book of Natural Healing*, a manual first published by the American writer Greg Brodsky in 1974 and concerned with living in accordance with the Kotodama Principle, a spiritual healing method developed by the Japanese martial artist Mutsurō Nakazono (1918–1994). *From Eden to Aquarius* combined Japanese and New Age ideas of healthcare and well-being, positing a spiritual, holistic 'Orient' that could serve as a correction to Brazil's materialistic 'Occidental' roots. Chapter 6 explores the role of mindfulness healing narratives in the meditative turn in contemporary American self-help culture and examines the ways in which writers reconfigured Buddhist mindful living into a modern art of being ill. Christina Lee shows that mindfulness healing narratives like Vietnamese American writer Sister Dang Nghiem's *Mindfulness as Medicine* (2015) do not reject but actively engage with biomedicine and neuropsychology to affirm the relevance of Buddhist spirituality and Asian practices of self-cultivation to healing in everyday life. In summary, Section 2 illustrates how 'East Asia' is not simply constructed against the 'Occident' or the 'West' but acquires value when it is shown to reaffirm what the 'Occident' is normatively associated with: modernity, materialism, and scientific medicine.

Following the enactment of therapeutic narratives in the legitimisation of East Asia-related therapies, Section 3 switches focus to processes of professionalisation and to how 'East Asia' remains a key factor in legitimising or, on the contrary, undermining such processes. Chapter 7 is a case study of the Colombian-born Alfonso Caycedo and his sophrology techniques as they are practised today in a Japanese birth clinic. Pamela Runestad analyses Caycedo's experiences in the East and how practitioners and healthcare media have interpreted them. She argues that sophrology in Japan complicates simple dichotomies of appreciation and appropriation, orientalism and occidentalism, professional and lay ways of knowing. She proposes a framework of 'critical bricolage' to explore the tensions between these ideas and to understand how concepts about health and well-being are constantly circulated and rearticulated to fit evolving ways of being in an increasingly transnational milieu. In Chapter 8, Fábio Stern describes how institutional and regulatory frameworks have since 1994 impacted the inclusion of Traditional Chinese Medicine (TCM) in Brazilian university curricula under the form of 'naturopathy' and 'natural healing'. The Brazilian Ministry of Education's initial rejection of courses in TCM owing to the use of the word 'medicine' in the title of such discipline led to a paradox by which naturopathy courses in Brazil ended up including TCM as one of their main subdisciplines, but as a result, do not offer enough content to meet international TCM qualification criteria. In Chapter 9, Nathan Jishin Michon discusses how two Buddhist Shingon priests, Ōshita Daien and Takayama Seiei, have combined esoteric Buddhist breathing techniques with contemporary psychology and chaplaincy, Western esoteric influences, and various world meditation techniques to form their own system of 'Clinical Meditation' and develop their own training programme to certify healthcare practitioners in using this system. Michon shows how their endeavours were encouraged by the contemporaneous influence of transpersonal psychology and professional chaplaincy in the Japanese Buddhist milieu, probing the two priests to systematise a technique stemming from a particularly rich pedigree of ideas yet officially associated with a quintessentially Buddhist setting. Section 3 thus demonstrates that imaginations about the East Asian identity of therapeutic techniques continue to play an important role in assisting or hindering their professionalisation in *milieux* where the established epistemic fields of religion and science act as discursive gatekeepers.

In the final section of this volume, Section 4, two authors tackle the primary effect that East Asian imaginaries have on the practice of alternative therapies: the reification and reformulation of national identities. In Chapter 10, Victoria Ten and Michael Wharton analyse an interview with Ch'oe Hyŏngsu, a trainee of *ki suryŏn* practice in contemporary South Korea. *Ki suryŏn* consists of a set of self-cultivation methods similar to yoga and *qigong*. The authors illustrate how Ch'oe and other practitioners connect their practices to an idealised image of 'old Korea' associated with childhood fairy tales and traditional images of mountain immortals. Ch'oe uses the term 'unscientific' in a positive sense, embodying a way to relate himself to the feeling of a disappearing old Korea and the arrival of Westernisation, globalisation, and modern science. Moving from a single case study in South Korea to a broader study of the role that TCM has played in Macau, Loretta Lou, in Chapter 11, illustrates how nationalism elevated the profile of TCM in postcolonial Macau and how TCM has provided the Macau SAR government and local TCM practitioners with a platform to showcase their patriotism to China while reinforcing Macau's self-imposed cultural identity as a bridge between 'Chinese' and 'Western' (bio)medicine.

This collection of chapters draws attention to the intellectual work involved in translation, appropriation, and innovation in the transnational development of therapies and spiritual techniques. It furthermore demonstrates the need for broader views of authority and influence in the worlds of holistic therapy and complementary medicine. The invocation of the language and trappings of the 'East' (and the 'West') has helped these techniques acquire not just popularity but also legitimacy, often drawing positive responses from institutions such as news media, universities, and medical faculties (cf. Harrington and Zajonc 2006). Narratives of modernisation and reenchantment, orientalism and occidentalism, and even self-exoticism have all been, for better or worse, strategically employed to situate healers and participants within their respective societies and a larger intertwined world. This volume offers critical insights for understanding and reconceptualising this state of affairs.

Bibliography

Andō, Reiji. 2020. 'Seimei to reisei 生命と霊性' [Life and Spirituality]. In *Kindai Nihon shūkyō-shi vol. 3: Kyōyō to seimei*, edited by Nishimura Akira, Ōtani Eichi, Sueki Fumihiko, and Shimazono Susumu, 60–70. Tokyo: Shunjūsha.

Asprem, Egil, and Julian Strube, eds. 2021. *New Approaches to the Study of Esotericism*. Leiden: Brill. https://doi.org/10.1163/9789004446458.

Asprem, Egil, and Kennet Granholm, eds. 2013. *Contemporary Esotericism*. London: Routledge. https://doi.org/10.4324/9781315728650.

Bernard, Léo. 2018. 'La médecine néo-hippocratique des années 1930: Le temps d'une rencontre'. *Histoire, Médecine et Santé* 14: 63–81. https://doi.org/10.4000/hms.1730.

Bivins, Roberta. 2008. *Alternative Medicine? A History*. Oxford: Oxford University Press.

Bogdan, Henrik, and Gordan Djurdjevic, eds. 2013. *Occultism in a Global Perspective*. London: Routledge. https://doi.org/10.4324/9781315728957.

Borup, Jorn, and Marianne Q. Fibiger. 2015. 'Introduction'. In *Eastspirit: Transnational Spirituality and Religious Circulation in East and West*, edited by Jorn Borup and Marianne Q. Fibiger, 1–10. Leiden: Brill.

Burke, Peter. 2015. *What is the History of Knowledge?*. Cambridge: Polity Press.

Bynum, William F., and Roy Porter, eds. 1987. *Medical Fringe and Medical Orthodoxy, 1750-1850*. London: Routledge.

Campbell, Colin. 1972. 'The Cult, the Cultic Milieu and Secularization'. *A Sociological Yearbook of Religion in Britain* 5: 119–36.

Campbell, Colin. 2007. *Easternization of the West: A Thematic Account of Cultural Change in the Modern Era*. London: Routledge. https://doi.org/10.4324/9781315635064.

Caplan, Eric. 2001. *Mind Games: American Culture and the Birth of Psychotherapy*. Berkeley: University of California Press.

Chang, Pang-yen. 2020. *Jingshen de futiao Jindai Zhongguo de cuimianshu yu dazhongkexue* 精神的複調：近代中國的催眠術與大眾科學 [Hypnotism and Popular Science in Modern China]. Taipei: Lianjing chuban gongsi.

Chen, Kuan-Hsing. 2010. *Asia as Method: Toward Deimperialization*. Durham: Duke University Press. https://doi.org/10.1215/9780822391692.

Chen, Tina. 2021. 'Global Asias: On the Structural Incoherence of Imaginable Ageography'. In *Asian American Literature in Transition, 1996–2020*, edited by Betsy Huang and Victor Román Mendoza, 311–30. Cambridge: Cambridge University Press.

Clart, Philip, David Ownby, and Wang Chien-chuan, eds. 2020. *Text and Context in the Modern History of Chinese Religions: Redemptive Societies and Their Sacred Texts*. Leiden: Brill. https://doi.org/10.1163/9789004424166.

Cohen, Elliot. 2021. *The Psychologisation of Eastern Spiritual Traditions: Colonisation, Translation and Commodification*. London: Routledge. https://doi.org/10.4324/9780429354922.

Davidann, Jon T. 2018. *The Limits of Westernization: American and East Asian Intellectuals Create Modernity, 1860-1960*. London: Routledge. https://doi.org/10.4324/9781315158204.

Fields, Rick. 1992. *How the Swans Came to the Lake: A Narrative History of Buddhism in America*. 3d ed. Boston: Shambhala.

Fuller, Robert C. 2001. *Spiritual, but Not Religious: Understanding Unchurched America*. Oxford: Oxford University Press. https://doi.org/10.1093/0195146808.001.0001.

Gaitanidis, Ioannis. 2022. *Spirituality and Alternativity in Contemporary Japan: Beyond Religion?*. London: Bloomsbury Academic. https://doi.org/10.5040/9781350262645.

Hanegraaff, Wouter J. 2006. *Dictionary of Gnosis & Western Esotericism*. Leiden: Brill. https://doi.org/10.1163/ejb1873-8338.

Hanegraaff, Wouter J. 2012. *Esotericism and the Academy: Rejected Knowledge in Western Culture*. Cambridge: Cambridge University Press.
https://doi.org/10.1017/cbo9781139048064.

Harding, Christopher, Iwata Fumiaki, and Yoshinaga Shin'ichi, eds. 2015. *Religion and Psychotherapy in Modern Japan*. London: Routledge. https://doi.org/10.4324/9781315773964.

Harrington, Anne, and Arthur Zajonc, eds. 2006. *The Dalai Lama at MIT*. Cambridge, MA: Harvard University Press.

Harrington, Anne, ed. 1999. *The Placebo Effect: An Interdisciplinary Exploration*. Cambridge, MA: Harvard University Press.

Harrington, Anne. 2008. *The Cure Within: A History of Mind-Body Medicine*. New York: W. W. Norton & Company.

Hickey, Wakoh S. 2019. *Mind Cure: How Meditation Became Medicine*. Oxford: Oxford University Press. https://doi.org/10.1093/oso/9780190864248.001.0001.

Holcombe, Charles. 2017. *A History of East Asia: From the Origins of Civilization to the Twenty-First Century*. Cambridge: Cambridge University Press. https://doi.org/10.1017/9781316340356.

Ichiyanagi, Hirotaka. 2021. *Saiminjutsu no Nihon kindai* 催眠術の日本近代 [Hypnotism in Modern Japan]. Tokyo: Seikyusha.

Jerng, Mark. 2021. 'The Asiatic Modal Imagination'. In *Asian American Literature in Transition, 1996–2020*, edited by Betsy Huang and Victor R. Mendoza, 173–99. Cambridge: Cambridge University Press. https://doi.org/10.1017/9781108914109.010.

Josephson-Storm, Jason Ā. 2017. *The Myth of Disenchantment: Magic, Modernity, and the Birth of the Human Sciences*. Chicago: University of Chicago Press. https://doi.org/10.7208/chicago/9780226403533.001.0001.

Junqueira, Luis Fernando B. 2023. 'The Science of the Spirit: Psychical Research, Healthcare and the Revival of the Occult in a Modernising China, 1900–1949'. PhD thesis, University College London.

Lüddeckens, Dorothea, Philipp Hetmanczyk, Pamela E. Klassen, and Justin B. Stein, eds. 2022. *The Routledge Handbook of Religion, Medicine, and Health*. London: Routledge. https://doi.org/10.4324/9781315207964.

Magee, Glenn A. 2016. *The Cambridge Handbook of Western Mysticism and Esotericism*. Cambridge: Cambridge University Press. https://doi.org/10.1017/CBO9781139027649.

Moreira-Almeida, Alexandre, Bruno P. Mosqueiro, and Dinesh Bhugra, eds. 2021. *Spirituality and Mental Health Across Cultures*. Oxford: Oxford University Press. https://doi.org/10.1093/med/9780198846833.001.0001.

Mori, Kazuko, and Kenichiro Hirano, eds. 2007. *A New East Asia: Toward A Regional Community*. Singapore: National University of Singapore Press.

Nehring, Daniel, Ole J. Madsen, Edgar Cabanas, China Mills, and Dylan Kerrigan, eds. 2020. *The Routledge International Handbook of Global Therapeutic Cultures*. London: Routledge. https://doi.org/10.4324/9780429024764.

Otmazgin, Nissim. 2016. 'A New Cultural Geography of East Asia: Imagining a "Region" through Popular Culture'. *The Asia-Pacific Journal* 14, no. 7.

Palmer, David A. 2007. *Qigong Fever: Body, Science, and Utopia in China*. New York: Columbia University Press. https://doi.org/10.13140/2.1.2859.9680.

Partridge, Christopher H. 2005. *The Re-Enchantment of the West: Alternative Spiritualities, Sacralization, Popular Culture, and Occulture*. London: Bloomsbury T & T Clark.

Peng-Keller, Simon, Fabian Winiger, and Raphael Rauch. 2022. *The Spirit of Global Health: The World Health Organization and the 'Spiritual Dimension' of Health, 1946-2021*. Oxford: Oxford University Press. https://doi.org/10.1093/oso/9780192865502.001.0001.

Platvoet, Jan G., and Arie Molendijk, eds. 1999. *The Pragmatics of Defining Religion*. Leiden: Brill.

Pokorny, Lukas, and Franz Winter, eds. 2018. *Handbook of East Asian New Religious Movements*. Leiden: Brill.

Revel, Jacques. 1996. *Jeux d'échelles. La micro-analyse à l'expérience*. Paris: Gallimard-Le Seuil. https://doi.org/10.7202/015443ar.

Rudbog, Tim, and Erik Sand, eds. 2020. *Imagining the East: The Early Theosophical Society*. Oxford: Oxford University Press. https://doi.org/10.1093/oso/9780190853884.001.0001.

Said, Edward W. 1978. *Orientalism*. New York: Pantheon Books.

Sax, William, and Claudia Lang, eds. *The Movement for Global Mental Health: Critical Views from South and Southeast Asia*. Amsterdam: Amsterdam University Press. https://doi.org/10.2307/j.ctv1kgdfk8.

Scheid, Volker, and Hugh MacPherson, eds. 2011. *Integrating East Asian Medicine into Contemporary Healthcare*. London: Churchill Livingstone.

Sigolo, Renata P. 2022. 'Healing through Plants: Relationships among Knowledge Systems in the Brazilian Press of the 1970s'. In *Herbs and the Evolution of Human Societies*, edited by Yue Yue and Molly Chatalic, 75–96. Newcastle upon Tyne: Cambridge Scholars Publishing.

Sigolo, Renata P., and Luis Fernando B. Junqueira. 2021. 'Entre agulhas e mãos: a "medicina chinesa" no Brasil da década de 1970'. *Locus* 27, no. 1: 122–51. https://doi.org/10.34019/2594-8296.2021.v27.32716.

Smith, Wendy, Hirochika Nakamaki, Louella Matsunaga, and Tamasin Ramsay, eds. 2019. *Globalizing Asian Religions: Management and Marketing*. Amsterdam: Amsterdam University Press. https://doi.org/10.1515/9789048531097.

Stein, Justin B. 2023. *Alternate Currents: Reiki's Circulation in the Twentieth-Century North Pacific*. Honolulu: University of Hawai'i Press. https://doi.org/10.1515/9780824896409

Suzuki, Daisetsu Teitaro. 1944. *Japanese Spirituality*. Translated by Norman Waddell, 1972. Tokyo: Japan Society for the Promotion of Science.

Taves, Ann, and Michael Kinsella. 2013. 'Hiding in Plain Sight: The Organizational Forms of "Unorganized Religion"'. In *New Age Spirituality: Rethinking Religion*, edited by Steven J. Sutcliff and Ingvild S. Gilhus, 84–98. Sheffield: Equinox.

Toniol, Rodrigo. 2016. 'Cortina de fumaça: terapias alternativas/complementares além da Nova Era'. *REVER* 16, no. 2: 31–54. https://doi.org/10.21724/rever.v16i2.29281.

Vargas-O'Bryan, Ivette M., and Zhou Xun, eds. 2015. *Disease, Religion and Healing in Asia: Collaborations and Collisions*. London: Routledge. https://doi.org/10.4324/9781315776262.

Voas, David. 2009. 'The Rise and Fall of Fuzzy Fidelity in Europe'. *European Sociological Review* 25, no. 2: 155–68. https://doi.org/10.1093/esr/jcn044.

Woodhead, Linda. 2010. 'Real Religion and Fuzzy Spirituality? Taking Sides in the Sociology of Religion'. In *Religions of Modernity: Relocating the Sacred to the Self and the Digital*, edited by Stef Aupers and Dick Houtman, 31–48. Leiden: Brill. https://doi.org/10.1163/ej.9789004184510.i-273.13.

Woods, Matthew. 2007. *Possession, Power and the New Age: Ambiguities of Authority in Neoliberal Societies*. London: Routledge. https://doi.org/10.4324/9781315601588.

Yoshinaga, Shin'ichi, ed. 2004. *Nihonjin no mi-shin-rei – Kindai minkan seishinryōhō sōsho* 日本人の身・心・霊——近代民間精神療法叢書 [Body-Mind-Spirit in Japan: A Collection of Books on Modern Folk Mind-Cure Methods] (2 vols.). Tokyo: Kuresu shuppan.

Yoshinaga, Shin'ichi. 2005. 'Daisetz to Swedenborg 大拙とスウェーデンボルグ' [Daisetz and Swedenborg]. *Shūkyōtetsugaku kenkyū* 22: 33–50. https://doi.org/10.20679/sprj.22.0_33.

Yoshinaga, Shin'ichi. 2014. 'Suzuki Daisetsu and Swedenborg: A Historical Background'. In *Modern Buddhism in Japan*, edited by Hayashi Makoto, Otani Eiichi, and Paul L. Swanson, 112–43. Nagoya: Nanzan Institute for Religion and Culture.
Zhan, Mei. 2009. *Other-Worldly: Making Chinese Medicine through Transnational Frames*. Durham: Duke University Press. https://doi.org/10.2307/j.ctv1198xrp.
Zheng, Guo. 2018. *Biandong shehui xia de Xinyang fenhua: Shanghai Lingxuehui yanjiu* 變動社會下的信仰分化:上海靈學會研究 [A Study of the Shanghai Society for Spiritualism]. Beijing: Zhongguo shehui kexue chubanshe.

Biographies

Ioannis Gaitanidis is associate professor at the Graduate School of Global and Transdisciplinary Studies, Chiba University (Japan). His research focusses on alternative therapies and contemporary religion in Japan. He has recently authored *Spirituality and Alternativity in Contemporary Japan: Beyond Religion?* (2022, Bloomsbury Advances in Religious Studies).

Luis Fernando Bernardi Junqueira (PhD, University College London) is a D. Kim Foundation Postdoctoral Fellow at the Department of History and Philosophy of Science, University of Cambridge. He is a global historian specialising in the intersections of science, medicine and religion in 19th- and 20th-century China, with extended interests in the histories of esotericism, psychology and mental health in modern East Asia and the history of alternative medicine in South America (https://luisfbj.com/).

Avery Morrow is a PhD candidate in Religious Studies at Brown University. His research broadly covers new religious movements and occultism in Japan from 1868 through the present day. He is currently preparing a book chapter on Shinto and hypnotism in the Meiji period.

Sangyun Han is a PhD candidate at the Graduate School of International Cultural Studies, Tohoku University. From August 2023 to July 2024, she was a visiting research student at the Centre for History of Hermetic Philosophy and Related Currents, University of Amsterdam. Her research focuses on the history of modern Japanese religion, especially the relationship between the 'Occult Boom' of the 1970s and Japanese esoteric Buddhism.

Part 1

Circulation of 'East Asian' Concepts

In his book-length examination of Reiki's history across the North Pacific – 'neither an American practice in Eastern trappings nor a Japanese practice that successfully adapted to meet the needs of Western practitioners' (Stein 2023, 202) – Justin Stein employs Bruno Latour's concepts of network and particular universalism to describe how 'transnational spiritual therapies' arise out of transnational networks all the while affording their practitioners 'a kind of imagined "citizenship" in a nonterritorial nation that collectively desires a home that both is and is not the geographical place attributed as the practice's origin' (Stein 2023, 198–99). The multidirectionality of the flow of concepts identified as 'East Asian' by therapists, clients, and a plethora of commentators and specialists does not thus preclude their transnational 'making'; rather, it seems to be the very energy that propels such movements across the globe. While the three chapters in this section are perfect illustrations of Stein's observations, they each also emphasise an as-of-yet understudied dimension in the transnational flows and making of the 'East Asian' concepts used in alternative therapies.

More specifically, all three chapters unveil the significance of the sociohistorical context in which such concepts are translated, localised, and interpreted. While the political dimension of the act of translation is not a new topic of discussion, the therapeutic environment in which these translations happen means that we ought to consider not only the textual and linguistic aspects of these concepts but also their embodiment. Indeed, the evidence presented in these chapters points to the role that a (sometimes radically) empiricist interpretation of therapeutic ideas plays in opening possibilities for the translingual practice of concepts associated with a real or imagined 'East Asia'. If concepts flow through complex networks of texts, peoples and territories, they also flow through bodies and machines that are keen on verifying, correcting, and sometimes subverting these ideas for new practitioners and clients alike.

Stein, Justin B. 2023. *Alternate Currents: Reiki's Circulation in the Twentieth Century North Pacific*. Honolulu: University of Hawai'i Press.

1 How *Qi* Became Energy

Parapsychology, Soviet Science, and Chinese Acupuncture in the 1970s

Emily Baum

Abstract: *Qi* has long been a thorny concept, presenting both translational and conceptual difficulties for scholars working within and beyond Asia. In English today, *qi* is most often translated as 'vital energy', but this was not always the case. This chapter focuses on one moment in the conceptual transformation of *qi* into energy. In the 1970s, a group of parapsychologists in the United States and Russia began to use Kirlian photography to document so-called 'energy flows' within organic matter, an undertaking that coincided with the rising global interest in acupuncture. This unlikely convergence of phenomena reinforced the correlation between energy and *qi*, a definition that has become the normative interpretation of *qi* today.

Keywords: Acupuncture, Chinese medicine, energy, Kirlian photography, parapsychology, *qi*

The Chinese concept of *qi* 氣 is one that has long befuddled translators. Despite being an essential facet of Chinese medicine, Daoist philosophy, and bodily practices like *qigong*, *qi* itself defies simple translation. This complexity stems from several sources. On the one hand, *qi* encompasses multiple meanings, ranging from 'breath', 'air', and 'gas' to a person's 'spirit' and 'manners'. In vernacular Chinese, the character for *qi* also forms part of hundreds of compound phrases related to ideas as disparate as emotions, weather, atmospheric conditions, flavours, temperaments, customs, physical exercises, and arts of self-cultivation. On the other hand, *qi* itself is not the 'unitary, singular substrate of the material universe' that it is often believed to be (Stanley-Baker 2022, 24). Early medical texts like the *Yellow Emperor's Inner Canon* distinguish between various forms and typologies of *qi*, and in

---

Gaitanidis, Ioannis, Luis Fernando Bernardi Junqueira, Avery Morrow, and Sangyun Han (eds), *Therapy, Spirituality, and East Asian Imaginaries*. Taylor & Francis Group 2025
DOI: 10.5117/9789048559015_CH01

practice *qi* can assume different traits, arise from different origins, and act on different parts of the body. The difficulty, or perhaps even impossibility, of condensing *qi* into a single translation therefore reflects the ontological diversity of the concept (Stanley-Baker 2022; Rogaski 2019).

Despite *qi*'s epistemic disunity, one translation has remained essentially ubiquitous throughout the last quarter of the 20th century. In medical textbooks, philosophical tracts, and handbooks on Chinese culture, *qi* is almost always glossed as a form of 'vital energy' – or simply 'energy' for short. Today, the equation of *qi* with 'energy' is so pervasive that it can be easy to forget that the translation is neither semantically obvious nor even particularly accurate. As a relatively modern facet of physics and chemistry, energy does not have an indigenous corollary in traditional Chinese conceptions of vitality. 'The core Chinese concept of *ch'i* [*qi*]', the medical historian Paul Unschuld has written, 'bears no resemblance to the Western concept of "energy" (regardless of whether the latter is borrowed from the physical sciences or from colloquial usage)' (Unschuld 1986, 5). *Qi*, instead, is much more slippery to pin down, since it does not conform to Western scientific paradigms that distinguish substance from process or matter from immateriality (Kaptchuk 1983). Indeed, *qi*'s very vagaries have left it open to a variety of competing translations – as well as hostage to facile oversimplification.

To be sure, the association of *qi* with 'energy' has not always existed. Throughout the 19th century, Chinese-to-English dictionaries used a variety of terms to render the character intelligible to non-native speakers, but energy was not among them. In his 1892 dictionary, Herbert Giles, professor of Chinese at Cambridge University and the man whose name would later become associated with the Wade-Giles system of romanisation, defined *qi* as 'the vivifying principle or *aura* of Chinese cosmogony [...] the thing in the universe [which] permeates all things and makes them what they are' (Giles 1892, 102). A dictionary published by the American Presbyterian Mission Press in 1896 succinctly described *qi* as 'ether' and 'aura', terms that hearkened back to classical Greek beliefs about the quintessential elements of the physical world (Poletti 1896, 163). And the Australian missionary Robert Henry Matthews, in a 1,200-page dictionary first published in 1931, translated *qi* as 'manner, demeanour, temper, force, [and] life-giving principle', thereby underscoring the concept's epistemic range (Matthews 1931, 73).

Given both the ontological diversity of *qi* and the many forms its translations have taken, how and why did *qi* come to be so closely equated with energy in the Western imagination? While the process was neither swift nor straightforward, this chapter suggests that a critical moment in the reinvention of *qi* as energy occurred in the early 1970s, at a time when the concept of energy itself had acquired a new significance and urgency. During this decade, a global energy crisis had facilitated the migration of discussions about energy from the scientific laboratory to the everyday household, a process that was bolstered by the concurrent counterculture movement in the United States. Unfolding at least partly in response to the ongoing war in Vietnam, the counterculture movement precipitated conversations about 'alternative' forms of healing practice, many of which – Chinese medicine, *reiki*, and Ayurveda among them – were understood as involving enigmatic flows of energy throughout the body (on Reiki, see Stein 2019; on healing and counterculture, see Saks 2003; Kaiser and McCray 2016; cf. Chapters 3 and 5). These views were aggressively championed by parapsychologists in both the United States and the Soviet Union, who were convinced that somatic and mental processes could not be explained by materialist biomedical paradigms alone. The intersection between these imagined forms of energy as both crisis and possibility, alongside the heightened attention to alternative forms of medical and bodily practices, coalesced to reinforce the notion that *qi* and energy were synonymous concepts.

Becoming Energy

Prior to the 1930s, Western translators had seen no obvious correlation between energy and *qi*. Indeed, throughout most of the 19th century, energy itself was a fairly novel scientific concept, one that had not yet been incorporated into everyday parlance. A scientific term for energy was only introduced in 1807, when the physicist Thomas Young borrowed the Greek word *energeia*, roughly meaning 'being at work', to describe forces that could not be observed by the naked eye. The word, however, did not become widely used in academic circles until the last third of the century, in tandem with the evolution of theoretical physics (Harman 1982). This process was primarily driven by the British Association for the Advancement of Science, which was largely responsible for replacing an older paradigm of mechanical physics with a physics based on the conservation of energy (Smith 1998). From the 1860s onwards, this science of energy began to precipitate a wider epistemological shift within physics as a whole, which, as the historian Crosbie Smith has argued, enabled energy to 'form the core of a science with universal character and universal marketability' (Smith 1998, 3).

When Sinologists first attempted to translate the Chinese concept of *qi*, they naturally were not thinking in terms of emerging constructs like energy. Instead, as Ruth Rogaski has observed, missionaries and scholars who were interested in mediating between Chinese ideas and Western sciences tended to translate *qi* as a form of 'air' or 'gas' (Rogaski 2019). Particularly as laboratory chemistry began to take shape in the 19th century, and as European chemists became more successful at isolating different gases like oxygen, air progressively took shape as a valid object of inquiry – and as a logical analogue for *qi*. Semantically, the correlations between air and *qi* were numerous. Both were omnipotent, invisible forces that pervaded the natural universe, and both could adopt alternately salutary or malignant forms. Both, moreover, transcended the physical world and could be used linguistically to refer to manners, affects, and emotions ('an air of sadness'). Thus, despite the many forms that *qi* took in the Chinese intellectual tradition, its omnipotence in the natural environment and its ability to flow in and out of human bodies made it a logical corollary for Western conceptions of air.

By the early decades of the 20th century, however, energy had begun to seep from the laboratory into society at large, encompassing metaphysical concepts like vitality, vigour, and strength alongside its purely technical usage. At around the same time that the colloquial use of energy was becoming increasingly ubiquitous, Georges Soulié de Morant, a scholar working in the French diplomatic corps in China, became interested in acupuncture. Morant first developed a fascination with the 'miraculous' practice during a cholera outbreak in Beijing. Impressed at how acupuncture appeared to cure patients more effectively than Western treatments, Morant embarked on a study of the procedure and eventually became skilled in its application. When he returned to France in the 1920s, his knowledge of acupuncture was at first met with scepticism, if not outright rejection. Nevertheless, upon the encouragement of his friend and physician Paul Ferreyrolles, Morant decided to introduce the practice more widely to Western readers through the first French-language text on the subject (Morant 1957; cf. Candelise 2010). The result, *Précis de la vraie acuponcture chinoise* (Introduction to the Real Chinese Acupuncture), was published in 1934.

In his effort to render Chinese concepts into an intelligible French form, Morant quickly ran into a problem. What was he supposed to do with *qi*? It was impossible to describe acupuncture without it, and yet no suitable French translation seemed to exist. For Morant, *qi* was most certainly not the 'air' of his missionary predecessors. The type of *qi* he was describing was not the stuff we breathe in or the stuff we emit; it was something even less tangible, something even more abstract – a type of incorporeal force that permeated our bodies yet defied simple explanation. 'The ancients asked what this "thing" was that they felt so often flowing in the meridians', he wrote in his 1934 treatise, 'and they called this energy *tsri* [*qi*]' (Morant 1934, 28). For Morant, then, energy became a simple shorthand for an otherwise obscure, opaque, and somewhat impenetrable idea.

Morant recognised that energy was not a flawless translation for *qi*, or even a particularly accurate one; he used it, quite simply, 'for lack of a better word' (Morant 1939, 46). In a later text, he elaborated on this authorial decision. It was even more difficult, Morant opined, to define *qi* than to define electricity – another invisible force that circulated in mysterious, yet occasionally manipulable, ways. And yet, it was for this very reason that 'energy' worked so well as a semantic shorthand. Readers did not have to understand the 'exact nature' of *qi* to 'recognize its existence' or 'appreciate its intensity' (Morant 1939, 46). Just like electricity, all that readers needed to know was that *qi* existed in the natural world, and that it could be channelled toward powerful, if unfathomable, ends. The very slipperiness of energy, in other words, matched the slipperiness of *qi*. It was their mutual inscrutability that made them a useful pair.

The Parapsychological Embrace of Acupuncture

Despite Morant's efforts to systematically expose Chinese acupuncture to Western readers, it would not be until the early 1970s that the practice would gain widespread attention beyond France. In the intervening decades, a hodgepodge of texts was published on the tenets of Chinese medicine, not all of which appropriated Morant's translations. Indeed, well into the 1960s, authors continued to treat *qi* as a polysemous concept, one that could only be understood through long strings of conflicting definitions and winding musings about the abstruse nature of Chinese cosmology. The British-based acupuncturist Felix Mann, who published the first English-language text on acupuncture in 1962, likened *qi* to the *prana* of Hindu philosophy and the 'etheric body' of theosophy. While describing *qi* as 'life energy', Mann went on to elaborate that *qi* could also be understood as 'the manifestation of any invisible force, whether it be the growth of a plant, the movement of an arm or the deafening thunder of a storm' (Mann 1962, 46–47). And in his 1962 volume on *Science and Civilization in China*, the British Sinologist Joseph Needham hearkened back to classical Greek medicine when he offered the concept of 'pneuma' as a logical equivalent for *qi* – a concept that, much like *qi* itself, could just as easily signify 'air' or 'breath' as it could the vital force required for all forms of life to exist (Needham 1962, xxiv).

Texts such as these, however, were few and far between. Throughout most of the 20th century, Western interest in acupuncture – alongside Chinese medicine more broadly – was sporadic, having not yet captured widespread attention outside of Asia. This began to change at the turn of the 1970s. At the time, the ageing Mao Zedong, chairman of the Chinese Communist Party, shocked the world when he decided to tentatively reopen the People's Republic of China to the capitalist bloc. Selected delegations from the United States, Canada, England, and elsewhere received coveted invitations to travel behind the Bamboo Curtain, where they were given the opportunity to tour the mysterious country for the first time since the PRC had closed its doors over two decades earlier. As part of their guided expeditions, Western delegations were brought to hospitals and clinics, where they were introduced to recent innovations in acupunctural therapy, including the use of acupuncture for analgesic purposes. Acupuncture anaesthesia, a technique developed in 1958, was one such procedure that shocked foreign visitors and immediately galvanised Western attention to Chinese medicine (cf. Chapter 4). Involving the use of acupuncture needles in place of medicinal anaesthetics, acupuncture anaesthesia appeared to be a radically transformative discovery in surgical therapeutics (Baum 2021).

Acupuncture and its surgical applications transfixed foreign audiences, who were persuaded to experiment with the procedure domestically. But despite the fervour with which Westerners scrambled to learn more about the technique, one problem that prevented its wider application in Europe and the United States was the fact that it could not be explained in a biomedical language. As a medical modality that functioned by manipulating the flow of *qi* as it moved through invisible channels called meridians (*jingmai* 經脈), acupuncture did not operate within the same epistemological universe as Western science. From a scientific perspective, acupoints (*xue* 穴) – areas on the surface of the skin where the insertion of a needle would most effectively alter the movement of *qi* through the body – did not correspond to any known physical structure, and *qi* itself had no analogue within biomedicine. Consequently, many establishment physicians argued (and continue to argue today) that until the point at which science could explain acupunctural techniques, the procedure had no place in conventional medicine (Baum 2021; Jones 2018).

If biomedical doctors were largely content to relinquish claims to acupuncture, healers on the fringes of establishment medicine were equally happy to appropriate the practice for themselves. One of the earliest groups to lay claim to the procedure was a hodgepodge mix of psychologists, physicists, and new-age gurus who happened to coalesce around a single mutual interest: parapsychology. From its inception in Europe in the late 19th century, parapsychology tottered on the edges of science. Concerned with supernatural phenomena like extrasensory perception, telekinesis, hypnosis, and telepathy, the discipline appeared to defy rational explanation. This did not prevent its earliest advocates from seeking to explain it through rational means. The first generation of parapsychologists, including the psychologist William James, maintained a firm conviction that they could apply scientific methods toward understanding the mystical world (Baum 1935). Throughout their investigations, they remained steadfast in their use of empirical experimental designs, mimicking the forms and structures of other scientific disciplines and occasionally blurring the lines between the two (Gordin 2021).

Over the course of the 20th century, the fate of parapsychology waxed and waned until it reemerged in the early 1970s with full force. Thanks in part to the counterculture fascination with psychedelic and occult phenomena – a fascination which, not unrelatedly, culminated in the CIA's covert attempts to deploy mind control against the Soviet Union[1] – parapsychology managed to temporarily bridge the gap between orthodox laboratory-based researchers and those who questioned the omnipotence of science. One field of inquiry that gradually came to attract the attention of the parapsychology community was acupuncture. At first, American parapsychologists were just as sceptical of acupuncture as biomedical physicians. As the psychologist Thelma Moss recalled, she had always considered the practice 'an ancient Chinese superstition' and something 'on the lunatic fringe' (Moss 1979, 70). The more she began to learn about it, however, the more she began to stake a claim to it, endeavouring to uncover a way to bridge the *qi* of Chinese medical philosophy with materialist scientific tenets.

Parapsychological researchers were not intimidated by acupuncture's position beyond the scope of conventional biomedicine. If anything, the fact that acupuncture operated within an epistemic universe that had nothing to do with establishment science was part of its appeal. Since parapsychologists intrinsically assumed that heretofore-unobserved and immaterial forces form a part of the natural world, acupuncture and its related ideas – including *qi* – were consistent with their underlying point of view. Seeking to draw on, but also go beyond, conventional scientific research, parapsychologists approached acupuncture as the perfect vehicle through which to discover and explore a *universal* medicine: one that was

1 For documents related to Operation Stargate, see the declassified materials at https://www.cia.gov/readingroom/search/site/stargate.

hostage neither to a particular culture nor to the assumptions of a specific time and place. If they could ascertain a scientific rationale for *qi*, then this would bring them one step closer to discovering the principles governing all phenomena in the natural world.

Toward a Theory of Energy

American parapsychologists like Moss were not the first to become captivated by acupuncture and the potential insights it could reveal about a universal body. In China, Japan, and Korea, scientists and physicians had been attempting to align acupuncture with biomedical principles for several decades.[2] Yet, for the American parapsychological community, it was the research being undertaken in the Soviet Union that proved most alluring. At the time, the American government had become increasingly concerned about apparent Soviet discoveries in parapsychology, including the rumour that the Russians had made striking advances toward determining a scientific mechanism for extrasensory perception and telekinesis. Fearing that the United States was falling behind in a critical field of research, American parapsychologists began travelling to the USSR in 1969 to learn more about Soviet discoveries in the field (LaMothe 1972; Lewis 1977). Their travels not only opened their eyes to innovations in Soviet science but also to the intersection between parapsychology, acupuncture, and the emerging discipline of bioenergetics.

The hypothesis underlying Soviet parapsychology was that mind and matter were inextricably linked through invisible flows of 'energy'. By gaining control over these energetic currents, individuals could channel their psychic processes toward physical ends, such as the telekinetic movement of objects through space. According to the American parapsychologists Lynn Schroeder and Sheila Ostrander, who visited the USSR in 1969 as part of a parapsychology study group, the Soviets had devised methods to study the 'energetic capabilities' of human thought. Russians, they noted, talked about the mind as a 'new form of energy', one that could effect changes in the physical universe through sheer force of will. (The magician Uri Geller, ostensibly providing evidence for this theory, similarly claimed that he could channel his psychic energy toward bending metal spoons.) 'The discovery of energies associated with psychic events', Ostrander announced in a

2 This work was most famously being carried out by Kim Bong-Han in North Korea, Yoshio Nakatani in Japan, and Cheng Dan'an in China. See, for instance, Kim 1964; Andrews 2014.

1971 talk, 'will be as important, if not more important, than the discovery of atomic energy' (Schroeder and Ostrander 1971). For Soviet scientists, in other words, energy powered the mental world in just the same way as it powered the material world.

If the discourse of energy proved persuasive to Americans like Ostrander and Schroeder, it was likely because they were already predisposed to thinking of physical processes in energetic terms. Indeed, at the time that parapsychologists had begun travelling to the Soviet Union, the populations of Europe and the United States were transfixed by a wholly different type of global conundrum: a crisis of energy. By the 1960s, American consumption of oil had outpaced domestic supply, causing an increasing dependence on oil production from the Middle East. This reliance on foreign oil was severely undermined in the early years of the following decade when an oil embargo was imposed by the Organization of Petroleum Exporting Countries (OPEC). The effects were felt immediately. Gas prices spiked across the United States and Europe, and politicians implemented drastic measures to reduce energy consumption. Suddenly, 'energy' was a word on everyone's lips, as it appeared that the world was both powered and connected by a global energetic output (Jacobs 2016).

In the Soviet Union, energy meant more than just oil and gas, and it was therefore not strictly the purview of physicists or environmentalists. More importantly, energy had also become the domain of physicians and biophysicists, who were attempting to prove that energetic flows drove psychosomatic processes in the exact same way that they powered physical ones. A major breakthrough in the field of bioenergetics was facilitated by the use of Kirlian photography, a technique that was believed to capture, in vibrant colour and exacting detail, the human aura. Kirlian photography derived its name from the husband-and-wife duo Semyon and Valentina Kirlian who, earlier in the century, had discovered a photographic process that appeared to capture electrical discharges as they were emitted from living organisms. These discharges, the Kirlians alleged, changed shape and hue in accordance with the subject's moods, emotions, and vital states. Hence, an image of the coronal discharge of a tense finger was unlike that of a relaxed finger, while a recently watered plant would appear differently than a parched one when photographed using Kirlian techniques (Kirlian and Kirlian 1973, 16–17). Through the use of the Kirlians' photographic method, the previously invisible (and unknown) energetic properties of the natural world had suddenly been thrown into sharp focus.

Although Kirlian photography had first been discovered in the 1930s, it would not be until the 1960s that Soviet researchers would begin to understand its implications for scientific knowledge. Rather than approaching the coronal effect as a trivial byproduct of the Kirlian technique, some physicists began to assert that the electrical discharges revealed by this photographic method were actually a new form of energy – one that had the potential to completely upend their understanding of somatic functioning. The Russian biophysicist Viktor Inyushin referred to this new energy as 'bioplasma' (Moss 1974, 479–85).[3] According to Inyushin, bioplasma was a type of energy exuded through the metabolic processes of living organisms. As a 'fourth state of matter', one that interacted with solids, liquids, and gases and could even mutate into them, bioplasma emitted electrical discharges that manifested visually as an aura, a pulsating matrix of colour that reflected an organism's vitality and mood (Krippner 1980, 171).[4]

What made the discovery of bioplasma so exhilarating to both Soviet scientists and the American parapsychology community was that it appeared to unlock the mystery of how the mind communicated with the body. If individuals could learn how to control and manipulate their bioplasmatic energies, then they could channel those forces toward both internal and external events: healing an injury, bending a spoon using only their mind, or sending psychic messages across great distances. Bioplasma, in other words, represented no less than a paradigmatic shift in how science understood mental function. If parapsychologists could harness the energetic properties of the mind, they could reveal the secrets of telekinesis, extrasensory perception, and all manner of phenomena that 'science' had historically been unable to explain. Energy, in its bioplasmatic form, had become the newest frontier in human knowledge.

Energy, Acupuncture, and *Qi*

At first glance, the discovery of bioplasma did not appear to have anything in common with the new acupunctural techniques being promoted in the PRC. But just as bioplasma was being celebrated as a great leap forward in parapsychological experimentation, so too would it be channelled toward the investigation of Chinese medicine and other 'alternative' medical modalities. As previously discussed, one of the reasons that biomedical physicians

3 Inyushin was not the originator of the concept. Rather, he was building on an idea previously developed by the Soviet engineer and physicist V. S. Grischenko in the 1940s.

4 Some sources referred to bioplasma as a 'fifth' state of matter, alongside solids, liquids, gases, and plasma. See White and Krippner 1977.

in the United States were so quick to dismiss acupuncture was because they had been unable to explain its efficacy in a scientific language. The conceptual breakthroughs engendered by Kirlian photography and the concomitant isolation of bioplasma in the 1960s, however, would enable Russian researchers to offer a significant new perspective on a medical procedure that had long been inexplicable to Western science.

The first attempt to link acupuncture to bioplasma was proposed by a Leningrad surgeon named Mikhail Kuzmich Gaikin. One day, Gaikin happened to be looking at a series of Kirlian photographs when he was struck by the pattern of light they formed on the body. The pattern did not appear to correspond to nerve endings or any other biological structure with which he was familiar. But it *did* remind him of something else: something he had seen while he had been serving as a surgeon on the Transbaikal Front during the Second World War. Specifically, the map of coronal discharges that had been rendered visible through Kirlian techniques reminded Gaikin of the Chinese system of meridians and acupoints – the invisible grid through which *qi* flowed and the points on the surface of the skin at which *qi* could most effectively be manipulated (Ostrander and Schroeder 1970, 226).

From this observation, Gaikin made a significant conceptual leap. Perhaps, he surmised, *qi* was simply bioplasma by another name. To put this differently, Gaikin was suggesting that *qi* was not just the *metaphorical* energy that George Soulié de Morant had invoked as an imprecise shorthand in his 1934 treatise. Gaikin was proposing instead that *qi* was a *literal* type of bioenergetic current: a physical property that could be rendered visible using Kirlian photography, and one that had the potential to be measured and channelled toward both therapeutic and parapsychological ends.

Gaikin shared his idea with the Kirlians, and the three set off to learn as much about acupuncture as possible (Ostrander and Schroeder 1970, 227–29). Proceeding from the assumption that *qi* was interchangeable with bioplasma, the trio experimented with aiming laser beams at critical acupoints to measure their somatic effects. Their experiments, which were taken up by later physicians as well, reportedly achieved marvellous results. In the case of grand mal seizures, a laser beam directed at an acupoint on the nasal septum halted the seizure and returned the patient to a state of rest (Krippner and Davidson 1972; Krippner 1980, 278). And in the case of sexual dysfunction, the physician Yuri Vassilchenko used mild electrical pulses along key meridians to ease frigidity and impotence (Krippner, Davidson, and Peterson 1973, 84). Thus, unlike their Chinese counterparts who were still practising acupuncture through needling, Soviet scientists had applied their belief in bioplasma toward pioneering new energetic modes of stimulating *qi*.

What made the association of *qi* with energy so convincing was the development of new technologies that appeared to establish an empirical link between the two concepts. In 1972, the Russian physicist Viktor Adamenko invented a device he referred to as the 'Tobiscope', a tiny machine about the size and shape of a pencil that lit up when it encountered points of low resistance on the surface of the skin (Moss 1979, 66). These points, Adamenko argued, correlated to the 695 acupoints that had already been mapped by the Chinese (Gris and Dick 1978, 280). Using blinded studies, Russian researchers told their test subjects to run the Tobiscope over their skin and stop whenever the device lit up. Researchers then made note of the precise locations at which the Tobiscope was triggered and correlated these areas to Chinese acupunctural maps. The findings generated by the Tobiscope were further corroborated by Kirlian photography, which showed alterations in the aura in the vicinity of the acupoints (Tiller 1976, 217).

The Russians were not the first to develop a device intended to map the acupoints using electrical resistance. Two decades before the Tobiscope had even been a kernel in Adamenko's imagination, a Japanese physician named Yoshio Nakatani had already invented an analogous instrument that he referred to as the Ryōdōraku 良導絡, a term which roughly translated to 'good conductive pathway'. Created in 1950, the Ryōdōraku likewise measured the electrical activity of the acupoints. Using this information, Nakatani went on to develop a diagnostic method that correlated certain bodily symptoms to either deficient or excessive electrical conductivity in that given region (Nakatani 1977). In Germany, likewise, the physician Reinhold Voll developed a method now known as Electroacupuncture According to Voll (EAV), a technique in which a small apparatus called the 'Dermatron' measured electrical resistance at the acupoints (Helmstädter 2001, 139). Despite Nakatani and Voll having published on the subject, however, it is unclear if the Russians were aware of their work. Soviet scientists thus claimed that they were forging an entirely new field of study, and the Soviet government even went so far as to display the Tobiscope at the 1967 World Expo in Montreal (Ostrander and Schroeder 1970, 230).

Within the Soviet Union, the Tobiscope was quickly directed toward the diagnosis and treatment of disease. Like Nakatani and Voll, Russian scientists had also determined that the strength of the electrical discharge emanating from any given acupoint was directly related to the state of health or illness in the corresponding organ; when the Tobiscope passed over a particular point, its bulb would either glow brightly or weakly depending on the force of the electrical emanation therefrom (Gris and Dick 1978, 281). Using this information, physicians asserted that they could diagnose the type, location, and intensity of the patient's condition. Even more intriguingly, Adamenko hypothesised that the information provided by the Tobiscope could be used to *predict* an illness before its symptoms had even begun to manifest; it was, in a sense, a telepathic tool, something that could identify a bodily phenomenon before it had materialised in the physically observable world. As Sheila Ostrander and Lynn Schroeder put it, the 'energy body' could manifest symptoms before they were reflected in the 'physical body', and acupuncture could thus become a mechanism through which to preemptively identify changes or disruptions in one's bioplasmic circulations, preventing disease before it had set in (Ostrander and Schroeder 1970, 231–32).

As it was described, the Tobiscope seemed to have the potential to revolutionise medicine, and American parapsychologists were thoroughly convinced by what they had observed in their travels abroad. Stanley Krippner, director of the Maimonides Dream Laboratory in New York and one of the first Americans invited to give a lecture on parapsychology in the Soviet Union, was struck by how much progress the Russians had already made in acupuncture research by the early years of the 1970s. While American physicians were still twiddling their thumbs over the procedure and turning up their noses at parapsychology, the Soviets had managed to bridge the two fields in ingenious ways (Krippner and Davidson 1972). Hoping to bring these discoveries back to the United States and galvanise scientific interest there, some American visitors asked to purchase a Tobiscope for further study at home. Their Russian hosts turned them down. The Tobiscope, they were told, was not for commercial purposes, and in any case they only had a limited number to spare (Gris and Dick 1978, 281). Undaunted, American parapsychologists set out to forge ahead on their own. Their ultimate goal, like that of their Soviet counterparts, was to legitimise a radically new understanding of human functioning: one that would not strictly be premised on visible, physical properties like organs and skin but more importantly on the channels of energy that flowed within and throughout them.

Energetic Acupuncture in the United States

Inspired by the advances that had been made by researchers like Gaikin and Adamenko, members of the American parapsychology community threw themselves with gusto into energetic research. At UCLA, the psychologist

Thelma Moss used Kirlian photography to document how energy flowed through the body along roughly the same pathways as Chinese meridian networks. Working with an acupuncturist, Moss used electrical stimulation to manipulate an acupoint on the right index finger of her research subject and then photographed the effects using Kirlian technologies. When she compared the before-and-after images, Moss noticed that the 'bright emanation' ordinarily enshrouding the finger was replaced with a 'blotch'. This change, Moss concluded, seemed to indicate that 'there is, in fact, an invisible channel (or meridian) conducting energy' throughout the body (Moss and Johnson 1976, 249–51).

At Stanford University, the materials scientist William Tiller worked on a similar study using a mocked-up version of a Tobiscope that he had recreated in his lab. Applying Soviet ideas about bioenergetics to Chinese advances in acupuncture anaesthesia, Tiller surmised that the insertion of a needle into a particular acupoint 'divert[ed] the flow of energy into other subsidiary channels', thereby blocking painful neurological information from travelling to the brain (Tiller 1976, 221). Through his work with the Tobiscope, Tiller began to reconceive of the body in energetic terms, referring to the 'deep inner circuitry' that connected the acupoints (Tiller 1973, 95). Tiller was not alone in his efforts to replicate Soviet technologies in order to interrogate the energetic properties of acupuncture. One of Moss's graduate students, Kendall Johnson, rigged his own version of a Tobiscope, one that he referred to as an Acuometer. Working with Moss, the two attempted to measure energetic movement as it pulsed along the meridians (Moss 1979, 75–89).

Some members of the parapsychology community had even bigger plans. Not content to strictly investigate the energetic properties of *qi* within their own laboratories, they attempted to make their discoveries accessible to the general public – and make a profit while doing so. At the University of California, Santa Barbara, a professor of physics named David Phillips saw the commercial possibilities of the Tobiscope. Constructing his own version of the device, which he marketed under the name 'Acupointer', Phillips promoted the apparatus via letters to individual physicians and through advertisements in medical magazines (Mody 2016). 'Pocket-sized instrument accurately locates tiny low resistance points of the skin at the control points of Chinese Medicine', one advertisement boasted, while another claimed that the Acupointer was an 'essential tool for studying acupuncture' and an instrument that could scientifically confirm that the 'acupuncture points are real'.[5]

5 UCSB Special Collections, Parapsychology Collection, ARC MSS 48, 'Acupointer'.

By the middle of the 1970s, the association between acupuncture and energy had become so ingrained that parapsychologists did not think twice about the semantic elision that had occurred between them. At a 1972 conference at Stanford University hosted by the Academy of Parapsychology and Medicine, the physician William McGarey described how psychics had long described 'a flow of energy through the body', one that was 'in many respects parallel to the energy movement the Chinese have written about... in the Chinese concept of life energy which they call "Qi"' (Academy of Parapsychology and Medicine, 1972, 12). The parapsychologist Hiroshi Motoyama, who developed his own device for measuring bioenergetics, likewise characterised *qi* as a 'type of energy' that mediated between 'the nonphysical and the physical aspects of the human organism' (Motoyama 1978, 125, 105). Moss and Johnson described *qi* as a 'flow of energy' that 'travel[ed] along meridians' (Moss and Johnson, 1976, 252), while Tiller, at a 1973 conference on Kirlian photography and acupuncture, explicitly revealed the extent to which energetics had infiltrated his understanding of *qi*. 'The energy "Chi" [*qi*] is thought to flow in the meridian circuitry', he noted. 'Think of it, if you like, simply as a fluid flowing along a river bed' (Tiller 1973, 107). For each of these researchers, *qi* was not some inscrutable or superstitious force that existed only within Chinese medicine. It was a universal property, equivalent to an energetic current, and one that was empirically measurable through new technologies that charted electrical resistance within the body.

The parapsychology community worked overtime to disseminate their findings on a broad scale. Aiming their efforts at both establishment physicians and the general public, they sought to generate interest in their discoveries by tapping into existing enthusiasm over acupuncture anaesthesia, rising curiosity about alternative methods of healing, and persisting lacunae in scientific knowledge. At the American Medical Association's 1972 annual convention, the Academy of Parapsychology gave a lecture and demonstration of acupuncture on the closed-circuit television network (American Medical Association Archives 1972). In the *Saturday Review*, Stanley Krippner co-authored a five-page spread on parapsychology and acupuncture, complete with images of bioplasmatic auras and feats of psychokinesis (Krippner and Davidson 1972, 56–60). In *Time* magazine, Thelma Moss discussed how she used Kirlian photography and acupuncture to render visible the human aura (*Time*, 1972, 73). And in *Prevention* magazine, acupuncture was linked to energetics and the laying on of hands, a combination that had rendered the aura 'perceptible as an amazing field of activity' (Jones 1973, 58).

What these articles and presentations collectively sought to communicate was that acupuncture, bodily energies, and auras had 'graduated from the mystic' and entered 'the scientific halls of our country' (Jones 1973, 62). There was, it seemed, nothing magical or superstitious about traditional Chinese concepts like *qi* or the meridians. Kirlian photography had made acupunctural channels visible to the naked eye; technologies like the Ryōdōraku, Tobiscope, and Acupointer had confirmed that the acupoints were simply areas of low electrical resistance; and Russian advances in bioenergetics had persuasively shown that electrical fields and laser beams possessed healing properties that worked by targeting energetic currents within the body. Through their explorations into the mysteries of human physiology and the natural environment, parapsychologists had come to the consensus that the enigmatic life force known to the Chinese as *qi* was intelligible to, and entirely consistent with, the scientific property of energy.

Conclusion

It did not take long for the parapsychology bubble to burst. Despite having enjoyed a moment of notoriety during the early 1970s, the American parapsychology community had begun to face widespread scepticism, if not outright hostility, by the close of the decade. The CIA, after determining that research into paranormal activity was futile, abandoned its attempts to use mind-reading and telekinesis against the Soviet Union. The illusionist Uri Geller became a target of attack when his apparent telekinetic powers were exposed as nothing more than sleight of hand (Randi 1975). And certain members of the parapsychological community, including the UCLA psychologist Thelma Moss, were forced out of their academic posts when university administrators lost confidence in the validity of their research (Greene 2010). The momentary enthusiasm that the parapsychologists had generated, alongside the seemingly paradigm-shifting theories they had proposed, had been extinguished almost as quickly as they had been advanced.

Yet one thing that endured from their experiments was the notion that *qi* and energy were one and the same: two phenomena that could be elided not just metaphorically but literally. As China once again began to open its doors to foreign visitors, and as more and more Westerners were able to travel to China to study acupuncture for themselves, they nearly unanimously retained 'energy' as a shorthand for the ineffable stuff that pulsated within and beyond the body. The American physician David Eisenberg, who studied

Chinese medicine in Beijing in the 1980s, unhesitatingly described *qi* as 'vital energy' in his popular monograph *Encounters with Qi* (Eisenberg 1985). The psychiatrist and anthropologist Arthur Kleinman likewise appropriated this language in his pathbreaking study of neurasthenia in China (Kleinman 1986).[6] And unlike their fin de siècle counterparts, contemporary Chinese-English dictionaries, almost without exception, tend to translate *qi* as some variant of 'energy', 'vital energy', or 'energy of life'. From the last quarter of the century on, *qi* and energy have been so wholly entangled that the tenuous conceptual relationship between them has become irrelevant.

What did *not* persist from the brief encounter between parapsychology and acupuncture, however, was the potential destabilisation of existing scientific paradigms. As the parapsychology community so passionately elucidated in their writings, their explorations into *qi* and bioenergetics had opened a door onto a completely new way of envisioning human physiology – if not the entire relationship between humanity and the natural world. Taking a cue from both Chinese medical philosophy and the writings of Soviet physicists, parapsychologists encouraged an epistemic shift within biomedicine; rather than thinking of disease as being localised in a single part of the body, they asserted instead that the patient should be treated as a 'bioenergetic whole' (Krippner 1980, 281).

Beyond medicine, as well, parapsychologists championed a model of natural philosophy in which 'energetic processes' formed the foundation of all types and manifestations of life (Inyushin and Chekerov 1976). This new epistemology based on energy would do more than just shift our understanding of organic functioning, the parapsychologists claimed. More crucially, it would also serve as a nexus through which to bridge the heretofore divergent philosophies of biomedicine, Chinese medicine, and other healing systems, like Ayurveda. If energy, *qi*, and *prana* were simply different words for the same concept (cf. Chapter 5), then Soviet discoveries into bioenergetics could forge a new 'universal understanding of what life and death are all about, offering [...] a new scientific explanation to many miracles of past centuries' (Gris and Dick 1978, 82). Energy, in short, was a way of bridging East and West and past and present, bringing the unsolved mysteries of bygone ages into scientific focus.

These optimistic aspirations for future scientific inquiry would all but go unheeded. By the dawn of the 1980s, in tandem with biomedicine's increasing embrace of a chemically oriented understanding of human

6 Kleinman's gloss of *qi* as 'energy' represents a terminological shift from some of his earlier writings, where he referred to *qi* as 'vital essence'.

physiology, the calls of the parapsychologists faded to little more than a whisper. And beyond the walls of the academy, as well, the goals of the international parapsychology community – to bridge Chinese medicine and bioenergetics with establishment science – failed to leave an indelible imprint. Indeed, for most champions of acupuncture in the Western world, the very allure of the procedure was its *distance* from conventional biomedicine, rather than its compatibility with it. Ironically, then, while the association of *qi* with energy was easily absorbed among the general public, the type of 'energy' they envisioned had little to do with the scientific stuff of laboratory physics or electrical circuitry. Acupuncture, instead, has almost consistently been perceived among Western consumers as a *mystical* art, one in which energy functions less as a concrete scientific principle than as a metaphor for the ineffable and unmeasurable workings of a universe beyond empirical grasp. To the extent that energy medicine has been retained within contemporary treatment regimens, it has been relegated almost entirely to 'holistic' or 'integrative' programs (Stein 2022). Thus, while the association of *qi* with energy continues to persist, the very implications of what 'energy' entails has lost both the conceptual and the practical significance that the parapsychologists once intended for it to have.

Bibliography

Academy of Parapsychology and Medicine. 1972. *Transcript of the Acupuncture Symposium.* Los Angeles: Academy of Parapsychology and Medicine.

American Medical Association Archives. 1972. 'Official Program for the AMA Closed Circuit Television Network', 18–22 June.

Andrews, Bridie. 2014. *Traditional Medicine in Modern China.* Honolulu: University of Hawaii Press.

Anonymous. 1972. 'Faith, Hands, and Auras'. *Time*, October 16.

Baum, Emily. 2021. 'Acupuncture Anesthesia on American Bodies: Communism, Race, and the Cold War in the Making of "Legitimate" Medical Science'. *Bulletin of the History of Medicine* 95, no. 4: 497–527. https://doi.org/10.1353/bhm.2021.0055.

Baum, Maurice. 1935. 'William James and Psychical Research'. *Journal of Abnormal and Social Psychology* 30, no. 1: 111–18. https://doi.org/10.1037/h0054396.

Candelise, Lucia. 2010. 'George Soulié de Morant: Le Premier Expert Français en Acuponcture' (George Soulié de Morant: The First French Acupuncture Expert). *Revue de synthèse* 131, no. 3: 373–99. https://doi.org/10.1007/s11873-010-0126-z.

Eisenberg, David. 1985. *Encounters with Qi: Exploring Chinese Medicine.* New York: Norton.

Giles, Herbert A. 1892. *A Chinese-English Dictionary, vol. 1.* Shanghai: Kelly & Walsh.

Greene, Sean. 2010. 'UCLA Lab Researched Parapsychology in the 1970s'. *Daily Bruin*, 26 October.

Gris, Henry, and William Dick. 1978. *The New Soviet Psychic Discoveries.* New York: Prentice-Hall.

Gordin, Michael. 2021. *On the Fringe: Where Science Meets Pseudoscience.* Oxford: Oxford University Press.

Harman, Peter. 1982. *Energy, Force and Matter: The Conceptual Development of Nineteenth-Century Physics.* Cambridge: Cambridge University Press. https://doi.org/10.1017/CBO9780511665394.

Helmstädter, Axel. 2001. 'Recharging the Battery of Life'. *Pharmacy in History* 43, no. 4: 134-43.

Inyushin, V.M., and P.R. Chekerov. 1976. 'Biostimulation through Laser Radiation and Bioplasma'. https://www.cia.gov/readingroom/docs/CIA-RDP96-00787R000500080001-0.pdf.

Jacobs, Meg. 2016. *Panic at the Pump: The Energy Crisis and the Transformation of American Politics in the 1970s.* New York: Hill and Wang.

Jones, Carol. 1973. 'Photos Show How Faith Can Heal'. *Prevention,* December.

Jones, Kelly H. 2018. 'Ancient Art Meets Modern Science: American Medicine Investigates Acupuncture, 1970–1980'. *Asian Review of World Histories* 6, no. 1: 68–97. https://doi.org/10.1163/22879811-12340026.

Kaiser, David, and W. Patrick McCray. 2016. *Groovy Science: Knowledge, Innovation, and American Counterculture.* Chicago: University of Chicago Press. https://doi.org/10.7208/chicago/9780226373072.001.0001.

Kaptchuk, Ted. 1983. *The Web That Has No Weaver: Understanding Chinese Medicine.* London: Rider.

Kim, Bong-Han. 1964. *On the Kyungrak System.* Pyongyang, NK: Foreign Languages Publishing House.

Kirlian, Semyon D., and Valentina Kh. Kirlian. 1973. 'Photography by Means of High-Frequency Currents'. In *Galaxies of Life: The Human Aura in Acupuncture and Kirlian Photography,* edited by Stanley Krippner and Daniel Rubin, 13–27. New York: Gordon and Breach.

Kleinman, Arthur. 1986. *Social Origins of Distress and Disease: Depression, Neurasthenia, and Pain in Modern China.* New Haven, CT: Yale University Press.

Krippner, Stanley, and Richard S. Davidson. 1972. 'Humanistic Psychology & Parapsychology: Parapsychological Research in the Soviet Union'. Recorded on 8 September in Squaw Valley, CA. Accessed at the Library of Congress, Washington, DC.

Krippner, Stanley, and Richard S. Davidson. 1972. 'Parapsychology in the USSR'. *Saturday Review,* 18 March.

Krippner, Stanley, Richard Davidson, and Nancy Peterson. 1973. 'Psi Phenomena in Moscow'. *Journal of Contemporary Psychotherapy* 6, no. 1: 79–88. https://doi.org/10.1007/bf01796038.

Krippner, Stanley. 1980. *Human Possibilities: Mind Exploration in the USSR and Eastern Europe*. New York: Anchor Press.

LaMothe, John D. 1972. *Controlled Offensive Behavior – USSR*. Defense Intelligence Agency Classified report, July.

Lewis, Flora. 1977. 'Emigre Tells of Research in Soviet [Union] in Parapsychology for Military Use'. *New York Times*, 19 June.

Mann, Felix. 1962. *Acupuncture: The Ancient Chinese Art of Healing and How it Works Scientifically*. New York: Vintage.

Matthews, Robert H. 1931. *Chinese-English Dictionary*. Shanghai: Presbyterian Mission Press.

Mody, Cyrus. 2016. 'Santa Barbara Physicists in the Vietnam Era'. In *Groovy Science*, edited by David Kaiser and W. Patrick McCray, 70–106. Chicago: University of Chicago Press. https://doi.org/10.7208/chicago/9780226373072.003.0003.

Morant, George Soulié de. 1934. *Précis de la Vraie Acuponcture Chinoise* [Introduction to the Real Chinese Acupuncture]. Paris: Mercure.

Morant, George Soulié de. 1939. *L'Acuponcture Chinoise* [Chinese Acupuncture]. Paris: Lafitte.

Moss, Thelma. 1974. 'Psychic Research in the Soviet Union'. In *Psychic Exploration: A Challenge for Science*, edited by Edgar D. Mitchell, 469–86. New York: Cosimo.

Moss, Thelma. 1979. *The Body Electric: A Personal Journey into the Mysteries of Parapsychological Research, Bioenergy, and Kirlian Photography*. New York: St. Martin's Press.

Moss, Thelma, and Kendall Johnson. 1976. 'Letter'. *Psychoenergetic Systems* 1, no. 3.

Motoyama, Hiroshi. 1978. *Science and the Evolution of Consciousness*. Brookline, MA: Autumn Press.

Nakatani, Yoshio. 1977. *Ryodoraku Acupuncture*. Tokyo: Ryodoraku Research Institute.

Needham, Joseph. 1962. *Science and Civilization in China*. Cambridge: Cambridge University Press.

Ostrander, Sheila, and Lynn Schroeder. 1970. *Psychic Discoveries Behind the Iron Curtain*. Englewood Cliffs, NJ: Prentice-Hall.

Poletti, P. 1896. *A Chinese and English Dictionary*. Shanghai: American Presbyterian Mission Press.

Randi, James. 1975. *The Magic of Uri Geller*. New York: Ballantine Books.

Rogaski, Ruth. 2019. '"Air/Qi" Connections and China's Smog Crisis: Notes from the History of Science'. *Cross-Currents* 30: 55–77. https://doi.org/10.1353/ach.2019.0007.

Saks, Mike. 2003. 'Medicine and the Counter Culture'. In *Medicine in the Twentieth Century*, edited by John Pickstone and Roger Cooter, 113–23. New York: Routledge. https://doi.org/10.4324/9781003078456-8.

Schroeder, Lynn, and Sheila Ostrander. 1971. *Parapsychology in Communist Countries*. Accessed at the Library of Congress, Washington, DC.

Smith, Crosbie. 1998. *The Science of Energy: A Cultural History of Energy Physics in Victorian Britain*. Chicago: University of Chicago Press.

Stanley-Baker, Michael. 2022. 'Qi: A Means for Cohering Natural Knowledge'. In *The Routledge Handbook of Chinese Medicine*, edited by Vivienne Lo and Michael Stanley-Baker, 23–50. London: Routledge. http://doi.org/10.4324/9780203740262-4.

Stein, Justin. 2019. 'Universe Energy: Translation and Reiki Healing in the Twentieth-Century North Pacific'. *Asian Medicine* 14: 81–103. https://doi.org/10.1163/15734218-12341436.

Stein, Justin. 2022. 'Energy Healing: Reiki, Therapeutic Touch, and Healing Touch in the United States and Beyond'. In *Routledge Handbook of Religion, Medicine, and Health*, edited by Dorothea Lüddeckens, Philipp Hetmanczyk, Pamela E. Klassen, and Justin B. Stein, 115–41. New York: Routledge.

Tiller, William A. 1973. 'Some Energy Field Observations of Man and Nature'. In *Galaxies of Life: The Human Aura in Acupuncture and Kirlian Photography*, edited by Stanley Krippner and Daniel Rubin, 71–112. New York: Gordon and Breach.

Tiller, William A. 1976. 'Field Effects, Acupuncture Points, and Meridians'. *Psychoenergetic Systems (An International Journal)* 1: 217–21.

Unschuld, Paul. 1986. *Nan-ching: The Classic of Difficult Issues*. Berkeley: University of California Press.

White, John, and Stanley Krippner. 1977. *Future Science: Life Energies and the Physics of Paranormal Phenomena*. New York: Anchor Books.

Biography

Emily Baum is associate professor of modern Chinese history at UC Irvine, where she researches and teaches on the social and cultural history of 20th-century China and the history of medicine. She is the author of *The Invention of Madness: State, Society, and the Insane in Modern China* (University of Chicago Press) and the co-editor of *Uncanny Beliefs: Superstition in Modern Chinese History* (Harvard Asia Center).

2 Finding *Kyo* in *Shiatsu* Spaces

Sensing the Global Movement of Embodied Knowledge

Peter Skrivanic

Abstract: This chapter utilises ethnographic engagements with practitioners of *shiatsu*, a form of manual therapy developed in Japan in the 20th century, to shed light on two issues relevant to the study of globalised East Asian spiritualities and therapies. First, it adopts a 'worlding' approach within the author's multi-sited, transnational field site, as a way of mapping the spatiality of global movements of ideas and practices without utilising and reinforcing dichotomies such as East/West, while nonetheless attending to how such notions can remain salient within informants' discourses and imaginaries. Second, by attending to the sensory dimensions of knowledge translation in *shiatsu* diagnostic practices, the study models one way for scholars of globalised East Asian spiritualities and health movements to engage with underexplored dimensions of how such knowledge practices work on and through the local minds and bodies who carry them into new environments.

Keywords: *shiatsu* therapy, senses, globalisation, worlding, cultural translation

Therapies that have been characterised as 'East Asian' in origin have remained fixtures within the medical marketplace of North America and Europe since at least the 1970s, and interest in them, among both consumers and researchers, continues to expand. Yet their position – as 'complementary' or 'alternative' to biomedicine, and as knowledges that are held to be 'traditional', 'spiritual', and 'Eastern' – marks them with powerful and historical meanings that can obscure a clear vision of their ongoing developments and transformations and of the shifting local and global connections that are constituted through the social worlds of their practice. Scholars thus need

Gaitanidis, Ioannis, Luis Fernando Bernardi Junqueira, Avery Morrow, and Sangyun Han (eds), *Therapy, Spirituality, and East Asian Imaginaries*. Taylor & Francis Group 2025
DOI: 10.5117/9789048559015_CH02

to find ways to reimagine the spatialities and movements of 'East Asian' medicines such as *shiatsu*.

At the same time, why is it that such medicines were able to *stick* in the Euro-American landscape? While the New Age movement's valorisation of 'Eastern' spiritualities and healing modalities surely helped to chart trajectories for the extension of such practices into North American communities, to address such a question fully, macro-level answers alone are insufficient. Instead, by attending to the 'local minds and bodies' of those who inhabit social worlds of *shiatsu* ideation and practice, different scales and textures of knowledge might emerge which can fill in the picture.

This chapter addresses both of these issues by unfolding in two movements. First, after a short introduction to *shiatsu*, highlighting its emergence in early 20th-century Japan and its links with circulating discourses of science, esotericism, and traditional medical knowledge within that milieu, I will discuss *shiatsu*'s global extension outside of Japan. I then describe an analytic approach of 'worlding' (Zhan 2009), as a way both of conceptualising knowledge production and movement and of structuring the author's translocal research field, which included sites in Canada and Japan, in order to avoid imposing East-West (and other) dichotomies upon the material. Next, I introduce the innovative *shiatsu* therapist and author Masunaga Shizuto 増永静人 (1925–1981), founder of a globalised system of *shiatsu* practice termed 'Zen *Shiatsu*', and consider the meaning of the term *kyo* 虚 (deficiency) as he deployed it in his writings, before turning to examine how contemporary students, practitioners, and teachers of *shiatsu* in Canada and Japan variously enact this idea within their embodied practices of *shiatsu* training and treatment. I will argue in closing that the cultural translation of globalised therapeutic knowledge frequently has embodied sensorial dimensions that are important to the knowledge's localisation and transformation.

Culturally Translating Japanese Manual Therapy

Shiatsu[1] is a form of manual therapy that emerged in Japan in the early 20th century and which has been recognised as a nationally regulated healthcare modality there since the 1950s. Beginning in the late 1960s, *shiatsu* began to be

1 *Shiatsu* 指圧, composed of the ideograms for 'finger' and 'pressure', is a form of whole-body, pressure point massage. Its principal technique consists of the therapist providing stationary, sustained pressure using the thumbs and palms to points distributed across the whole of the

taught and practised beyond Japan's borders, and it has since become a part of the global wellness industry, with a modest presence in spas and alternative medical treatment centres across North and South America, Europe, Oceania, Taiwan, Vietnam, and elsewhere. While in these settings, it is sometimes described as an 'ancient' or 'traditional' form of Japanese medical practice, this section will demonstrate instead that *shiatsu* is better thought of as a novel reformulation of longstanding healing practices, produced through processes of global encounter, local innovation, and cultural translation (for a similar example, cf. Chapter 4). Cultural translation (Bhabba 1984, Spivak 2000) assumes that some degree of incommensurability between domains is a feature of all knowledge movements. The result is that translations are not simple one-to-one transfers of concepts across boundaries but instead are power-laden processes of appropriation and recontextualisation that give rise to new uses and nuances. The following brief excursion into Japanese medical history will illustrate how *shiatsu* emerged in a milieu in which the institutional and epistemological power of scientific medicine contributed to the cultural translation of existing modes of medical practice, prompting transformations that were theoretical, practical, and perceptual. This background will help to frame the subsequent discussion on how we might fruitfully approach questions related to *shiatsu*'s global 'movement'.

Prior to the 20th century, massage had long been a feature of healthcare in Japan. *Kanpō* 漢方, the medical system of Chinese origin which had been introduced to Japan in the Asuka Period (528–710 CE), had included medical massage as one of its modalities, in addition to herbal medicine, acupuncture, and moxibustion.[2] Massage remained a feature of courtly medicine for several centuries, where its practice was organised in accordance with *kanpō*'s notions of illness and its particular ontological vision of the human body. The *kanpō* 'mind-breath-body complex'[3] was sustained and animated by *ki* 気 (pronounced *qi* in Chinese), the 'constituent material of living things' (Drott 2010, 255), sometimes translated as 'material force' or 'vital material force' (cf. Chapter 1). When a practitioner massaged a patient,

patient's body; this is frequently supplemented with stretching and joint mobilizations. Patients typically remain clothed during treatment.

2 'Moxibustion' refers to the burning of dried mugwort herb on or close to the body for therapeutic effect.

3 Received categories trouble our efforts to speak appropriately about the body as it was understood in early and medieval Japan. Winfield (2012, 467) proposes instead the combinatory phrase 'mind-breath-body complex' as a way to decenter assumptions based on the biomedically informed categories of the contemporary West, and to signal an enduring basis of Japanese medical ontology from the Asuka period (528–710 CE) onwards.

the object of ministration was the body's *ki*, with the massage aimed at alleviating 'blockages' and thereby encouraging its unrestricted free flow.

By the Edo Period (1603–1868), acupuncture and massage had become separated from the more elite practice of herbal medicine, and *anma* 按摩 massage had become a popular modality in urban centres such as Edo. *Anma* was commonly practised by blind masseurs who were trained and organised within a large guild and who treated both elite and non-elite clientele (Groemer 2001, 361). Practitioners applied various techniques of pressing, rubbing, and pounding to soft tissues and of stationary or swirling rotational pressure to specific points. Originally a practice imported from China, medical massage had undergone centuries of local development and reformulation, coming to occupy its own niche within the medical marketplace of late preindustrial Japan. Yet strong traces of its *kanpō* origins remained, and the medical body of *anma* remained something that housed quasi-material forces that were constantly moving and transforming.

It has been suggested that 'medical modernity' arrived in Japan first in the form of an illustrated volume of anatomy: *Kaitai shinsho* 解体新書 (1774) was a Japanese translation of a Dutch anatomy text[4] which became an influential tome, precipitating important shifts in Japanese medicine and in the medical body as a domain of knowledge and experience (Kuriyama 1992). While we might not wish to set one historical moment apart as marking the definitive pivot point between successive 'cultural ages', *Kaitai shinsho* was much copied and discussed at the head of a new wave of resources – discourses, technologies, and techniques – entering Japan, prompting further changes to come. Fifty years after its publication, the smallpox vaccine was introduced to Japan for the first time. The study and practice of anatomical medicine[5] soon came into ascendancy, and within a few decades the Prussian model of medical education was formally adopted as the state-endorsed model for the training and licensing of physicians. In the Meiji period (1868–1912), public health campaigns were launched to combat outbreaks of cholera, while the population was educated on the need for hygiene according to scientific principles. The modernising Japanese state made use of biomedical models and technologies to help shape its new political order (Kitanaka 2012, 41);

4 Actually, it was a Dutch translation of the German text *Anatomische Tabellen* by Johann Adam Kulmus, 1725.

5 I refer to the Prussian medical practices imported to Japan in the 18th and 19th centuries as 'anatomical medicine' (when referring to the practice) or 'scientific medicine' (when referring to the discourse), and to the technological and pharmaceutically driven practices of the post-WW2 era as 'biomedicine' to acknowledge the significant differences between them, despite their threads of historical continuity.

meanwhile, restrictions began to be placed upon the practice of *kanpō* and other indigenous medical practices.

Thus, through the Meiji and Taishō (1912–1926) periods, practitioners of manual therapy found themselves in a social environment that was becoming increasingly science-literate and in which scientific medicine was establishing a hegemonic political power within the modernising state. These developments posed challenges to massage practitioners that were political as well as epistemological, as they needed to contend both with the institutional power of the new medicine, as well as with its conceptual categories (Skrivanic 2016, 2018).

By this time, *anma* had become largely associated with the blind in the popular imagination and was assumed to be mainly for the purpose of relaxation. Many sighted practitioners, however, held it to have therapeutic potential beyond that. Increasingly, proponents of this latter position looked to the anatomical and physiological discourses of scientific medicine to explicate their approaches, even as they appropriated and mixed numerous techniques, of both foreign and indigenous origin, into their styles of practice. Many of these sighted practitioners sought to distance their practices from *anma* and called their therapies by different names. '*Shiatsu*' was one such name that began to circulate as the heterogeneous movement continued to grow, until in 1939 Tamai Tenpeki 玉井天碧 published *Shiatsu-hō* 指圧法 (*Shiatsu* Method). The name caught on, and several subsequent publications by other practitioners also used the term; the new movement now had a name. *Shiatsu* thus emerged as a distinctly modern reformulation of *anma* massage, a 'scientific' therapy that its proponents argued had retained effective and essential resources from the long history of Japanese manual therapy, while purifying them of premodern superstitions.

Yet medical modernity did not only assume the form of scientific medicine. With the expansion of literacy in Japan and a boom in the translation and publication of foreign texts, by the early 20th century, books and pamphlets on a variety of heterodox Euro-American medical modalities, from chiropractic to hypnotherapy, had achieved a wide readership. Particularly in the Taishō era, in the face of widespread epidemic disease and other disasters, alternatives to scientific medicine became attractive and there emerged a movement of *seishin ryōhō* 精神療法, or 'psycho-spiritual therapies' (Stein 2023). These therapies culturally translated the ideas of mesmerism, Theosophy, New Thought, and more into the idiom of *ki* healing. The *kanpō* notion of *ki* was itself culturally translated in multiple ways through such global encounters, taking on moral-spiritual associations in some contexts, while being reimagined as a premodern apprehension of the nervous system in others (cf. Chapters 1, 3, and 5). Being amenable to multiple readings, the unsettled nature of *ki* would later come to haunt efforts to articulate the proper clinical object of *shiatsu* therapy, even as different processes of cultural translation would serve to establish *shiatsu*'s legitimacy as a scientifically validated, state-regulated 'anatomical' therapy in the postwar era (Skrivanic 2018, 208–9).

This unsettled meaning would become especially evident as *shiatsu* began to globalise in the 1960s and '70s. By this time, the predominant model of *shiatsu* in Japan was that of a rationalised therapy whose benefits could best be understood via the biosciences. Such biomedical knowledge was an essential element of the national licensing examinations, and therefore in the curricula of the vocational schools that prepared their students to sit these exams. Yet there remained numerous therapists who felt that *shiatsu*'s effects could be better understood with reference to the clinical models of *kanpō* and classical *anma*, as well as to the models of *ki* that had first emerged among practitioners of *seishin ryōhō*, and who presented their cases in published writings or in study groups they offered for graduates of the vocational schools.[6] On the ground, there was abundant movement between these conceptual poles, with different theorists proposing creative and innovative models for synthesising these diverse streams of *shiatsu* knowledge. Yet as *shiatsu* globalised, this multiplicity became reified in terms of two representative models of the therapy: the 'neuromuscular' approach of the therapist Namikoshi Tokujiro 浪越徳治郎 (1905–2000) and the *ki* and meridian (or 'Zen *Shiatsu*') approach of Masunaga Shizuto 増永静人 (1925–1981).[7] The former was understood to be the predominant model in Japan, while the latter would soon find a large, welcoming audience in Europe and North America.

Theorising *Shiatsu*'s Global Extension

The above-mentioned reification of *shiatsu* into two competing models of therapy, one 'scientific' and the other 'traditional', is itself a social effect

6 This mode of instruction itself hearkened back to the apprenticeship model of teaching, which had been the fundamental method for the transmission of *anma* in the Edo period. The formation of vocational schools with licensing examinations was itself a reflection of how *shiatsu* knowledge was being shaped by its institutionalisation within a biomedical state regime of healthcare.

7 The 'neuromuscular' or anatomical approach to *shiatsu* is simply referred to as '*shiatsu*' within contemporary Japan, having become hegemonic upon *shiatsu*'s legal regulation in the 1960s. Masunaga's approach is known as *ki to keiraku shiatsu* 気と経絡指圧 in Japanese.

of the epistemology of biomedical categories and their instantiation as a form of state power. This movement was also in alignment with a wider stream of nationalist discourse in which the salvage of knowledge resources from the past, and their 'purification' (Latour 1993) through science, would help to produce a healthy, modern nation.[8] Yet there were countervailing discourses too, not of salvage but of loss, in which the embrace of the modern and scientific were held to occlude and displace important values and resources from the past. As has been documented elsewhere with respect to diverse forms of traditional medicine (Langford 2002; Alter 2005), the purported holism of these systems can be contrasted with the reductionism of biomedicine, bolstering the claim that they account for aspects of health and illness that biomedicine overlooks (cf. Chapter 5). In the case of *shiatsu*, both kinds of imaginaries would come to have discernible effects upon its practice, and on the self-understanding of its practitioners. (More on this second point later). Further, they would also engage particular affinities overseas, impacting how *shiatsu* became reproduced in the global field.

Accounts of the globalisation of East Asian medicines have frequently noted how such medicines, while rationalised in their countries of origin, are often spiritualised or psychologised in the West (Barnes 1998, Janes 2002, Warrier 2009; cf. Chapters 3, 4, and 5). This is in part due to the Orientalist assumptions that Heelas (1996, 2005) and others have noted as a key feature of the New Age movement, and which have helped to drive consumption of such practices. In the late 1970s, when on account of such imaginaries, Euro-American interest in Zen and the 'Zen Arts' (Cox 2003) was still high, Masunaga Shizuto's book *Zen Shiatsu* was published in English. Originally entitled simply *Shiatsu* in Japanese, the book made explicit reference to Zen only in its preface, but its influence was significant. Masunaga's style became known as 'Zen *Shiatsu*' globally, and the book – which includes generalised accounts of East-West difference and what some might term 'auto-Orientalism' (e.g., Befu 2001) – became a must-have item for many of those in Europe and North America who sought to learn a spiritualised form of the newly-available therapy. Thirty years after its publication, a survey of *shiatsu* practitioners in Europe found that almost 90% of them claimed to practise Zen *Shiatsu* or a derivative form of it (Long 2007b, 6).

While the work of Orientalist imaginaries doubtlessly contributed to the patterning of *shiatsu*'s global extension, such macro-level analyses alone are insufficient descriptions of this process. On the one hand, they

8 This movement took on a pronounced new life in the postwar era. See Igarashi 2000; Skrivanic 2018.

invoke a smoothness to patterns of a global movement that would be belied by careful attention to the local productions of difference unfolding within specific settings (see, e.g., Adams 2002; Warrier 2009); and on the other hand, they structure the global field in terms of cartographies of contrast, thereby subtly importing East-West, tradition-science dichotomies into the background of scholars' accounts of their mobile medicines. Such assumptions, as mentioned above, frequently *do* factor into how informants such as *shiatsu* practitioners may understand and articulate their own practices, but they risk obscuring much if they are imported into scholarly analyses.

In an effort to avoid such problems in my own fieldwork, which focused on trainee *shiatsu* therapists in Canada and Japan, I drew inspiration from Mei Zhan's notion of 'worlding'. In her ethnography of Chinese medical knowledge-building in Shanghai and San Francisco, Zhan writes against the 'out of China narrative that seems to haunt the mapping of Chinese medicine' (2009, 19), choosing instead to think *through* her two settings, attending to localised productions of difference that are continually being negotiated. The worlding of Chinese medicine, she writes,

> is not about how a local system of therapeutic knowledge expands into other corners of the world by transcending geopolitical limits and cultural boundaries. The routes of Chinese medicine resemble nothing like a seamless circuit; rather, they take many unexpected turns, burst at the seams, and carve out new landscapes while recharting old ones. (2009, 7)

Rather than as bounded objects that travel, Zhan invites us to conceive of East Asian spiritual and therapeutic practices as forms of knowledge that are entangled within translocal networks of actors and institutions, within discourses and histories through which their meanings are continuously reimagined and reproduced. Through processes of translation, contestation, and negotiation, and through movement, dislocation, and disjuncture, such forms of knowledge become involved in processes of meaningful 'world-making'.

The metaphor of 'travelling knowledge' breaks down when seen through a worlding lens because, as the product of such translocal actor networks, East Asian spiritualities and therapies emerge within worlds that are already globally enmeshed. In the case of *shiatsu*, we can see that Japanese manual therapists were situated within discursive worlds of translated and locally reproduced discourses of scientific knowledge, when *shiatsu* emerged as a distinctive modality in the early 20th century. Similarly, later individuals living in North America or Europe who began learning about *shiatsu* in the 1970s from books, or as patients or students of travelling *shiatsu* teachers, were themselves entangled in discursive worlds wherein the traditional medicines and religions of East Asia had long been imagined as cyphers for the ills of the Western self (Clarke 1997), and had more recently emerged as attractive means for self-production within New Age projects of 'self-spirituality' (Heelas 1996). It is less the case that these forms of knowledge 'travel' than that they are the focus of world-making projects that create linkages between diverse networks of actors and infrastructures through which their meanings are continually renegotiated.

Such a view also invites us to reconceptualise the appropriate means of framing research sites, away from assuming a global field that is already structured and fixed with meanings (e.g., East-West), or from comparisons between bounded local sites (e.g., Tokyo and Toronto), to recognising and charting emergent forms of connection and disjuncture across a variety of scales. It brings into focus new questions: not, 'How did *shiatsu* make its way to the West?' but rather, 'Why did Toronto emerge as a major *shiatsu* training hub, but not Montreal?' Such questions bring into focus specific actors – their mobility, their creative translations of *shiatsu* knowledge, their interactions with clients, students, licensing officers, business partners, communal migration histories, and immigration law, as well as their personal stories of struggle and setbacks, of serendipity and success. What comes into view is their activity within diverse networks and infrastructures as they pursue their world-making *shiatsu* projects.

Among my informants, their worlding projects possessed their own spatio-temporalities. An East-West mapping could be a prominent feature of such mappings in one instance, while being less important in another. Take for example one informant, Takeda-sensei, a Japanese national who studied under Namikoshi Tokujiro, who was the popular 'face' of (neuromuscular) *shiatsu* in Japan, before emigrating to Toronto for the express purpose of opening a satellite school of his teacher's own institution. The dream of bringing 'authentic Japanese *shiatsu* as taught by its "founder"' to the West was a prominent feature of his thinking and writing, and motivated the tremendous efforts he made over a period of years, as well as the political disputes he engaged in with other Toronto-based Japanese *shiatsu* teachers who were teaching meridian *shiatsu*. Meanwhile, Fernanda, a Brazilian-born immigrant to Toronto who first encountered *shiatsu* at a wellness fair in a park near her home in Toronto, would go on to study a hybridised neuromuscular-meridian *shiatsu* style at a local school. She would then become a travelling teacher in her own right, creatively adapting the style she had learned by adding her own innovations as well as techniques drawn from an eclectic mix of other therapies, to aid in her method's appeal to her students in São Paulo (cf. Chapters 5 and 8).

Within a project that involves multiple such participants, the *shiatsu* 'movement' becomes far too unwieldy to map onto static categories of East and West. My attention turns instead to how depictions of East-West differences are variously formulated and invoked in the biographies, practices, and models of my informants. Thus, while my research is grounded in such a way that it includes sites in Tokyo and Kyoto (Japan) as well as sites in and around Toronto (Canada) – thus spanning 'East' and 'West' – the meaningful productions of difference or continuity that my informants articulate do not necessarily fall along those lines. Instead, '*shiatsu* spaces' are created between multiple actors who are linked through their shared participation in networks of meaning that enable their diverse projects of worlding and to the connections or forms of disjuncture that they produce. These spaces may cut across a given local site even as they span between Kyoto and Toronto.

One such space that I will consider below is the 'Zen *Shiatsu* Space' within my research site, composed of the networks of *shiatsu* teachers, researchers, and practitioners – and the discourses, practices, institutions, and alliances they were involved in – that were all engaged in an ongoing worlding of the 'Zen *Shiatsu*' approach associated with Masunaga Shizuto.

So far in this chapter, my examples of *shiatsu* worlding have focused predominantly on the work of imaginaries and models, which is too disembodied an approach for something like *shiatsu*, in which therapists train their bodies to be therapeutic tools to apply to the bodies of others (cf. Chapters 4 and 10). Why do some imaginaries seem to take root in certain locales, while others never do? A part of the answer to this question has to do with how imagined worlds create meanings that not only attract individuals but that 'stick' (Tsing 2015). As one meridian *shiatsu* stylist in Toronto told me bluntly, 'Look, the theory is all very nice, but this stuff has to *work*'. Part of the 'work' of Zen *Shiatsu* training and practice that was of most interest to me was its embodied practices: how students and therapists trained their senses and cultivated forms of clinical perception that seemed to trouble the powerful sensory models implicit in the biosciences, and in much of what we might describe as 'everyday ontology'. Below, I introduce a disjuncture into the body of this chapter, turning to the role of the senses in knowledge production, before proceeding with an ethnographic account of sensory worlding in the above-mentioned Zen *Shiatsu* space.

Sensory Ways of Knowing

Scholarship in the field of sensory studies has demonstrated that the senses are always culturally elaborated (Classen 1998; Howes 2003; 2005; Howes and Classen 2014). Not only do cultural categories shape how the senses are imagined relative to one another, but implicit models of the senses help to ground lived practice, facilitating the emergence of particular sensory dispositions and capacities among a society's members. Cultural values determine what senses are emphasised and what are downplayed, which in turn influences what potentials get developed and extended, and in what directions (Bendix 2005, 13). Attention to this process of social and cultural elaboration of the senses undermines the tendency to think of the senses as being 'naturally given', and hence unworthy of problematisation. It also opens up analytic space to consider how the senses are imagined, developed, and utilised within situated practices of knowledge production.

This in turn further invites us to recognise that a potent dimension of the encounter between European and Japanese medical knowledge was a sensory one. Trained vision was of primary importance in the development of medicine and the biological sciences in 17th- and 18th-century Europe (Foucault 2003; Daston and Galison 2010), and its primacy had the effect of marginalising the role of touch and other senses within scientific knowledge practices (Classen 2012). Yet the primary sensory emphasis in *kanpō* was upon touch (Kuriyama 1997, 138) and upon the tactile discernment of subtle indications of change. No realist, ocular metaphors encapsulated the discrimination of patterns through pulse or abdominal diagnosis. Rather, accurate medical perception in *kanpō* was produced through a subjective engagement with fluid and changing patterns of the patient's *ki*, as registered through touch. Such an attitude towards medical perception would be overtly challenged by the new modality of visual praxis that was brokered by *Kaitai shinsho* and other scientific works that followed it.

Thus, as the Japanese medical body began to change in response to the powerful discourses and technologies of scientific medicine throughout the Edo and Meiji Periods and after, the sensory practices that interpreted that body were likewise impacted. As the ethnographic section to follow will demonstrate, however, such changes were not solely hegemonic but were also productive of novel ways of elaborating and engaging sensory potentials, processes that I would find continuing to unfold with the present-day globalised space of Zen *Shiatsu*.

Sensing *Kyo* in Zen *Shiatsu* Spaces

The term 'Zen *Shiatsu*' (a.k.a. 'meridian *shiatsu*') has been used to refer to a diverse set of *shiatsu* practice styles that developed from the teachings and writings of Masunaga Shizuto. As mentioned earlier, Zen *Shiatsu* has attained a greater prominence outside of Japan than inside it, although its most well-known innovators have all been Japanese-born therapists who studied with Masunaga before the latter's passing in 1981.

In this section, I consider the sensory dimensions of Zen *Shiatsu* training by focusing on its practices of diagnosis, which in different ways involve attending somatically and affectively in order to enact connective modes of touch. These practices reveal features of bodies and senses distinct from biomedical ones, and I argue that they become important to practitioners in part because of how they facilitate novel experiences of their own embodied subjectivity. There are three local sites that comprise this *shiatsu* space: a three-day seminar held at an ecological retreat centre north of Toronto; the Tokyo clinic of a senior practitioner and former associate of Masunaga's; and an intermediate-level class at a school in Kyoto founded by a Buddhist priest. In each of these sites, practitioners all sought to find *kyo*, the quality of deficiency which Masunaga proposed was equivalent to finding the root of a patient's health imbalance. They all approached this task differently, and their findings and descriptions were also diverse. And yet individually and collectively, they provide compelling examples of how reimagined East Asian spiritual therapies create possibilities for novel modes of sensory subject formation.

Before commencing with the ethnographic examples, I first provide a brief introduction to the founder of this approach, Masunaga Shizuto.

Masunaga Shizuto: Shiatsu Diagnosis as 'Feeling the Echo of Life'

Masunaga Shizuto (1925–1981) was an innovative *shiatsu* practitioner and theorist. He integrated diverse sources into his presentation of *shiatsu*, from classical literature on Chinese medicine and contemporaneous discourses on *ki*, to neurological research and the psychoanalytic teachings of Carl Rogers. He described *shiatsu* as a therapy that addressed the mind and body of the patient through clinical practices that likewise addressed the mind and body of the practitioner. For Masunaga, *shiatsu* was both a therapy and a form of embodied self-cultivation (cf. Chapters 3 and 10). He taught his students to develop an awareness of *ki* in their patients and in themselves through practices that married meditative self-awareness with clinical touch.

A key element of Masunaga's *shiatsu* was its diagnostic practice, which emphasised empathic touch. He taught his students to contact the patient's abdomen while also attending *internally* to their own lower abdomen, the *tanden* 丹田, as in meditation and martial art techniques. By bringing attention away from discursive thought, he held that a *shiatsu* practitioner could 'tune in' to subtle perceptions that would enable them to ascertain the quality of *kyo* in the patient's *ki*. *Kyo* represented deficiency and was seen as the fundamental energetic root of the body's illness and discomfort.

Discerning *kyo* was a major challenge. Hidden by nature, an expression of the patient's vulnerability, *kyo* was seldom something that was perceived directly. Students were given an audio metaphor: they were feeling for an 'echo', what Masunaga termed *seimei no hibiki* 生命の響き (echo of life). Their touch was likened to a form of compassionate listening. The therapist's fingers connected to the patient's body; the 'feeling' was something that happened not at the fingertips but at the centre of the therapist's own body-mind, in the *tanden*. Masunaga further explained this as a movement away from ordinary, discriminative awareness, towards a felt sense of 'oneness' with the patient. By cultivating empathy for one's patient, one could share in the patient's pain. This consubjective state, which Masunaga contrasted with the objectifying gaze of biomedicine, enabled one to perceive *kyo*.

While some have argued that Masunaga was 'recovering' lost knowledge from the classical East Asian medical tradition (Endo 2014), it is more accurate to say that he was innovatively reproducing it through cultural translations that were textual but also, in a sense, embodied.[9] Through his physical presence when teaching, and via exercises that he developed and demonstrated, he held out an embodied example for his students which inspired many of them to devote themselves to cultivating the subtle sensory capacities he described. Thirty years after Masunaga's death, I found *shiatsu* students and practitioners in Japan and Canada still engaging with his theoretical and clinical models – and with freshly embodied examples that were carried by a new generation of teachers – as they continued going about creatively cultivating diverse modes of sensory subjectivity.

Sensing Kyo at Shiatsu Summer Camp (*Barrie, Ontario*)

Learning this mode of connective touch and finding *kyo* was not easy, as the quality might be masked by the physical presentation of the soft tissue and could be 'drowned out' if students attended to their tactile sense.

9 Internal concentration on the *tanden* has long been a feature of Daoist self-cultivation practices in China (see Stanley-Baker 2012). Such practices also featured prominently in the methods and teachings of numerous healers in the broad *seishin ryōhō* movement of early-modern Japan (see, e.g., Kurita 2016).

Ikeda-sensei, a former student of Masunaga's, now a senior teacher in his own right who was leading a session at the *Shiatsu* Summer Camp in Ontario, told me,

> Masunaga was great. He would touch one part of your leg and say, 'See? The *ki* is blocked here. While over here [pointing elsewhere on the leg], the flow is normal'. But when I touched the same spots, I couldn't feel any difference. Nothing at all! It took me a long time to understand what he was showing me. (Field interview, August 2012)

Teachers of Zen *Shiatsu* whom I spoke with at the summer camp used different methods to instruct their students in this subtle mode of sensing, often highlighting an affective dimension of touch and bodily comportment, combined with attention to one's lower abdomen.

Randall, a male therapist in his mid-30s who had taught at a well-known *shiatsu* school in Toronto for several years before branching out on his own, told me that his committed practice of meditation was an essential part of his *shiatsu* practice, as it helped him to cultivate a sense of inner spaciousness and stillness, which he felt was necessary in order to connect with the patient and to perform *kyo* diagnosis. He mentioned that students new to *shiatsu* had a tendency to 'be in their heads, caught up in models and theories'. Part of his job, he felt, was to bring them 'down into their bodies' and to get them to trust their own feelings. Doing so would guide them on where to go in their treatments. He said that he tried to impart this in his teaching, and offered an example, describing how in a practice class he had asked a new student to treat her partner's headache without touching her partner's head. The student did not yet know a lot of theory, so did not know what areas she should focus on in her treatment. Randall said he told the student to 'just connect' by bringing attention to her *tanden* and trusting her hands. Her successful result that day gave her confidence in her own ability to diagnose and treat.

What did practitioners notice when they worked in such ways? What did *kyo* feel like? I received a perplexing diversity of answers to this question from Zen *shiatsu* practitioners. Emma, an instructor from another school, described her process as 'looking for the point that will relax the whole body'. As she scanned the patient's body while cultivating a feeling of empathy for the patient, certain points would 'stand out' for her, her eyes either coming to rest there, or the point exhibiting a momentary vividness or brightness.

Others described their perception of *kyo* in more kinesthetic terms, for example as a subtle pulling, as though their thumbs or fingers were being magnetically drawn to a point or area, or as simply noticing a hollow space that needed to be filled. Others described detecting subtle ripples or vibrations. The kinesthetic language frequently shaded into the poetic language of metaphor or simile:

> Sometimes tissues are hard and congested; but *kyo* hardness is different, like pressing on something like glass that's fragile [...]. you don't want to go too hard, or you'll break it, so you just hold gently and let the warmth of your hands soften it up.

For some, images were not only useful for explaining somatic perceptions but were actually the medium through which such perceptions were apprehended. Tanya, a female therapist in her late 20s based in a suburb of Toronto, gave me a short treatment during one of the workshops. Afterwards, she mentioned that while she had been treating my legs, she had received a strong visual impression of me sitting with my feet towards a fire, which she interpreted to mean that my legs were deficient in *ki* and thus needed 'warming up' through longer-than-normal periods of holding.[10]

As *shiatsu* practitioners attended inwardly, to their own internal abdomens, they often described to me that they were simultaneously discerning something of the deeper layers of the patient's 'energy'. Many held to some form of the notion that the body-mind had a material front but an 'energetic' core, where currents could flow or become stuck (cf. Chapters 1 and 5). Reaching 'through' the surface texture of clothing, skin and soft tissue was often said to be best accomplished by conjoining an internal awareness of one's own body with some form of compassion or empathy for the patient. One might then perceive images, kinesthetic sensations, or alterations to one's vision. One might even 'tune into' and help to release a patient's 'blocked emotions' (cf. Chapter 4). Several practitioners described to me how this was a dimension of their clinical experience. I would receive a taste of this myself when I visited the clinic of a longtime Zen *Shiatsu* practitioner in Tokyo, whom I call Shirakawa-sensei.

A Treatment with Shirakawa-sensei

I met Shirakawa-sensei at his '*Shiatsu* Gakuen' ('*Shiatsu* Academy'), a six-tatami-mat room in the small apartment he shared with his wife, very close

10 Interestingly, this particular piece of feedback – that my legs were deficient in *ki* – was something I heard from a number of therapists at different times during my fieldwork, even though their individual processes were all quite different.

to a major railway station located on Tokyo's loop line. I had arranged to meet him for a treatment and an interview, and he suggested we start with the treatment first. I lay down on the treatment futon and he began right away, without doing any intake, just pressing upon my abdomen and then beginning a whole-body treatment. I found Shirakawa-sensei's pressure gentle, and his pace unhurried. In several places on my body, he held his pressure for a duration of several seconds. I was quickly lulled into a slightly dreamy state, where his pressure sometimes seemed to have a spreading quality.

At the end of the treatment, there were two notable occurrences. First, he asked me to lay on my back, and while sitting behind my head he lifted both of my arms and supported them each at the elbows with a gentle grip. I could notice a slight asymmetry in how easily my arms rested in this position. Suddenly, and quite unexpectedly, my pelvis and right leg gave a large involuntary twitch, which was followed by a few deep breaths and long sighs that seemed to come of their own accord. I laughed and asked him what had just happened, to which he replied, 'It's hard to explain'.

Then he laid my arms back down at my side and, taking a kneeling position beside me, began palpating my abdomen again. I assumed he was assessing which organ he thought was *kyo* and asked him if he could tell me what he was discerning. After a short pause, he began to press with the fingertips of his right hand softly but steadily under my rib cage on the right side, while his left hand rested upon my lower abdomen. Then he spoke in a quiet voice, saying that my body was a bit tense (*chotto katai* ちょっと硬い), that this was due to stress which was not only emotional but also 'spiritual', and that it was showing in my liver system. He maintained his pressure after he finished speaking. Suddenly I experienced a rush of recent memories pertaining to my son, who had undergone some bullying at his new daycare and had started showing troubling psychological symptoms. The images were vivid and coincided with strong emotions on my part, and my eyes began to tear up.

After a minute or so, I had recovered enough to explain to Shirakawa-sensei what I was experiencing and mentioned my worries about my son. 'Give *shiatsu* to him. Every day', was his immediate response. 'When you touch with a warm heart, this is acceptance, this is communication'. Later, when I asked him to confirm that he had found my liver meridian to be *kyo*, he said that while it was true that *kyo* was the 'hidden part, the root' of a patient's condition, too much attention to this made things complicated. When he taught students, he said, he encouraged them to practise *shiatsu* simply, and to try to let go of their expectations and desire for results. 'You find *kyo*', he said, 'by not looking too hard' (cf. Chapter 3).

The Body is the Shadow of Ki

While Masunaga did not elaborate any formal connections between the theology or practice of Zen Buddhism and the practice of *shiatsu*, the name 'Zen *Shiatsu*' had stuck to his system, and as in the case of Randall, above, there were many practitioners who felt that some form of meditation was an important support for effective Zen *Shiatsu* practice. The Sangha School (pseudonym),[11] however, made this Buddhism-*shiatsu* connection central to their approach (although it was Pure Land Buddhism, not Zen, which was the basis of the teachings). In this school, located at the end of a narrow lane in the Gion district of Kyoto, *shiatsu* was expressly described as a kind of spiritual training, the goal of which was to actualise an enlightened state of selflessness. Students worked at this through a mode of sensory training, in which they activated what I term 'affective senses' – tuning in to the sensations that accompanied their own strong expressions of affect, which came in the form of compassionate wishing for others. When they had actualised a deep enough practice of wishing, the *ki* of their fellow students became sensible to them, and they could find *kyo* either by feel or by sight.

During my fieldwork, I took part in an intermediate-level course at the school, the goal of which was to move students to a place where they could perceive the effects of *ki* via subtle senses. Learning to shift one's *kokoro* 心 ('heart-mind')[12] was essential to this endeavour. This training involved an affective practice of wishing the best for others or for one's partner (*sesshin* 接心[13]), along with an interiorly-directed somatic scanning and introspection (*naikan* 内観). Students would endeavour to wish with such intensity that they felt pain or discomfort arise in their own *kokoro*, which was usually felt in the chest region. The pain was understood to be the pain of their own deep-rooted negativity which had been triggered in response to the powerful wish: it was their ego reacting to an effort at selflessness. Students attuned to this sensation and tried to recognise the particular form of selfish inclination that was generating such resistance, which they did by noticing

11 *Sangha* is a Buddhist term denoting a spiritual community.

12 In the Japanese language, the term *kokoro* is suited to both affective and embodied connotations, as well as to notions of gradual development. It is a polysemic term which is suggestive of English notions such as mind, psyche, emotion, feeling, wish, intention, sympathy, and care: it also possesses a more corporeal dimension, as the character with which it is written (心) was used to refer to the bodily heart within *kanpō*, which was simultaneously the seat of intention and emotion. In Sanga School practices, when students attended to their *kokoro*, they noted affective sensations that were typically felt in the chest region, close to the anatomical heart.

13 This *sesshin* 接心 was a Buddhist term implying focused concentration on the well-being of others; such was needed to practise the *sesshin* 切診 of *kanpō* touch diagnosis, within Sangha *Shiatsu*.

the tenor of thoughts that arose in its wake (was it doubt? vanity?). By feeling the discomfort in their *kokoro*, investigating and accepting the negativity behind it, and then intending to shift beyond it into a fuller expression of wishing the best for others, students could attain a still deeper level of this selfless, 'Giving Heart', which enabled unique forms of clinical perception.

Before trying to diagnose *kyo* or to treat others, students undertook different kinds of practice exercises in order to help them recognise a subtle, nonphysical body termed the '*ki* body' (*ki no karada* 気の体). The *ki* body was understood to be a subtle energetic field that extended for more than one metre around the periphery of the physical body but that also interpenetrated it. Meridians, and the quality of *kyo* itself, were held to be features of *this* body, not the physical one. This body was held to be a truer, more essential expression of the whole person; in contrast, the physical body of daily experience was held to be only the 'shadow of *ki*', and the common understanding of people as being 'only' their physical bodies was held to be a misperception. Yet learning to 'see through' this illusion required extensive practice and commitment (cf. Chapters 5 and 10).

One mode of practice was as follows: students would sit on the tatami-matted floor, back-to-back with a partner. One partner would concentrate on cultivating a strong expression of their Giving Heart by wishing intensely for their partner's happiness; the 'receiver' would sit quietly and pay attention to what they felt in their own body-mind. When they noticed a 'shift', they were to indicate it verbally. These shifts often took the form of their physical body suddenly relaxing, of a tingling feeling or a feeling of lightness, even bliss. Occasionally some would report that a headache or other ailment was relieved or reduced in intensity.

The idea of this practice was that by wishing sincerely, one could activate one's *busshō* 仏性 (Buddha Nature), and this would result in a very pure form of *ki* (*seiki* 正気) starting to flow from one's own *kokoro*. This would permeate one's own *ki* body and that of one's partner, bringing feelings of upliftment to the latter. The verbal feedback from the receiver helped the first partner to correlate their own inner sensation (of painful wishing) with the successful activation of their *ki* body. Conversely, feedback that nothing had changed, or that the receiver's body was feeling 'heavy', was an indication that the first partner's wishing practice was not sufficient and that they needed to apply themselves more earnestly. In this way, trainee therapists were exposed to how their own affective states were transmissible and perceivable to their partners, and thus developed a somato-affective yardstick for recognising what sort of effect their heart state was having on others. Advanced students could accomplish the same result without being in direct physical contact with a partner, while the instructors claimed to be able to identify the particular mode of egoic resistance arising in the one wishing while standing across the room. In this classroom, students were developing and training nonmaterial sensory skills that reworked their experiences of body and mind.

Once students had demonstrated a facility with shifting into the mode of the Giving Heart, they were ready to begin diagnosing *kyo* on their partner. In these exercises, the receiving partner would lay on their back upon a futon, and the acting therapist would begin by cultivating their wish. The receiver would indicate when the wish was positively impacting their *ki* body, and then the therapist would gaze at the arm, inwardly asking, 'Where does the receiver most wish to be pressed?' while continuing to deepen their wishing. This would help the *kyo no tsubo* (虚のツボ; 'point', as in pressure point or acupuncture point) become discernible – to both the therapist and the receiver. The therapist would find *kyo visually*: my fellow students described seeing localised areas of brightness or of a small region that magnetically attracted their vision. Some reported momentarily seeing white or pale blue lines shining through the receiver's clothing. Meanwhile, the receiver would notice the *kyo no tsubo somatically*, via an internal sensation of hollowness, emptiness, achiness, or a feeling of 'wanting to be pressed here'. The therapist would touch the point first before treating it and check it in with the receiver. If the point that the therapist had selected coincided with what the receiver had felt – which it very often did, especially when senior students were in the therapist role – then the therapist could proceed to treatment, applying pressure to the point while deepening their wish. (If not, they needed to pull back and start over). Pressure delivered in this way was reported to be deeply satisfying, and receivers often reported perceiving an 'echo' – a sensation of achiness somewhere distal to the point of pressure, where it was understood that stagnant *ki* was exiting the *ki* body.

Sangha School practices thus represented a significant extension of Zen *Shiatsu* ideas. Masunaga's statements about compassion as being fundamental to the act of medical diagnosis had here been culturally translated through ideas and practices from the Pure Land Buddhist meditation tradition, as well as from the head teacher's own textual and embodied innovations. Applying themselves to these practices, students enacted strong expressions of compassionate affect and learned that affect was not only somatically sensible to themselves but to others as well (cf. Chapters 4 and 6). In diagnosis, these practices rendered the 'material surface' of the body momentarily transparent, so that features of the '*ki* body' could shine through. This body was not bounded as was the physical body; it interpenetrated the *ki* bodies of others, creating shared affective spaces and 'consubjective' modes of attention (Csordas 1993). Sangha School students thus found that their *shiatsu* training to be a radical means of overcoming the material ontology of everyday life, while also a means of producing themselves as certain kinds of ethical actors. While this training was difficult, students all reported finding it deeply meaningful.

Conclusion

This chapter has engaged with two of the questions that motivate the present collection. The first is as follows: While entangled imaginaries of 'East Asia' – as an origin point of and epistemic frame for therapeutic/spiritual practices such as *shiatsu* – may hold a particular salience for our research subjects, how might scholars avoid letting them structure our analyses of the global movement and transformation of these practices?

In answer, this chapter has argued that adopting an analytic approach of 'worlding' helps to reconfigure implicit cartographies that might structure our analyses of global forms of knowledge. In a worlding approach, claims about 'East Asian-ness' emerge *within* the field, rather than structuring it a priori. Spiritual or healing practices are always already enmeshed within complex translocal networks (of actors, institutions, economies, communities, regulatory and discursive regimes, etc.), and their meanings and routes of movement are continuously remade. Thus, they are continuously reformulated and reproduced through the enactment of meaningful 'worlds'. Recognising that even at their time and point of origin, practices were already enmeshed within multiple forms of global connection helps to destabilise any essentialist power that 'East Asia' might hold as an epistemic frame. Instead, the category becomes one more feature whose culturally translated meanings can be traced within translocal spaces that are connected through particular worlding projects.

The second question invites us to shift analytic scales, to see whether attending to 'local minds and bodies' (Asprem and Strube 2021) might help us to better understand why practices that are labelled 'East Asian', and which make use of concepts such as *ki*, have become so widely adopted and adapted by individuals across the globe.

With regard to this second question, this chapter has proposed that while an analysis of Orientalist East Asian imaginaries can tell us something about how a modality such as Zen *Shiatsu* has come to 'stick' in places across the globe, attention to the embodied practices of teachers and practitioners can provide additional textures to such an answer. In particular, Zen *Shiatsu* practices of diagnosing *kyo* involve *shiatsu* practitioners in the production of novel forms of sensory subjectivity and experience. For many practitioners, they enable glimpses or tastes of mutualistic forms of subjective expression and can galvanise potent expressions of positive affect. Such experiences not only offer practitioners a basis from which to critically reflect upon the hegemonic models (of body and mind, and of the therapeutic relationship itself) within biomedicine, but also hold out resources for reworking individuals' everyday ontologies of being-in-the-world. While such transformations and translations of sensory subjectivity can be difficult to locate and track, they enable Zen *Shiatsu* practitioners to produce themselves as embodied, ethical actors in novel sensory worlds. Such 'sensory worlding', I suggest, is an important dimension of the broader worlding of Zen *Shiatsu* therapy and is likely to be salient to the study of other modalities of bodily movement, healing, and religious practice.

Bibliography

Adams, Glyn. 2002. '*Shiatsu* in Britain and Japan: Personhood, Holism and Embodied Aesthetics'. *Anthropology and Medicine* 9, no. 3: 245–68. https://doi.org/10.1080/13648470216334.

Alter, Joseph. 2005. 'Introduction: The Politics and Culture of Medicine'. In *Asian Medicine and Globalisation*, edited by J. Alter, 1–20. Pittsburgh: University of Pennsylvania Press. https://doi.org/10.9783/9780812205251.1.

Asprem, Egil, and Julian Strube, eds. 2021. *New Approaches to the Study of Esotericism*. Leiden: Brill. https://doi.org/10.1163/9789004446458.

Barnes, Linda. 1998. 'The Psychologizing of Chinese Healing Practices in the United States'. *Culture, Medicine and Psychiatry* 22: 413–43. https://doi.org/10.1023/A:1005403825213.

Befu, Harumi. 2001. *Hegemony of Homogeneity: An Anthropological Analysis of Nihonjinron*. Melbourne: Trans Pacific Press.

Bendix, Regina. 2005. 'Introduction: Ear to Ear, Nose to Nose, Skin to Skin – The Senses in Comparative Perspective'. *Senses—Special Issue of Etnofoor, Anthropological Journal* 18, no. 1: 3–14. https://doi.org/10.2307/25758082.

Bhabha, Homi. 1984. *The Location of Culture*. London: Routledge.

Classen, Constance. 1998. *The Color of Angels: Cosmology, Gender and the Aesthetic Imagination*. London: Routledge. https://doi.org/10.4324/9780203007594.

Classen, Constance. 2012. *The Deepest Sense: A Cultural History of Touch*. Chicago and Springfield: University of Illinois Press. https://doi.org/10.5406/illinois/9780252034930.001.0001.

Clarke, J.J. 1997. *Oriental Enlightenment: The Encounter Between Asian and Western Thought*. London and New York: Routledge. https://doi.org/10.4324/9780203004388.

Cox, Rupert. 2003. *The Zen Arts: An Anthropological Study of the Culture of Aesthetic Form in Japan.* London: RoutledgeCurzon, in association with The Royal Asiatic Society of Great Britain and Ireland. https://doi.org/10.4324/9781315028910.

Csordas, Thomas. 1993. 'Somatic Modes of Attention'. *Current Anthropology* 8, no. 2: 135–56. https://doi.org/10.1525/can.1993.8.2.02a00010.

Daston, Lorraine, and Peter Galison. 2010. *Objectivity*. New York: Zone Books.

Drott, Edward. 2010. 'Gods, Buddhas, and Organs: Buddhist Physicians and Theories of Longevity in Early Medieval Japan'. *Japanese Journal of Religious Studies* 37, no. 2: 247–73. https://doi.org/10.18874/jjrs.37.2.2010.247-273.

Foucault, Michel. 2003 [1973]. *The Birth of the Clinic: An Archaeology of Medical Perception*. New York: Pantheon.

Heelas, Paul. 1996. *The New Age Movement*. Oxford: Blackwell.

Howes, David. 2003. *Sensual Relations: Engaging the Senses in Culture and Social Theory.* Ann Arbor: University of Michigan Press. https://doi.org/10.3998/mpub.11852.

Howes, David, ed. 2005. *Empire of the Senses: The Sensual Culture Reader.* Oxford: Berg.

Howes, David, and Constance Classen. 2014. *Ways of Sensing: Understanding the Senses in Society*. London: Routledge. https://doi.org/10.4324/9781315856032.

Groemer, Gerald. 2001. 'The Guild of the Blind in Tokugawa Japan'. *Monumenta Nipponica* 56, no 3: 349–80. https://doi.org/10.2307/3096791.

Janes, Craig. 2002. 'Buddhism, Science and the Market: The Globalization of Tibetan Medicine'. *Anthropology and Medicine* 9, no. 3: 267–89. https://doi.org/10.1080/13648470216337.

Kitanaka, Junko. 2012. *Depression in Japan: Psychiatric Cures for a Society in Distress.* Princeton: Princeton University Press. https://doi.org/10.2307/j.ctt7rrvo.

Kurita, Hidehiko. 2016. 'Fukushiki kokyū no kindai: Fujitashiki sokushin chōwahō o jirei toshite腹式呼吸の近代: 藤田式息心調和法を事例として' [Modernity in Japanese Breathing Techniques: Fujita Reisai and his Activities]. *Studies in Religions East and West* 43:1–24.

Kuriyama, Shigehisa. 1992. 'Between Mind and Eye: Japanese Anatomy in the Eighteenth Century'. In *Paths to Asian Medical Knowledge*, edited by Charles Leslie and Allan Young, 21–43. Berkeley: University of California Press. https://doi.org/10.1525/california/9780520073173.003.0002.

Kuriyama, Shigehisa. 1997. 'The Historical Origins of Katakori'. *Japan Review* 9: 127–49.

Langford, Jean. 2002. *Fluent Bodies: Ayurvedic Remedies for Post-colonial Imbalance.* Durham: Duke University Press. https://doi.org/10.1215/9780822384113.

Latour, Bruno. 1993. *We Have Never Been Modern*. Cambridge, MA: Harvard University Press.

Long, Andrew. 2007a. *The Effects and Experience of Shiatsu: A Cross-European Study.* Leeds: University of Leeds School of Healthcare.

Long, Andrew. 2007b *The Practitioners within the Cross-European Shiatsu Study. Their Characteristics and an Insight into Their Practice*. Leeds: University of Leeds School of Healthcare.

Masunaga, Shizuto (translated by Wataru Ohashi). 1977. *Zen Shiatsu: How to Harmonize Yin and Yang for Better Health*. Tokyo: Japan Publications, Inc.

Scheid, Volker. 2002. *Chinese Medicine in Contemporary China: Plurality and Synthesis*. Durham: Duke University Press. https://doi.org/10.1215/9780822383710.

Screech, Timon. 2002. *The Lens within the Heart: The Western Scientific Gaze and Popular Imagery in Later Edo Japan*. 2nd ed. Richmond: Curzon.

Skrivanic, Peter. 2016. 'Worlding *Shiatsu* Therapy: Circumventing the East-West Dichotomy in a Comparative Ethnographic Project'. *Inochi no mirai* 1: 193–216. https://doi.org/10.14989/203146.

Skrivanic, Peter. 2018. 'Medicine and Religion are Not-Two: Sensory Economies of Knowledge in "Zen *Shiatsu*"'. *Studies in Religion/Sciences Religieuses* 47, no. 2: 210–22. https://doi.org/10.1177/0008429817733140.

Spivak, Gayatri. 2000. 'Translation as Culture'. *Paralax* 6: 13–24. https://doi.org/10.1080/135346400249252

Stanley-Baker, Michael. 2012. 'Palpable Access to the Divine: Daoist Medieval Massage, Visualization and Internal Sensation'. *Asian Medicine* 7, no. 1: 101. https://doi.org/10.1163/15734218-12341245.

Stein, Justin. 2023. *Alternate Currents: Reiki's Circulation in the Twentieth-Century North Pacific*. Honolulu: University of Hawaii Press.

Tamai, Tenpeki玉井天碧. 1939 (Reprint 2008). *Shiatsu-hō furoku: Shiatsu ryōhō jibyō higaki* [指圧法 付録・指圧療法治病秘鍵*Shiatsu* Method with Appendix: The Secret Key to *Shiatsu* Therapy Treatment]. Tokyo: Hachiman Shoten.

Tsing, Anna. 2015. *The Mushroom at the End of the World: On the Possibility of Life in Capitalist Ruins*. Princeton: Princeton University Press.

Warrier, Maya. 2009. 'Seekership, Spirituality and Self-discovery: Ayurveda Students in Britain'. *Asian Medicine: Tradition and Modernity* 4: 423–51. https://doi.org/10.1163/157342009x12526658783691.

Zhan, Mei. 2009. *Other-Worldly: Making Chinese Medicine through Transnational Frames*. Durham: Duke University Press. https://doi.org/10.1215/9780822392132.

Biography

Peter Skrivanic is a graduate student at the Department of Anthropology, University of Toronto. His research focuses upon the cultivation of sensory skills among trainee *shiatsu* therapists in Canada and Japan.

3 Capturing the Moment of *Kimochi-ii*

Transnational Flows and the Transformation of *Qigong* in Japan

Huang Xinzhe

Abstract: This paper focuses on the practice of *qigong* and aims to analyse its localisation and transformation in contemporary Japan. Instead of solely examining how *qigong*'s theories and knowledge originated in China and were adapted to the Japanese context, this chapter highlights the significance of bodily experiences, including affect, senses, and imagination, to describe the generation and transformation of specific feelings during Japanese *qigong* classes. When discussing 'transnational *qigong*', I suggest that it is also crucial to consider how the sharing, generation, and transformation of sensory and affective experiences through *qigong* practice preserves its vitality in the local context and constructs a local *qigong* culture.

Keywords: *qigong,* affect, bodily experience, feeling

I still vividly remember my first time conducting fieldwork for Amano-sensei's *qigong* 气功 (pronounced *kikō* 気功 in Japanese) class five years ago (2018). Although I was not a *qigong* practitioner at the time, I was confident that I could understand *qigong* better than most beginners due to my six years of training in Traditional Chinese Medicine (TCM). I thought to myself, '*qigong* is part of TCM, and I am an experienced practitioner who has studied it at an accredited Chinese university'.[1] However, when I arrived in my first class, my convictions were quickly replaced by a culture shock.

1 I studied TCM at Shanghai University of Traditional Chinese Medicine for six years and obtained a medical license to work as a TCM doctor in hospitals in China.

Gaitanidis, Ioannis, Luis Fernando Bernardi Junqueira, Avery Morrow, and Sangyun Han (eds), *Therapy, Spirituality, and East Asian Imaginaries.* Taylor & Francis Group 2025
DOI: 10.5117/9789048559015_CH03

After listening to a lecture by Amano-sensei lasting an hour and a half, my original views on *qigong* were completely overturned. Amano-sensei made no reference to TCM, *qigong* theories, meridians, or acupoints – all topics that I was initially expecting to hear about. Instead, he delved into topics I was entirely unfamiliar with, such as the body's *kyūsho* 急所 and *katsuten* 活点.[2] Occasionally, he also spoke enthusiastically about Buddhism, the unconscious, and even the concept of *harai* 祓い (purification) from Shinto. Although I was struck by how Amano-sensei's approach to *qigong* differed from my expectations, I was most surprised by the practical part of his lecture. When Amano-sensei and his students practised *qigong*, I was struck by their facial expressions more than their movements or postures. Almost every student seemed to be making an expression of intense joy. I was surrounded by smiles. Occasionally, I would hear someone say, 'Oh... that feels so good' (*aa... kimochi-ii* あ...気持ちいい). Amano-sensei also seemed to be wholly immersed in this world of 'feeling good' (*kimochi-ii*). With each movement, he expressed his *kimochi-ii* in various ways. He used verbal expressions, such as 'feeling good' (*kimochi-ii*), 'feeling comfortable' (*kokochi-ii* 心地いい), 'feeling better' (*raku ni naru* 楽になる)', and 'feeling lighter' (*karuku naru* 軽くなる). He raised the corners of his smile just a little higher and gently opened his eyes – which, to my surprise, had been closed – leaving the students in the classroom with a feeling of his genuine delight in the moment.

His teachings contrasted with what I had previously learned at the field site in Shanghai, where *qi* was understood to be the core concept of *qigong* and the 'feeling of *qi*' (*qi gan* 气感) was an important junction between *qigong* and other health exercises (Huang 2022; cf. Chapter 1). For Amano-sensei, learning to feel *kimochi-ii* is the gateway to *qigong* practice. In fact, the 10 movements of Amano-sensei's most well-known *qigong* technique, referred to as the 'simple way to calm your mind',[3] are actions meant to induce *kimochi-ii* and similar bodily experiences. Moreover, as I became more familiar with Amano-sensei's conception of *qigong*, I gradually realised that *kimochi-ii* was not merely a physical sensation that he wanted his students to experience by themselves: it was also intertwined with the therapeutic effects and unique bodily experiences of *qigong* practice. Put differently,

2 Both concepts refer to vital locations on the body and are often associated with *Noguchi Seitai*, a Japanese therapy that encompasses osteopathy, massage, and chiropractic (see later sections of this chapter).

3 In Japanese, *kokoro ga ochitsuku yasashii kikō* こころが落ち着くやさしい気功. The English translation is Amano's. Based on his personal *qigong* experience, these 10 movements are the simplest way to get the feeling of *kimochi-ii*, whether one practices in group or alone.

in Amano-sensei's class, all aspects of *qigong* experiences should begin by learning and mastering the feeling of *kimochi-ii*.

How can *kimochi-ii* emerge and be transformed into other *qigong* experiences through practices and techniques in Amano-sensei's class? Indeed, perhaps an even more basic question is: How did people feel *kimochi-ii* while participating in Amano-sensei's *qigong* practice? With these research questions in mind, this chapter will describe and analyse Amano-sensei's classes of *qigong* at his Qigong Association (Kikō Kyokai 気功協会) in Kyoto.

The Globalisation and Localisation of *Qigong*

Many people think of *qigong* as a traditional Chinese bodily practice. Although the theories and practices of *qigong* consist of various elements from Daoism, Buddhism, and other traditional cultural contexts, it is also partially an 'invented tradition' that emerged in modern times (Palmer 2003; cf. Chapter 4). In the early 1950s, Liu Guizhen (刘贵珍), a cadre of the Chinese Communist Party, brought together various ancient movement practices into what he later called '*qigong*'[4], subsequently developing a so-called '*qigong* therapy' (*qigong liaofa* 气功疗法). That is to say, *qigong* as a category has existed for only approximately 70 years. Nevertheless, *qigong* has since then been practised and researched by numerous people worldwide, including scientists and medical doctors. This is perhaps due to *qigong*'s healing effects and the mysterious experiences (such as the feeling of *qi*) that practitioners claim it induces. However, although there is extensive research on the therapeutic benefits of *qigong*, its benefits are often explained with reference to psychological and psychiatric concepts, such as the 'placebo effect' or the 'suggestibility effect' (Murakawa 2015). Modern societies, particularly advanced industrialised nations such as Japan, tend to emphasise evidence-based medicine. Yet, practices such as *qigong*, which lack concrete scientific validation but emphasise bodily experiences such as sensation and affect, are accepted by the population at large.

In fact, similar to yoga, *qigong* continues to expand globally (Hsu 2008). Sociological and anthropological studies on *qigong* have examined this international expansion – the phenomenon of 'transnational *qigong*' – from the macro perspectives of politics and economics (Chen 2003; Chen 2005). There exist, however, no specific studies looking at how 'transnational

4 The term *qigong* is a combination of two Chinese characters, *qi* 气 and *gong* 功. *Qi* is often translated as 'breath', 'spirit', or 'vital energy', and *gong* means 'practice', 'skill', or 'ability'.

*qigong*s' have been localised and transformed within specific cultural contexts. Meanwhile, anthropological studies focusing on other religious and spiritual healing practices have examined how therapies are shaped by interactions between local and imported 'traditional medicines', as well as by the interplay between traditional medicines, religious healing, and biomedicine in the context of ongoing globalisation (Kate and Samuel 2013; Zhan 2009). For example, Zhan's (2009) research on the development of TCM in the United States shows that different paths of knowledge inflow have led to differences in the understanding of TCM between the East and West Coasts of the United States. Moreover, Palmer and Siegler (2016) examine issues related to authority and legitimacy that arise when religious healing practices cross borders, which the authors illustrated by analysing the contact between American Daoist practitioners and Chinese Daoist ritual specialists. The above studies describe how therapeutic practices have been transformed when interacting with local knowledge and how theoretical frameworks have been modified during the interrelated processes of globalisation and localisation. However, most works have primarily been written from the perspective of medical professionals, therapists, and other authorities in the field. As a result, the experiences of those receiving treatment and engaging in these practices have been largely marginalised, creating a significant gap that my study aims to address and bridge.

The teachings and practices of *qigong* in Japan have undergone significant changes over the past 40 years. In the beginning, *qigong* masters from China were often invited to Japan to teach. Eventually, Japanese practitioners established their own *qigong* organisations and therapy centres founded on their own ways of thinking and understanding *qigong*. In response to this phenomenon, which could be described as the 'Japanisation of *qigong*', in their book *Kikō: Sono shisō to jissen* 気功：その思想と実践 (Qigong: Its Philosophy and Practice), the Liao brothers, renowned Chinese *qigong* masters and scholars, criticised the so-called 'absence of thought' and 'opportunism' (*gotsugō shugi* 御都合主義) of Japanese *qigong*. They asserted that these deficiencies in traditional Chinese philosophy and traditional medical theory in Japanese *qigong* have been detrimental to the overseas development of the practice (Liao and Liao 2012).

The decrease in the authority of nationally established medical knowledge due to the rise of local alternatives is not a rare phenomenon. It is evident, for example, in Iida's (2006) research on Thai massage therapy as well as in Farquhar and Lai's (2021) research on medical practices within minority communities in China. Therefore, it is likely that a similar change has occurred in the adoption of *qigong* in Japan. This chapter does not address the accusations of 'opportunism' or 'absence of thought' directed towards Japanese *qigong*, nor does it examine the interactions between knowledge and theoretical systems of *qigong* in China and Japan. Instead, I delve into how the category of 'Japanese *qigong*' has been generated through specific bodily practices. Furthermore, as previous anthropological studies on religious and spiritual healing practice have highlighted, the bodily experiences of patients, especially the sensations and affects that arise through the practice of engaging with the environment, also have a powerful impact on the construction of the therapeutic effect of *qigong* (De Antoni 2022). That is, while comparing knowledge and theories and assessing the legitimacy and authority of practitioners are essential aspects of studying practices conducted under the label of *qigong*, equal attention must be given to the bodily experiences of *qigong* practitioners arising from their actual engagement in the practice.

Bodily Experiences and Affective Technologies in *Qigong* Practice

From 1980 to the end of the 1990s, *qigong* grew rapidly in China – a period known as the '*qigong* boom' or '*qigong* fever' (Palmer 2007). During this time, *qigong* practices became a subject of increased interest for sociologists and anthropologists. Studies from this period have primarily examined *qigong* from a macro perspective, considering the effects of *qigong* on the body in relation to politics, economy, education, and healthcare within the particular historical context that followed the Cultural Revolution during the post-Mao period (Chen 2003; Palmer 2007; Hsu 1999; Utiraruto 2009). Micro-scale studies that emphasise bodily experience have been conducted in the past. However, these studies often tended to concentrate solely on either the instructor or the learner, and, as a result, they frequently overlooked the interrelationships between *qigong* movements, postures, and the bodily experiences of those involved. They also overlooked how practice generates specific experiences and therapeutic effects (Ots 1994; Sagli 2008). A body that practices *qigong* is not an isolated entity, though, and it is thus necessary to take into account the interactive and intersubjective relationships between the bodies of the instructor and the learners in environments where *qigong* is practised. In this regard, Csordas (1994), who studied religious therapeutic practices in North America, posited the concept of 'somatic modes of attention', processes of culturally refining attention through bodily practice in an intersubjective environment. This notion can also be used when studying the bodily experiences of *qigong*.

Similar to other anthropological studies of the senses (cf. Chapters 2 and 4), this chapter is also concerned with the problem of how sensory experience can construct the social practice of *qigong* (Howes 2005; Pink 2009). To better understand the prelinguistic and ambiguous bodily experiences of *qigong* practices, I will examine the concept of affect (Massumi 2002; cf. Chapter 2), understood as the precognitive, presymbolic, prelinguistic, and prepersonal lived intensities that constitute the realities from which subjects emerge. Because *qigong* experiences cannot be reduced into either sensations or emotions, this chapter adopts a broader conception of affect that encompasses both sensation and emotion while focusing on 'practices of feeling with the world' (De Antoni and Dumouchel 2017). This approach is based on Ingold's (2000) notion of 'enskilment', understood as the active involvement of affect and bodily perception in acquiring bodily techniques. This acquisition is facilitated by the emergence of the social within the practice, as well as through coordination, attunement and correspondence with the environment.

For example, existing anthropological research on *qigong* contains many descriptions of practitioners utilising their imagination to memorise *qigong* techniques (Chen 2003; Palmer 2007; Hsu 1999; Sagli 2008). However, there is no description linking the imagination to the bodily experiences that are induced by *qigong*. In anthropology, imagination is often used as a template to link practice and thinking, and anthropological studies often demonstrate how imagination limits experience. Here, the notion of 'technologies of imagination', which posits the imagination in processual terms (Sneath, Holbraad and Pedersen 2009), is helpful for analysing the *qigong* experiences that emphasise the importance of process. Meanwhile, according to Csordas's (1994) research on charismatic healing, embodied memories always interact with the imagination and contribute to the efficacy of healing through bodily practice. That is, embodied memories obtained from bodily healing practices can be understood as conditions that enable imagination. In the context of my study, this finding implies that the generation of *qigong* experiences can be described more clearly by analysing interactions between embodied memories and imagination. Furthermore, De Antoni (2023) suggests that ontologies of the spirit can be accessed by attuning oneself to and feeling with affective technologies together with others in the field. In this context, De Antoni is implying that the bodily experience of *qigong* can also be captured by the ethnographer. In other words, describing the moment of capturing a *qigong* experience is a direct approach to understanding the local practices of *qigong*. Therefore, during my fieldwork, I adopted the role of a student rather than just a researcher in order to shift my default mindset and approach to learning *qigong* (cf. Chapters 2 and 10 for similar approaches). Despite undergoing training for several months, it remained challenging to fully grasp the same feelings and experiences as the other participants in the field. Nonetheless, as a researcher, it was crucial for me to integrate myself within the community to gain a profound understanding of how emotions emerged, evolved, and were acknowledged as the wellspring of healing power.

Relativising *Qi* and Transcending *Qigong*: Amano-sensei's Qigong Association

Qigong is not an invention of Japan. *Qi*, on the other hand, has for centuries been a central element in Japanese medicine and self-cultivation. By the early Taisho Period (1912–1926), *qi* was restructured within the framework of spiritual therapy and merged with concepts from the Western intellectual tradition (Kurita 2019). Several spiritual healing techniques that emerged during that period, such as 'Okada-style sitting meditation' and *reiki*, were also seen as pioneering forms of Japanese *qigong* (Imura 1984). However, the most recognised form of *qigong* among veteran figures in the Japanese *qigong* community is Noguchi Haruchika's (野口晴哉,1911–1976) *Noguchi Seitai* 野口整体. Tsumura Takashi (津村喬,1948–2020), a leading figure in the Japanese *qigong* community, categorises Japanese body practices such as Noguchi *Seitai* as 'Japanese-style *qigong*'.

Although the invention of *qigong* and the emergence of the '*qigong* boom' first occurred in China, the concept of *qigong* was also gradually embraced in Japan. According to the findings of the Society for Mind-Body Science in Japan, which studies the history of Japanese *qigong*, the beginning of Japanese *qigong* can be traced back to the establishment of the Chinese Sports Research Association by Tsumura Takashi and Hoshino Minoru (星野稔,1947–2020) in 1978. As a result of their efforts, *qigong* organisations were subsequently established all across Japan. In 1987, Tsumura established the Kansai Qigong Association (*Kansai Kikō Kyōkai* 関西気功協会) in Kyoto, and Hoshino established the Japanese Qigong Health Research Association (*Nihon Kikō Eiseigaku Kenkyūkai* 日本気功養生学研究会) in Tokyo, both of which were important for the diffusion of *qigong* in Japan. Two years later, in 1989, the philosopher Yuasa Yasuo (湯浅泰雄,1925–2005) played a central role in founding the Society for Mind-Body Science, which focused on *qigong* research and worked to foster exchanges with China. Consequently, the number of *qigong* practitioners in Japan increased significantly. In addition, numerous academic organisations began conducting *qigong* research, leading to publications on the materiality of *qi* and the therapeutic benefits of *qigong*. Indeed, beginning in the early 1990s, *qigong*'s popularity peaked in Japan. However, the 1995 Aum Shinrikyō Incident and the 1999 Falun Gong Incident significantly hampered the development of *qigong* in the country. As a result, there is little contemporary research on *qigong* in Japan, and *qigong* practitioners belong increasingly to the elderly population.

My *qigong* teacher in Japan, Amano-sensei, has practised *qigong* for over 30 years. He graduated from Kyoto University and is currently the manager of the largest *qigong* organisation in the Kansai region. After graduating from the Faculty of Agriculture, Amano-sensei worked for a food processing company. During that time, he felt uncomfortable with the production of artificially processed foods and mechanised production techniques. Two years later, he quit his job and immersed himself in the world of *qigong*. He explained to me that during a period of personal frustration, he was introduced to *qigong* through the works of Noguchi Haruchika, in a bookstore in Kyoto.

At that time in Japan, influenced by the *qigong* boom in China, Tsumura had already established the Kansai Qigong Association. Amano was impressed by the practicality of *Noguchi Seitai* and he soon realised that *qigong* and *Seitai* were similar.[5] He and his wife joined the Kansai Qigong Association and diligently studied various *qigong* techniques. Afterwards, he was promoted to the position of the organisation's secretary general. Although the Kansai Qigong Association was dissolved in 2000, Amano-sensei currently carries on the association's legacy by offering qigong lessons under his own *qigong* association's name. In addition, he serves as a part-time lecturer at Kyoto University of the Arts, teaching a course on 'The Body'. Moreover, he has continued to write and has published eight books that draw on his teaching experience of *qigong*. Although Amano-sensei's Qigong Association inherited the traditions and legacy of the Kansai Qigong Association, its methods and philosophy differ from its predecessor's in several respects.

The former representative of the Kansai Qigong Association, Tsumura Takashi, had a tendency to directly translate Chinese *qigong* theories and

5 *Noguchi Seitai* also used *qi/ki* as the core concept for both its theories and practices. However, in *Noguchi Seitai*, *qi/ki* is not portrayed as a mysterious and invisible physical energy; instead, it represents a tangible sensation of connection and harmony among individuals, between individuals and society, and between individuals and the natural environment (Tanojiri 2019).

methods into Japanese and incorporate them into practice. In contrast, Amano-sensei seeks to revitalise the theories of *qigong* that were passed down from Chinese masters by appealing to the concept of 'nature' (*shizen* 自然) and the feeling of *kimochi-ii*:

> The tendency to drown in self-centred satisfaction is hidden in every spiritual practice and is surprisingly not well-known; this is more dangerous than pursuing material satisfaction. Moreover, *qigong* was certainly one of the breeding grounds [of this tendency]. Looking back now, it feels like the essential reason for the dissolution of the Kansai Qigong Association and the birth of a new Qigong Association lies here. Since the decision to disband [the Kansai Qigong Association], new encounters and learnings have arisen one after another, leading to the emergence of a significant trend of learning from nature. This 'nature' is an ever-changing world that exists independently of the rest. To reach this world, it is necessary to thoroughly eliminate unnecessary matters rather than add new matters. (excerpt translated from Japanese, from Amano's personal blog posted on 5 September 2008)

Amano-sensei emphasises following 'nature' as the fundamental philosophy of *qigong*. His intentions here transcend the existing framework of *qigong* to create a unique form centred around the feeling of *kimochi-ii*. However, as the name of this physical practice is not 'exercise' or 'gymnastics' but rather '*qigong*', where can the essence of *qi* and the crucial 'feeling of *qi*' within *qigong* practice be located? Eager to satiate my curiosity, I approached Amano-sensei one day after class and asked him this question directly:

Huang: How do you understand *qi* and the 'feeling of *qi*' in *qigong* practices?

> Amano-sensei: I'm not very interested in the external *qi*, the one that can be felt. Some people may feel it, yet others may not. If we focus excessively on that, the number of people who practise *qigong* will decrease. I believe it is more important to emphasise the internal *qi*. In Japan, there is an expression – '*ki wa kokoro*' – which means '*qi* is the heart/mind [*kokoro*]'. The natural state of the heart/mind is *kimochi-ii*.

Amano-sensei's response shows that he neither denies the existence nor undermines the value of *qi* but seems uninterested in the possibility of perceiving it from external sources (external *qi*[6]), because it is quite different from his goal of the *kimochi-ii*. Additionally, by stating that *qi* is the heart/mind, he appears to view *qi* as something internal. Medical anthropologist Kitanaka (2012) similarly discusses the psychologisation of *qi* in Japan when examining the concept of premodern depression or *kiutsu* 気鬱. She suggests that whereas in China the concept of *ki*/*qi* has retained its traditional and physical meaning, in Japan, the concept of *ki/qi* has gradually turned into a metaphor representing the heart/mind. This phenomenon can also be seen in the Japanese language, where *ki/qi* is used as a term for sense, emotion, and personality (Hamano 1987). That is to say, Amano-sensei is directly influenced by the Japanese usage of *ki*, adopting it as a metaphor for the heart/mind. On this basis, it can be argued that *kimochi-ii* is not only an internal and psychological expression but also an expression that indicates the 'feeling of *qi*' in the Japanese language. Nevertheless, Amano-sensei does not simply perceive *kimochi-ii* as a psychological state. Rather, he likely recognises *qi* as a wild force inherent to the body and mind and present from birth. This perspective diverges from the context of the functional, physiological, and metaphysical *qi* found in authoritative systems, such as Traditional Chinese Medicine and *qigong*, instead using expressions such as '*ki wa kokoro*' and *kimochi-ii*.

Practices Related to *kimochi-ii* in Anmano-Sensei's Class

Ethnographic examinations of *qigong* have often noted the role of 'feeling good' and similar sensations during practice. For example, the English-language terms 'pleasure' and 'pleasant' give meaning to the simple and repetitive movements and postures of *qigong* and serve as a guideline for describing the skills of *qigong* masters (Hsu 1999; Farquhar and Zhang 2012). However, the methods that enable practitioners to acquire this sense and similar experiences have not been described or analysed in detail. This section provides a comprehensive description of Amano-sensei's *qigong*, with a focus on the feeling of *kimochi-ii*. It also examines how this kind of feeling manifests itself in practitioners' bodies – including my own.

6 External *qi* (*waiqi* 外气) is the emission of *qi* from the body of the practitioner into others' bodies. It is often used as a medical skill for healing patients. The research on external *qi* through *qigong*, which was extremely popular in the period of the *qigong* boom, claimed that it was possible to materialise and objectively measure *qi*. This allowed *qigong* to become not only a part of Traditional Chinese Medicine (TCM) but also the primary research subject in the field of 'somatic science', leading to the '*qigong* boom' in China (Palmer 2007).

Unlike those in China, practitioners in Japan tend not to elaborate on their bodily experiences. For example, Dr Aka (52, male) is a chief physician in the gastrointestinal department of a public hospital in Osaka. He has been studying *qigong* under Amano-sensei for about six years. Because he and I practise near each other, I asked him multiple times how he felt immediately after his training. In general, he would smile in satisfaction and offer a reply similar to the following sentiment: 'I don't know. Hmm, it's hard to describe, but it felt really good'. When I would ask follow-up questions to learn more about when and how the practice functions, as well as how it feels and so on, his only response was, 'I don't really know what to say about that'. Whenever I asked other practitioners, I often received similarly unclear answers. In fact, some participants flatly refused, stating, 'That's a private matter'. Through my countless failures, I learned that, aside from practitioners who do not wish to share their experiences, most of them simply had difficulty finding the appropriate words to describe the sensations they felt. In the paragraphs that follow, to overcome this barrier regarding participants' abilities to express their experiences of *kimochi-ii*, I focus on my own experience of studying Amano-sensei's *qigong* techniques, with a particular focus on how affective states like *kimochi-ii* are taught, as well as how they emerge and are transformed through practice.

Standard Practice: The Manifestation of *Kimochi-ii*

The standard practices in Amano-sensei's lectures consist of a set of *qigong* movements that he himself compiled. It includes his original *qigong* practice, referred to as 'a simple way to calm your mind'. As the practice begins, prerecorded music fills the space with the sounds of nature and the wilderness.[7] At this point, Amano-sensei usually stands at the front of the classroom, facing his students while demonstrating *qigong* movements. Throughout this process, he keeps his eyes closed and refrains from checking the students' movements. Indeed, instead of merely teaching, he actively engages with the students by doing *qigong* movements with them. During these sessions, Amano-sensei not only verbally explains how to perform each movement but also openly shares his own feelings and emotions.

Amano-sensei describes the movements with a gentle intonation, often accompanied by a warm smile. He occasionally expresses his genuine

7 For example, Enya, an Irish singer known for her 'healing songs' in Japan. Her songs are edited as background music for Amano's *qigong* practices.

feelings in the moment, saying things like, 'Oh, it feels so good; it feels really good'. As he utters these words, his expression becomes even gentler and the corners of his mouth naturally turn upward. This reveals that he is not expressing the message of *kimochi-ii* to his students in a forced manner but is rather enjoying the sensations of his body, such that the words simply tumble effortlessly from his mouth. In the final stage of the series of movements, his gestures become more grandiose. Amano-sensei lifts his face toward the ceiling and opens his mouth wide while keeping his eyes closed, looking as comfortable as if he were yawning. From this moment forward, he offers no more verbal explanations of how to move one's body, and students are free to sway as they please. It is as if he has lost control of his body and moves spontaneously.

During my first days of attending lessons, I was extremely confused. I did not know whether I had performed the movements correctly, and there was no one to instruct me. The students surrounding me shook and stroked their bodies while holding their eyes closed and listening to Amano-sensei's instructions. Others appeared to proceed completely on their own, with their body movements and postures differing from Amano-sensei's. During the final stage, there were no more verbal instructions, and all the students swayed their bodies 'naturally' with their eyes closed. In this strange atmosphere, I was the only one observing the situation, as I had my eyes half open. I noticed that not only Amano-sensei but, in fact, most of the students had large, beaming smiles on their faces and looked comfortable as they performed the movements. Despite attending several lessons, I was still unsure whether my movements were correct, but I decided, for the time being, to imitate Amano-sensei's smile rather than his movements. As one female student in her 50s told me, 'If you imitate Amano-sensei's smile, your heart will become kinder, too'. Later, during casual conversations with other students, I discovered a surprising fact – like me, quite a few of them had also initially started their *qigong* practice by imitating Amano-sensei's smile rather than his movements.

As I became more acquainted with Amano-sensei's *qigong*, I found that when I practised it alone at home, the first thing that came to my mind was not the specific movements and postures but Amano-sensei's infectious smile, the soothing music, and his soft murmurs of 'Oh, it feels so good', 'It's so comfortable' and 'So nice'. As I continued attending more classes, I gradually became familiar with the flow of his *qigong*. Like other students, I learned to move and sway with my eyes closed, following the music and verbal instructions, and I started to worry less about the correctness of my movements. Over time, I noticed that my body seemed to move effortlessly, almost as if it had a mind of its own. It was as if I were floating in the air, experiencing a sense of natural harmony and unity with my *qigong* practice.

The Advanced Practice of *Zen Mitsu* 禅密: The Manifestation of 'Light'

Zen mitsu[8] lectures are advanced courses offered only to students who have studied the basic courses for at least two consecutive years. Although these lectures are called 'advanced courses', the movements themselves are not complicated. They focus on swaying and twisting the body back and forth and side to side while remaining grounded through one's spine. The most critical component here is to concentrate on the spine and the *missho* 密処[9] in order to obtain the specific *kimochi-ii* while swaying and twisting.

During the first *zen mitsu* lecture I attended, Amano-sensei stood behind me, swaying his body in sync with my rhythm, perhaps to allow me to reach the feeling of *kimochi-ii* faster. While doing so, he said in a low voice, 'Did you notice it? It is warm, and it feels good. It is in the *missho* now. Yeah, this feeling is just like going to pee'. After some time, he stated, 'Now the tailbone… the sacrum… lumbar… thoracic… cervical… thoracic vertebra… [and] cervical vertebra'. He announced the specific bodily locations where he experienced the given sensations during the *zen mitsu* practices with me. Furthermore, he described the specific *kimochi-ii* in his body as it moved up along his spine, using onomatopoeias, such as '*shu-to*', '*wa-to*', '*za-to*', '*hu-to*', and '*bwa-to*'.

Immediately following these physical movements, the students engaged in a form of meditation called *zen mitsu*. The feeling of 'warmth and *kimochi-ii*', as Amano-sensei referred to it, became 'light'. The 'light' in his body illuminated the *missho* and spine, moving up and down along the spine, penetrating deeper into his body and thereby creating a profound connection between heaven and earth. During meditation, Amano-sensei also utilised a variety of onomatopoeias to vividly describe the movements and changes of the light inside his body, effectively conveying his feelings to the students.

8 This practice originated in China, where it is pronounced Chanmi.

9 The position of *missho* is approximately at the midpoint between the genitals and the anus. In the theory of *zen mitsu*, it is the centre of the whole body's energy.

I was able to grasp such bodily sensations as warmth and *kimochi-ii*, but I could not understand the bodily sensation of light, as I had initially conceived of it as a visual phenomenon. Therefore, after class, I asked Amano-sensei about this directly:

> Huang: Why do you see 'light' when your eyes are closed?
> Amano-sensei: This 'light' is a subtle resonance between human beings and nature. Just as the sun, moon, and other planets emit light, we humans can interact with nature through our own light. It is the nature of our bodies, and it feels very good [*totemo kimochi-ii*].

I still did not understand what he meant, so I asked the other students attending the class the same question. Most of them gave only vague answers, using phrases such as, 'I don't know, but…'. However, Sei-san, a woman in her 30s, described in detail the bodily changes she experienced as a result of four years of practice:

> In my first year of *zen mitsu*, I enjoyed the feeling brought about by the wriggling movement of my body. The more I practised, the more often I found that the movement just occurred spontaneously. I don't know if this feeling can be described as *kimochi-ii*, but it is not clear exactly where or what sensations appeared in my body. In the second year, I learned that the *missho*, as Amano-sensei calls it, produces a warm sensation, and when my body trembled slightly, I could sense a little of that warmth scattered along my spine as well. And in the third year, the warmth of the *missho* and the spine grew even more, and I could even feel it moving up and down along my spine during meditation. This is my fourth year, and every time I practise *zen mitsu*, the *missho* feels like a gentle, dim candle that shines in the dark night, and my whole body feels as if I'm in a hot spring! (interview, 26 May 2019)

Unlike Sei-san, I have never experienced the warmth and light in either the *missho* or the spine. Each time I engaged in *zen mitsu* practice, I tried my best to concentrate on those two body parts and imagine that something was moving there. In particular, when I swayed my body slowly and paid attention to the spine and the *missho*, these two body parts – which I was not actively cognisant of in my daily life – would sometimes appear as a dim image. This experience made me realise that with consistent practice over many years, I might undergo similar sensory changes as Sei-san did.

Kimochi-ii in Japan: Feeling with the Japanese *Kikō* (*Qigong*)

As mentioned earlier, although Amano-sensei offers a variety of *qigong* lectures, their primary focus is on the techniques and theories of *Noguchi Seitai* and *zen mitsu*. *Noguchi Seitai* is a Japanese form of therapy, while *zen mitsu* is one of the over 3,000 forms of *qigong* that emerged during the *qigong* boom in China. Amano-sensei learned the practice and theories of *zen mitsu* directly from its founder in Dalian, China. It is important to note that *zen mitsu* contains elements of Zen Buddhism and esoteric Buddhism, both of which have had a significant and lasting influence on Japanese culture. On the other hand, it still remains unclear why Amano-sensei chose *zen mitsu* out of the 3,000 Chinese modalities of *qigong*.

At first glance, it may appear that Amano-sensei has placed his teaching in the category of '*qigong*', according to a strategy of 'opportunism'. However, he did not rely on theory to understand *qigong*; instead, he gradually and naturally led practitioners to feel the essence of what he considered a 'Japanese' culture through specific *qigong* practices. In the following section, I focus on the Qigong Association's 2020 Qigong Training Camp in order to demonstrate how 'Japanese *kikō*' was constructed through sensory and affective experiences.

While conducting fieldwork in Japan, I participated in two *qigong* training camps, in 2019 and 2020, organised by the Qigong Association. To be eligible for the two-day training camps, applicants were required to have completed a one-year course on *zen mitsu*. This means that all participants had studied *qigong* under Amano-sensei for at least three years. The first camp was held at Mount Kōya (Kōya-san 高野山), and the second camp was held at The Grand Shrine of Ise (Ise Jingū 伊勢神宮). Although I attended these two camps, I will focus on the second one, as the first location was chosen due to its association with Kūkai (774–835)[10] and the esoteric elements of Shingon Buddhism that were considered to have a special connection to *zen mitsu*. In *zen mitsu*, the term *mitsu* alludes to esoteric Buddhism (*mikkyō* 密教, where the first character is the same as the second character of *zen mitsu*). As a large temple settlement of the Shingon school of esoteric Buddhism, Mount Kōya consists therefore of an obvious choice of a location for *zen mitsu qigong* practice.

In contrast, The Grand Shrine of Ise, which enshrines Amaterasu Ōmikami,[11] has no apparent connection to *qigong*, and I speculated that

10 Kūkai was a Japanese Buddhist monk, who founded the esoteric *Shingon* school of Buddhism at Mount Kōya.

11 Amaterasu Ōmikami, is one of the most important deities in the Shinto pantheon. She is the goddess of the sun, and a direct descendant of the *kami* (deities) that emerged during the mythological creation of Japan.

choosing this site was part of a strategy to Japanise *qigong*. According to Teeuwen and Breen (2017)'s research, although the Ise Shrine's journey through history has been marked by numerous fluctuations, it never faded into obscurity. Especially today, the shrine has consistently and discursively stood as one of the most prominent embodiments of Japanese identity and Shinto. In other words, I suspected that Amano-sensei's aim was to let students combine their knowledge of *qigong* with that of Shinto or reinterpret *qigong* within what they considered to be the rules of etiquette of Shinto. However, after attending the camp, I soon realised that my previous assumptions had been rather shallow. This is because Amano-sensei's intention was not to teach a specific style or body of knowledge related to Japanese *kikō* but rather to make participants feel they were immersed in the environment that he believed represented 'the essence of Japan's nature'.

The main activities of the 2020 winter *qigong* camp were visiting and praying at various shrines according to a particular method known as 'instantaneous *zen mitsu*'.[12] One day, Amano-sensei took us to The Grand Shrine of Ise at 5:00 in the morning before the sun rose. According to him, 'instantaneous *zen mitsu*' refers to the process of experiencing the replication of the *kimochi-ii* that occurs during the practice of *zen mitsu*. However, if the primary goal was to interact with nature, then the location of the act should be irrelevant. I therefore asked Amano-sensei why he chose The Grand Shrine of Ise. His answer was as follows:

> The Grand Shrine of Ise, where imperial rituals are held, was nationalised during Japanese militarism; nevertheless, it is also a symbol of the 'nature worship' of ancient Japanese people. In other words, the location where The Grand Shrine of Ise was built represents the carefully chosen 'living nature of the land' by the ancient Japanese. Therefore, by practising *qigong* at this place, one's normal senses are enhanced. (12 December 2020)

According to Amano-sensei, the choice of The Grand Shrine of Ise for the *qigong* camp was not made because it symbolises Japanese identity. Instead, the decision was guided by Ise's natural surroundings, selected by the ancient Japanese for their capacity to cultivate a feeling of *kimochi-ii* among practitioners. This resonates with Amano-sensei's view of *kimochi-ii* as a natural state of the human body. Hence, rather than seeking to Japanize *qigong* through the symbolic significance of Ise, Amano-sensei directed attention towards

12 There are 125 shinto shrines, centered around Kotaijingu (Naiku), dedicated to Amaterasu-Omikami, and Toyo'uke-daijingu (Geku), dedicated to Toyo'uke-no-Omikami.

feeling *kimochi-ii* within a particular location embodying the essence of Japan's natural environment. On the same day, we also visited approximately 30 shrines of The Grand Shrine of Ise with him while concomitantly practising 'instantaneous *zen mitsu*'. As a beginner, I could not reproduce the instant *kimochi-ii* of *zen mitsu*; but as I swayed my body, I felt a sensation like the one I had experienced earlier during his lecture. This feeling emerged harmoniously with the tranquil ambience of the shrine during the early morning. The sound of trees swaying in the gentle breeze and of the leaves rustling created a serene backdrop that enhanced my meditative state of mind. All these elements combined to make the participants feel as if they were truly 'blending with the surrounding nature at this very moment'. Subsequently, about 20 participants, together with Amano-sensei, bowed, clapped, smiled, swayed, and repeated the act of worship and prayer about 30 times. Meanwhile, I had subconsciously forgotten that I was practising *qigong* and unintentionally continued to participate in the practice of invoking the sensation of *zen mitsu* along with others. I pondered that this might be what Amano-sensei wanted us to do in the first place. Rather than imposing 'his version of *kikō/qigong*' on practitioners in a top-down manner, he intended to guide practitioners to feel the '*kimochi-ii* of Japan' and thus build their own 'Japanese *kikō/qigong*'.

Through the practice of 'instantaneous *zen mitsu*', skilled practitioners are able to reproduce the elusive and difficult-to-verbalise *kimochi-ii* together with other sensations and affects that they have obtained through previous lectures and *zen mitsu* practices. This unique ability is fostered within the special and sacred 'nature' of The Grand Shrine of Ise. Here practitioners have the opportunity to access their past embodied experiences of bowing and clapping, which are traditional practices of Shinto worship, and merge them with the present moment of *zen mitsu* experience, creating a profound and spiritually enriching connection with their surroundings through prayer. All this is supposed to produce a specific feeling of 'Japanese nature'. At that time, any authoritative knowledge, such as ideology and theory, had already lost its importance. In short, the feeling of *kimochi-ii* obtained through the practice of *qigong* on Japanese soil served as a foundation for constructing a culturally unique form of *qigong*.

Discussion and Conclusion

This paper has focused on 'transnational *qigong*' in Japan and described how its practical application has transformed the category of *qigong*. By delving into the case study of Amano-sensei, the founder of the Qigong

Association in Kyoto, I have described his attempts to construct a new frame for *qigong* by placing emphasis on the feeling of *kimochi-ii* rather than Chinese *qi* (cf. Chapter 1). Part of my approach has consisted of analysing the inducement of *kimochi-ii* in Amano-sensei's *qigong* classes by examining my own experiences of learning *qigong*.

First, I immersed myself in Amano-sensei's world of *qigong* to experience the feeling of *kimochi-ii*, which is difficult to verbalise. Through the 'practices of feeling with the world' (De Antoni and Dumouchel 2017), which enabled me to interact with Amano-sensei, his students and healing music, I gradually deepened my experience of *kimochi-ii*. While I cannot claim to have attained a complete understanding thereof, my comprehension improved as I continued. Thus, the *kimochi-ii* feeling brought about by Amano-sensei's *qigong* cannot be reduced to mere physical movement; more importantly, it is generated by enskinment (Ingold 2000) through response to Amano-sensei's teaching and his *qigong* worldview.

Second, I failed to acquire the sensations of warmth and light in the *missho* and the spine, which are regarded as special feelings of *zen mitsu* in Amano-sensei's advanced class. From this practice, I can hypothesise that the change in the 'somatic modes of attention' (Csordas 1994) caused by focusing on specific body parts and the surrounding environment are entangled with the *kimochi-ii* embodied in the standard practices. Moreover, through repeated 'affective practices' (Wetherell 2012) or 'affective technologies' (De Antoni 2023), abstract concepts such as the flow of 'light' within the body may become embodied in a step-by-step procedure. Similarly, the images of the 'sun and moon's light', as well as 'the spine' and the *missho*, may also have contributed to the production of specific *kimochi-ii* of *zen mitsu*. That being said, it is no longer important to determine whether what is perceived is indeed the '*missho*' or 'light'. Rather, what matters are the practices of *zen mitsu*, which generate the imagery of 'light' and the '*missho*' and serve as 'technologies of imagination' (Sneath, Holbraad and Pedersen 2009). For example, some people, including Sei-san, can confidently state, 'This is the light' and 'This is the feeling of the *missho*'. On the other hand, numerous individuals, myself included, do not exhibit the same degree of certainty. For some of them, this initial sense of uncertainty can gradually transform into a feeling of certainty through consistent repetition – and it is also said that repetitive practice in *qigong* is inherently and pleasantly intertwined with a natural healing power.

Finally, accounts of the *qigong* training camp suggest that, superficially, the selection of Ise as a venue for *qigong* practice, as well as the incorporation of *zen mitsu* and *Noguchi Seitai* alongside various other *qi*-related practices into Amano-sensei's *qigong* teachings, appeared to be efforts aimed at

Japanising the practice of *qigong*, as if a sort of 'opportunism'. However, as elucidated in the preceding ethnographic depiction, Amano-sensei's focus does not predominantly reside in the theoretical underpinnings of these practices. He tends to select suitable 'tools' for his *qigong* according to what will best improve students' ability to feel *kimochi-ii*. Simultaneously, he also stresses communication with 'the surrounding nature' and 'the nature of the body'. This 'surrounding nature' pertains to the practice of 'now, in Japan', serving as a natural transformation of Chinese *qigong* into 'Japanese *kikō*'. Csordas (2002, 4–5) points out that 'portable practices' and 'transposable messages' are two commonly observed features of religions that are easily adopted across cultures. Although *qigong* might not be labelled a religion, it contains multiple religious elements, whether in its theory or practice. This chapter has investigated not only how the specific movements, techniques, theories, and knowledge (messages) of *qigong* have been 'easily' appropriated by a Japanese practitioner but also how sensory and affective experiences, such as *kimochi-ii*, derived from bodily practices in Japan, have contributed to a form of *qigong* distinct from that in China. My findings suggest that although it is essential to understand changes in the macro social context, such as political and economic conditions, it is equally important to take into account a micro-perspective when studying transnational religious and spiritual healing practices. In this case, I argued that it is critical to account for the sensory and affective experiences produced by these practices.

This chapter focused on the ongoing localisation process of *qigong* in Japan. What makes this study particularly unique is its approach. I did not employ the conventional 'cultural perspective' of globalisation to examine the interplay between an 'original Chinese *qigong* culture' and its local appropriations in Japan. Instead, I delved into affective and sensory interactions rooted in the practitioners' bodies and their bodily experiences. In contrast to being attracted to elements of traditional Chinese culture, Japanese practitioners seemed to be primarily driven by a common goal: to cultivate, generate, and transform sensory and affective experiences through *qigong*. Their goal was to maintain the essence of *qigong* and construct what they conceived of as a distinct Japanese *qigong* culture.

Bibliography

Amano, Takayasu. 2008. 'Kikō zyōhōkyoku 気功情報局' [Intelligence Department of Qigong]. Accessed on 21 July 2023. http://npo-kikou.cocolog-nifty.com/blog/2008/09/index.html.

Chen, Nancy. 2003. *Breathing Spaces: Qigong, Psychiatry, and Healing in China.* New York: Columbia University Press.

Chen, Nancy. 2005. 'Mapping Science and Nation in China'. In *Asian Medicine and Globalization*, edited by Joseph S. Alter, 107–20. Philadelphia: University of Pennsylvania Press. https://doi.org/10.9783/9780812205251.107.

Csordas, Thomas J. 1994. *The Sacred Self: A Cultural Phenomenology of Charismatic Healing.* Berkeley: University of California Press.

Csordas, Thomas J. 2002. 'Introduction: Modalities of Transnational Transcendence'. In *Transnational Transcendence*, edited by Thomas J. Csordas, 1–31. Berkeley: University of California Press.

De Antoni, Andrea. 2017. 'Sympathy from the Devil: Experiences, Movement and Affective Correspondences during a Roman Catholic Exorcism in Contemporary Italy'. *Japanese Review of Cultural Anthropology* 18, no. 1: 143–58. https://doi.org/10.14890/jrca.18.1_143.

De Antoni, Andrea, and Paul Dumouchel. 2017. 'The Practices of Feeling with the World: Towards an Anthropology of Affect, the Senses and Materiality – Introduction'. *Japanese Review of Cultural Anthropology* 18, no. 1: 91–98. https://doi.org/10.14890/jrca.18.1_91.

De Antoni, Andrea. 2023. 'The Ghosts That Haunt Me: Feeling with Affective Technologies and Doing Ethnography about Spirit Possession in Contemporary Japan'. In *Other Worlds, Other Bodies Embodied Epistemologies and Ethnographies of Healing*, edited by Alberto Groisman, Diana Espírito Santo, and Emily Pierini, 179–215. New York: Berghahn Books.

Farquhar, Judith, and Lai Lili. 2021. *Gathering Medicines: Nation and Knowledge in China's Mountain South.* Chicago: University of Chicago Press. http://doi.org/10.7208/chicago/9780226763798.001.0001.

Farquhar, Judith, and Zhang Qicheng. 2012. *Ten Thousand Things: Nurturing Life in Contemporary Beijing.* New York: Zone Books. https://doi.org/10.2307/j.ctv14gphrg.

Hampshire, Kate R., and Samuel Asiedu Owusu. 2013. 'Grandfathers, Google, and Dreams: Medical Pluralism, Globalization, and New Healing Encounters in Ghana'. *Medical Anthropology* 32, no. 3: 247–65. https://doi.org/10.1080/01459740.2012.692740.

Hamano, Kiyoshi. 1987. 'Seikakuyōgo ni tsukawareru "ki" no kenkyū 性格用語に使われる「気」の研究' [A Study of 'Ki' as Used in Personality Terms]. *Shinrigaku kenkyū* 58, no. 5: 295–301.

Howes, David. 2005. *Empire of the Senses: The Sensual Culture Reader.* Oxford: Berg.

Hsu, Elisabeth. 1999. *The Transmission of Chinese Medicine.* Cambridge: Cambridge University Press.

Hsu, Elisabeth. 2008. 'The History of Chinese Medicine in the People's Republic of China and Its Globalization'. *East Asian Science, Technology and Society: An International Journal* 2, no. 4: 465–84. https://doi.org/10.1007/s12280-009-9072-y.
Huang, Xinzhe. 2022. 'How Can Qi Be Felt? The Example of Qigong Practice in Shanghai'. *Japanese Review of Cultural Anthropology* 23, no 3: 305–12.
Iida, Junko. 2006. *Tai massāji no minzokushi: Taishiki iryō seiseikatei no shintai to jissen* タイ・マッサージの民族誌ー「タイ式医療」生成過程における身体と実践 [Ethnography of Thai Massage: Body and Practice in the Making of 'Thai-Style Medicine']. Tokyo: Akashishoten.
Imura, Hiroji. 1984. *Reijutsuka no kyōen* 霊術家の饗宴 [Feast of the Spiritualists]. Tokyo: Shinkōsha.
Ingold, Tim. 2000. *The Perception of the Environment: Essays on Livelihood, Dwelling and Skill.* London: Routledge. https://doi.org/10.4324/9780203466025.
Kitanaka, Junko. 2012. *Depression in Japan: Psychiatric Cures for a Society in Distress.* Princeton: Princeton University Press. https://doi.org/10.2307/j.ctt7rrv0.
Kurita, Hidehiko, Hotaka Tsukada, and Yoshinaga Shin'ichi, eds. 2019. *Kingendai Nihon no minkan seishin ryōhō* (*jō*)*: Fukashina enerugī no shosō* 近現代日本の民間精神療法（上）：不可視なエネルギーの諸相 [Folk Psychotherapy in Modern Japan (I): Aspects of Invisible Energy]. Tokyo: Kokushokankōkai.
Liao, Chihong, and Liao Chiyang. 2012. *Kikō*: *Sono shisō to jissen* 気功：その思想と実践 (Qigong: Its Philosophy and Practice). Tokyo: Shunjūsha.
Massumi, Brian. 2002. *Parables for the Virtual: Movement, Affect, Sensation.* Durham: Duke University Press. https://doi.org/10.1215/9780822383574.
Murakawa, Haruhiko. 2002. 'Phenomenology of the Experience of Qigong: A Preliminary Research Design for the Intentional Bodily Practices'. PhD thesis, Graduate Faculty of the California Institute of Integral Studies.
Otehode, Utiraruto. 2009. 'The Creation and Reemergence of Qigong in China'. In *Making Religion, Making the State: The Politics of Religion in Modern China*, edited by Yoshiko Ashiwa and David L. Wank, 241–66. Stanford: Stanford University Press. https://doi.org/10.1515/9780804771139-011.
Ots, Thomas. 1994. 'The Silenced Body: The Expressive Leib: On the Dialectic of Mind and Life in Chinese Cathartic Healing'. In *Embodiment and Experience: The Existential Ground of Culture and Self,* edited by Thomas J. Csordas, 116–36. Cambridge: Cambridge University Press.
Palmer, David A. 2003. 'Modernity and Millenialism in China: *Qigong* and the Birth of Falun Gong'. *Asian Anthropology* 2, no. 1: 79–109. https://doi.org/10.1080/1683478x.2003.10552531.
Palmer, David A. 2007. *Qigong Fever: Body, Science, and Utopia in China, 1949–1999.* New York: Columbia University Press. https://doi.org/10.13140/2.1.2859.9680.

Palmer, David A., and Elijah Siegler. 2017. *Dream Trippers: Global Daoism and the Predicament of Modern Spirituality*. Chicago: The University of Chicago Press. https://doi.org/10.7208/chicago/9780226484983.001.0001.

Pink, Sarah. 2009. *Doing Sensory Ethnography*. Los Angeles: SAGE. https://doi.org/10.4135/9781446249383.

Sagli, Gry. 2008. 'Learning and Experiencing Chinese Qigong in Norway'. *East Asian Science, Technology and Society: An International Journal* 2, no. 4: 545–66. https://doi.org/10.1215/s12280-009-9071-z.

Sneath, David, Martin Holbraad, and Morten A. Pedersen. 2009. 'Technologies of the Imagination: An Introduction'. *Ethnos* 74, no. 1: 5–30. https://doi.org/10.1080/00141840902751147.

Tanojiri, Tetsuro. 2019. 'Katsugenundō no rekishi: Noguchiseitai no shitekihenyō 活元運動の歴史—野口整体の史的変容' [History of *Katsugenundō*: Transformation of *Noguchi Seitai*]. In *Kingendai Nihon no minkan seishin ryōhō (jō): Fukashina enerugī no shosō*, edited by Kurita Hidehiko, Hotaka Tsukada, and Yoshinaga Shin'ichi, 191–216. Tokyo: Kokushokankōkai.

Teeuwen, Mark, and John Breen. 2017. *A Social History of the Ise Shrines: Divine Capital*. London: Bloomsbury Academic. https://doi.org/10.5040/9781474272780.

Wetherell, Margaret. 2014. *Affect and Emotion: A New Social Science Understanding*. Los Angeles: Sage.

Zhan, Mei. 2009. *Other-Worldly: Making Chinese Medicine through Transnational Frames*. Durham: Duke University Press. https://doi.org/10.2307/j.ctv1198xrp.

Biography

Huang Xinzhe is senior researcher at the Kinugasa Research Organization, Ritsumeikan University. He holds a PhD in Anthropology and is also a trained TCM (Traditional Chinese Medicine) doctor with a master's degree in Psychology. Huang's doctoral research is an anthropological study of *qigong* in contemporary China and Japan. His research interests include the use of various therapies within traditional Chinese medicine, Daoism, and folk psychotherapy.

Part 2

Circulation of Therapeutic Narratives

In his case study of Terry Hu (Hu Yinmeng 胡因夢), a Taiwanese movie star turned translator, author, spiritual guide, and New Age advocate, Paul J. Farrelly traces how Hu creatively tailored American New Age thought and practices for the evolving landscape of post-martial-aw Taiwan. Farrelly illustrates how Hu's works not only aimed to introduce American New Age as a viable spiritual path aligned with Taiwanese 'traditional' values such as Buddhism, but to present Hu herself as a tangible example of its transformative potential. This synthesis of the authority of foreign authors with personal experience allowed figures like Hu to craft their own religious authority. Hu's adept storytelling and personal journey narratives positioned her at the forefront of Taiwan's New Age movement, which, according to Farrelly, has been partly defined by 'the ability of authors and translators to write themselves into the milieu through spiritual auto-hagiographies where they augmented their own experiences with the authority of those they translated' (Farrelly 2019, 57).

Hu's story underscores the compelling nature of personal stories of healing and self-discovery in establishing credibility for alternative approaches to life, spirituality, and well-being. The three chapters in this section explore many individuals like Hu who have gained popular appeal not only by introducing novel ideas and practices from distant lands but also by demonstrating their commitment to these principles through the narrativisation of their own lives. This 'lived-experience' approach to storytelling establishes their authority in spiritual and therapeutic fields, authenticating the viability of their alternative lifestyles and offering a source for others to imagine their future lives. The authors in this section ultimately suggest, implicitly or explicitly, that an analysis of therapeutic narratives would gain significantly from a literature studies perspective.

Farrelly, Paul J. 2019. 'Terry Hu: Writing Her Transition from Actor to New Age Authority in Taiwan'. *Asian Ethnology* 78, no. 1: 53–73.

4 Five-Element Acupuncture in 1960–1980s Britain

In Pursuit of Alternative Treatment with Body-Mind-Spirit

Yang Yi

Abstract: This paper examines the history of Five-Element Acupuncture – a British reinterpretation of Chinese medicine that became prevalent in the Anglophone world during the second half of the 20th century – as a form of alternative medicine deployed by those seeking alternative lifestyles. It also sheds light on how this alternative medicine negotiated the boundaries between science and culture on the one hand and modernity and tradition on the other. Using oral history interviews with members of the counterculture and the New Age – some of whom embarked on a career as Five-Element acupuncturists – this paper shows the (re)invention and (re)construction of a Chinese medical tradition in late 20th-century British society, a process that embedded alternative values of antiestablishment and personalised holistic healthcare.

Keywords: Chinese Medicine, New Age, Counterculture Movement (CCM), Britain, Orientalism.

During the globalisation of the 20th century, acupuncture therapy gained popularity in Britain and the United States as a representative practice of Chinese medicine. Today, it is a household name in the English-speaking world as a form of Complementary and Alternative Medicine (CAM), alongside homoeopathy, which has grown in popularity in Europe as part of the same medical category. One study showed that, in 2009, registered members of major UK acupuncture associations provided a total of 4 million acupuncture treatments (Hopton et al. 2012). An earlier study showed that 4.1 million adult citizens in the UK (about 7% of the population) had received acupuncture

Gaitanidis, Ioannis, Luis Fernando Bernardi Junqueira, Avery Morrow, and Sangyun Han (eds), *Therapy, Spirituality, and East Asian Imaginaries.* Taylor & Francis Group 2025
DOI: 10.5117/9789048559015_CH04

treatment in the past year (Thomas, Nicholl, and Coleman 2001).[1] The factors that contributed to the success of acupuncture in the UK are multifaceted and intertwined with postcolonial and postmodernisation reflections, as well as social transformations that took place during the second half of the 20th century. Another significant driver was the increasing promotion of multiculturalism and the creation of a more diverse medical environment. These developments allowed for greater openness to different approaches to healthcare and well-being, leading to the emergence and flourishing of alternative medical practices, including acupuncture, in Britain. This pursuit of pluralism was partly driven by certain youth-subcultural movements in Europe and the United States from the 1960s onwards.

This chapter explores the rising popularity of acupuncture among young people in the UK during the 1970s and '80s. The first part provides a brief overview of the characteristics of the historical transmission of acupuncture in Europe. Then, through the case study of Five-Element Acupuncture (FEA), in which I combine oral history interviews with journal articles and archives produced by members of the movement, I reconstruct the body of acupuncture knowledge employed by FEA acupuncturists during the countercultural period. The aim is to demonstrate how the counterculture movement (CCM) and the unique British medical environment shaped the dissemination of acupuncture theories during that time. My analysis of this historical process reveals and embodies the influence of Orientalist thinking with countercultural characteristics among this professional group, and the inauguration of a new phase in the spread of acupuncture in contemporary Euro-American societies.

The Conventional Narrative of Acupuncture Transmission in Europe

According to the work of medical historian Rebecca Bivins (2000) and medical anthropologist Linda Barnes (2005), the earliest records of the spread of acupuncture in Europe date back to the late 17th century. However, until the mid-20th century, acupuncture was still poorly understood by most people

1 This means a total expenditure of 47.3 million pounds in today's value, as each session usually costs 50 pounds (British Acupuncture Council: https://www.acupuncture.org.uk/public-content/public-ask-an-expert/ask-an-expert-about-acupuncture/ask-an-expert-about-acupuncture-nhs-private-healthcare/2679-how-much-does-acupuncture-cost-and-how-many-treatments.html; accessed on 10 Feb 2020).

outside of Asia. One of my British interviewees, Janie, recalled moving to central England after graduating from an acupuncture school in 1981, and setting up a practice in a small town with a friend. When they introduced their profession to neighbours at a community event, she described how 'people looked at us like we were aliens, calling ourselves "acupuncturists"'. At that time, acupuncture was like an alien word to most Britons. Another, Canadian-born, interviewee, John, who studied acupuncture in the UK in the 1970s, recalls that when he expressed his desire to become a full-time acupuncturist to his mother, she confessed that she was ashamed to tell her friends that her son had changed careers from being a successful businessman to being an 'acupuncturist'. The practice of this unfamiliar profession was seen as wildly unorthodox in European and American societies at the time.

The popularity of acupuncture in the 20th-century Euro-American world is commonly attributed to a combination of certain political forces and events, beginning with propaganda by the Chinese government using acupuncture anaesthesia to build China's national image on the international stage since the 1950s (Taylor 2005, 138–41; Zhan 2009, 2–3; cf. Chapter 1). Later, at the dawn of a revived US-China relationship, an American journalist's experience with acupuncture analgesia in Beijing was reported on the front page of the *New York Times* (Reston 1971). The following year, the then President of the United States, Richard Nixon, observed an acupuncture analgesic procedure during his first visit to China. This series of media exposure of acupuncture successfully drew international attention to this medical technique and had a profound impact on the spread of acupuncture in the West. Following Reston's report and Nixon's visit, some Western doctors and scientists came to China in the 1970s and '80s to further study acupuncture analgesic procedures and, on their return, to explore possible mechanisms of such effectiveness. Subsequently, many of them published academic papers on the subject in leading English-language medical journals such as *The British Medical Journal*, *Science* and *The Lancet* (Hamilton et al. 1972; Cheng 1973; Bull 1973). Popular British newspapers such as *The Daily Telegraph* also reported on the analgesic use of acupuncture in China, which had just come out of the bamboo curtain (Hollingworth 1972).

However, influential as those events and historical actors were, professional publications of the time indicate that those political forces hardly induced much interest in acupuncture outside the sphere of medical scientists and professionals. Even reports in the press, which hardly caused a stir among the general public, were read merely as an exotic overseas story. In my recent study, of my 26 British and European interviewees who studied acupuncture in the 1970s and ‘80s, only one mentioned Nixon’s visit to China and the medical reports of its use for pain relief when responding to my question, ‘What made you interested in acupuncture in the first place?’ (Yang 2023). As this particular respondent explains, her initial interest in acupuncture was sparked during her undergraduate studies in physiology at university, more precisely, when a medical school professor mentioned the news about the analgesic use of the technique. Despite the small sample size, the responses from my respondents offer some support for my argument that the surge in interest in acupuncture for pain relief during its initial phase in the 1970s and early ‘80s was more pronounced among medical professionals than among the general public in the Anglophone world.

An Epochal Shift in the 20th Century: Counterculture and the (Re-)Construction of Acupuncture

If not the influence of political events or state propaganda, what factors contributed to the spread of acupuncture in Euro-American societies outside the narrow confines of the biomedical community? The local medical and economic environment, social and cultural attitudes, public health and health policies, the development of modern medicine and the boom of Chinese immigrants coming to the UK in the 1980s and ‘90s are all relevant elements to this historical process. My focus is on a group of young people in Britain during the 1970s and ‘80s who have been given many different names and actions in the academic and popular press, the most widely known of which is ‘hippies’. The post-World War II ideological shifts regarding capitalism, industrialisation, and the institutions of Western modernity initiated by these hippie youths became known as the counterculture movement and later the New Age movement.[2] The former began in the late 1960s as a protest against the homogeneity of people’s lives brought about by the so-called establishment, emphasising the importance of pluralism and personal choice (Nelson 1989, 27–29; Melville 1972, 2). The New Age movement originated in the 1980s, largely as an extension of the CCM. It emphasises the exploration and development of the ‘spiritual’ dimension of the individual, which was suppressed by the dominant ‘rationalism’ and

2 Sociologist Yinger (1960) indicates that the concept of ‘counterculture’ and ‘subculture’ were originally used in a criminal context, in relation to delinquent gangs typically found among adolescent males in lower-class areas of large urban centres. But in this context, counterculture refers to a much more middle-class revolution.

'mind-body dualism' that dominated the West after the Industrial Revolution (Campion 2015, 1–2; Heelas 1996, 18–20; cf. Chapters 5 and 8).

The Chinese medical historian Nathan Sivin has argued that successful medical practice results from an effective response to society's needs and values (Sivin 2011, 142). In the case of acupuncture, the question is then, how was a medical tradition that originated in China over 2,000 years ago rediscovered or reinvented in late 20th-century Britain? In order to understand the perception of Chinese medicine in the modern world and its reception and development outside of China, it is important to comprehend the different attitudes towards alternative medicine and contextualise its meanings over the last century. Simply put, with the ascendency of biomedicine and its power over individuals, an orthodoxy developed around what did and did not constitute mainstream and legitimate scientific medicine (Foucault 1972, 40). Other unorthodox medicines, including Chinese medicine, were styled as 'alternative' and, therefore, as a less legitimate means of healthcare (Salmon 1984, 2–3). By taking a social and cultural history perspective, one can uncover valuable insights into the utilisation of alternative therapies by individuals pursuing nontraditional or so-called alternative' lifestyles (Campion 2015, 2; cf. Chapter 8). A closer examination of the history of Chinese medicine in Europe and North America during the 1970s reveals the lasting connections and dynamic interactions it had with members of the CCM.

CCM is not a self-designation but a term that scholars (such as Theodore Roszak and Kenneth Leech) working on the 1970s have attributed to this transnational movement. Followers of the CCM espoused anti-industrialisation and antimaterialism. Many advocated a bucolic utopia, environmental protectionism, and going 'back to the land', living a simple and primitive life, practising organic farming in communes of like-minded people (Melville 1972; Nelson 1989). To oppose technocracy and the dominance and power of natural science, many young people also rejected the unquestioning pursuit and acquisition of scientific modernity (Roszak 1970, 4; Campion 2015, 121–28). Instead, they pursued alternative sources of energy, championing a technical philosophy of 'small is beautiful' while expanding their spiritual lives through psychedelic experiences and searching for wisdom in ancient Asian philosophies and religions (Schumacher 1999; Roszak 1970). According to Edward Said, since the Enlightenment, the Orient has been invoked by 'the Westerners' (initially Europeans, but later also North Americans) to designate an apparently homogeneous Asian culture as 'exotic', 'mysterious', and 'sexy', but at the same time 'undeveloped', 'backward', and 'Other' (Said 1979, 1–7, 51, 107). This kind of alterity had the dual effect of feminising and disempowering the East, thereby justifying the exploitation of colonies in underdeveloped Asian regions during the 19th and early 20th centuries. As society's priorities shifted, the concept manifested itself in various ways, legitimising alternative forms of knowledge ranging from Jungian psychotherapy and the *I Ching* divination oracle to mindfulness and yoga, all drawing on the perceived mystery and power of Eastern philosophy and religion (Leech 1973, 64–68, 86). In the postcolonial era of the late 20th century, there was still a strong tendency towards this kind of polarised characterisation between West and East, but with notable differences influenced by the counterculture movement.

As Bivins has observed, the early interest in acupuncture among Europeans prior to the CCM came mainly from social elites and scientists, who approached the method with a clear 'separation of theory from practice' (2000, 71). In other words, these pioneers were fascinated by acupuncture and Chinese medicine from a typically Orientalist perspective, as Said characterises it, imagining these knowledge and skills as a static cultural 'Other', both exotic and contemptible, unworthy of being an equally valuable medical system with its own techniques and theories. From a strong scientific and/or medical background, their study of acupuncture aimed to reduce it to a purely medical technique by analysing it through the lenses of modern science and medicine. They sought to understand the mechanisms behind the observed effects of acupuncture by using anatomy-based medical theories. Their primary goal was to confidently incorporate acupuncture as a simple technique into modern medicine. In a sense, the ongoing research on the anatomical and physiological foundations of acupuncture meridians, points, and their clinical effects (including analgesia), without addressing acupuncture theories, is a continuation of such an Orientalist approach.

In contrast, young students enrolled in British acupuncture colleges in the second half of the 20th century held a mentality which I label 'counterculture Orientalism'. With this term, I refer to their collective belief at the time of a 'golden past' when an authentic medical tradition was invented and passed on as a static unity within 'five thousand years' of Chinese history (Worsley 1984, 14–15). At the time, their limited proficiency in the traditional Chinese language and limited access to accurate translations of Chinese medicine theories and history likely contributed to such belief. This collective interpretation aligns with Said's definition of Orientalism, which perceives the East as an essentialised Other to Euro-Americans. However, for those who quested for alternatives from the dominance of the establishment, acupuncture appeared to be a 'hip' choice, because of the identities indicated by its title: 'traditional' and 'Chinese' (Mole 2021). In other words, 'counterculture Orientalism' differs from the original concept of Orientalism in that it adopts a respectful approach to the otherness of Chinese medicine, rather than the dismissive and superior attitude invoked by the pioneers who introduced acupuncture to Europe in previous centuries, as well as by some contemporary medical professionals.

According to my interviews with CCM acupuncturists, their motivation to study and practise traditional Chinese philosophy and medical theory as a lifelong pursuit stems from their desire to address the limitations of modern medicine and the medical establishment. Within this context, several schools of acupuncture have emerged in the UK since the 1970s. These include the Five-Element Acupuncture (FEA) taught by Jack Worsley (1923–2003), which is based on the Five Elements theory (*wuxing* 五行; sometimes translated as 'Five Phases' or 'Five Agents'), and the Acupuncture of Stems and Branches taught by Dick van Buren (1921–2003), which is based on the theory of *yin-yang* 陰陽 and the Heavenly Stems and Earthly Branches (*tiangan dizhi* 天干地支).[3] In the following, I use the FEA as an example to demonstrate how the counterculture movement has significantly influenced the popularisation and local practice of acupuncture in the UK over the late 20th century.

The Counterculture Generation of FEA Practitioners in Britain

To trace the history of the FEA in the 1970s and '80s, I collected the memories of FEA practitioners through semistructured, in-depth interviews. In this chapter, I quote from five of those interviewees. They were all once students of the founder of the FEA, J.R. Worsley, and later became acupuncture practitioners themselves. Three of them – John, David, and Janie – were trained at Worsley's College in Leamington Spa (southeast of Birmingham) in the 1970s, and the other two – Volker and Anna – studied there in the

3 *Yin-yang* and *wuxing* are two ancient Chinese philosophical concepts that have been integrated into the theoretical foundation of traditional Chinese medicine since the Han Dynasty (Yun-Ju 2022). Both concepts were developed into a systematic correspondence between natural substances/phenomena and human bodily functions in order to serve Chinese medical doctors to understand and explain the psychophysiology of the human body, the occurrence and development of illness, and the principles of effective treatments. *Wuxing* is commonly translated in English as Five Elements, Five Agents, or Five Phases. It consists of the characteristic activities of the five Elements (wood, fire, earth, metal, and water), their interrelationships, and their corresponding categories, ranging from sounds, colours, and flavours to viscera, sensing organs, and the emotions of human beings (See Table 1).

1980s. Although they all went on to practise acupuncture, John and Volker were more critical of the FEA style and integrated other styles into their practice after graduation; they also shared a more cynical attitude towards their teacher. In contrast, the other three – David, Janie, and Anna – remain loyal to their master and have practised 'pure' FEA as they learned it from Worsley; they hold warm memories of him, some even recalling the quality of his touch during pulse-taking and how it conveyed a special healing power.

When these participants studied with Worsley, they were in their 20s and early 30s. Now, the oldest of them is over 80 years old, and the youngest is in his 60s. In terms of chronological age, my respondents may not be considered to be of the same generation (Musgrove 1974, 8–9). All of them, however, are broadly representative members of the counterculture movement (henceforth: CCMers) in their early life: they were generally born and raised in white, middle-class families; they were interested and involved in arts and/or left-wing political and feminist campaigns (e.g., pacifism, social justice, and environmental causes); and before studying acupuncture, they had all chosen conventional life pathways as employees of, for example, major companies or hospitals, or as students in higher education. David studied architecture at a university in France and worked in an architecture firm during his 20s and 30s. John had a doctoral degree in philosophy and was a successful businessman. Janie identified herself as a left-wing activist for social equality and, in her 20s, worked for a feminist magazine before studying herbal medicine at college. Anne pursued graphic design at an art college, compromising with her parents who wanted her to study fine art and painting, and worked at an advertising company after completing her studies. Volker was an exception: he was born into a prosperous German herbalist family, which inspired him to learn alternative medicine from his teenage years. In search of freedom and creativity, they all opposed conformity and mainstream lifestyles. During the years of CCM, they abandoned conventional career paths to pursue an 'Oriental alternative medicine' (acupuncture) as their lifelong profession (on the concept of 'oriental medicine', cf. Chapter 5).

Alongside their backgrounds and occupations, other alternative CCM elements can also be spotted in their lifestyles. For example, at different points in their lives and in different ways, they all navigated the 'Way' of life wisdom (*dao* 道) through traditional Oriental wisdom – such as the divinatory oracle the *Yijing* 易經 (or *I Ching*, usually translated as the *Book of Changes*), and consulted Oriental religious classics, masters, and gurus from Daoism, Hinduism, and Zen Buddhism (or an eclectic mix of these) as an alternative to Christianity – looking for practical ways to enlightenment and transcendence with a reassessment of the value of life and spirituality (Leech 1973; Brink 1992; Oliver 2014). Among my respondents, Volker and John shared an interest in Indian and Classical Chinese philosophies; John, David, Anna, and Volker mentioned their practice of yoga and/or *taiji* (also known as *tai chi*) at the time. These are all pursuits that could mark them as typical members of the counterculture and New Age culture (Roszak 1970; Heelas 1996). They also shared an interest in a bucolic utopia centred on nature and environmentalism, reflected in a collective passion for an organic, healthy, and/or vegetarian diet (Melville 1972). Among my interviewees, David was a frequent customer of health shops; Anna mentioned her vegetarian diet in the 1970s and her love of brown rice. Thus, their reminiscences can be seen as representative of the CCM context in which FEA emerged and developed.

The Construction of Five-Element Acupuncture in Britain

FEA is considered by many the most popular style of acupuncture in Anglophone society of the second half of the 20th century. Taught and popularised in Britain since the late 1960s, FEA is a fascinating and highly influential transnational interpretation of Chinese medicine. According to the British Acupuncture Council (BAcC), half of currently active acupuncturists in the UK have been trained with FEA. The construction and development of FEA can be attributed to two generations: 1) the founder, J.R. Worsley, and 2) his early group of students influenced by the CCM.

Worsley was born in Coventry, England to a family of railway engineers (Eckman 2007, 171). His father had a passion for gardening and Eastern culture, both of which influenced Worsley's later career as an acupuncturist. After studying physiotherapy and naturopathy (cf. Chapter 8), he was introduced to acupuncture in the UK and Germany and trained with teachers in Korea, Japan, Taiwan, and Singapore in the 1940s and '50s (Eckman 2007, 165–75). In the 1960s, he returned to the UK and developed the FEA system inspired by the theory of the *wuxing* (commonly translated in the acupuncture community as 'Five Elements') and the knowledge of acupuncture meridians that he had learned from his teachers in East Asia. The College of Traditional Acupuncture (Figure 4.1), which Worsley founded with friends in 1971 in his hometown of Coventry, is considered one of the first acupuncture colleges in Europe. For Worsley's countercultural students, the knowledge of Chinese medicine taught at this college provided a humanistic and holistic approach to healthcare. With its ancient philosophy of the *wuxing* correspondence system connecting nature and the human body,

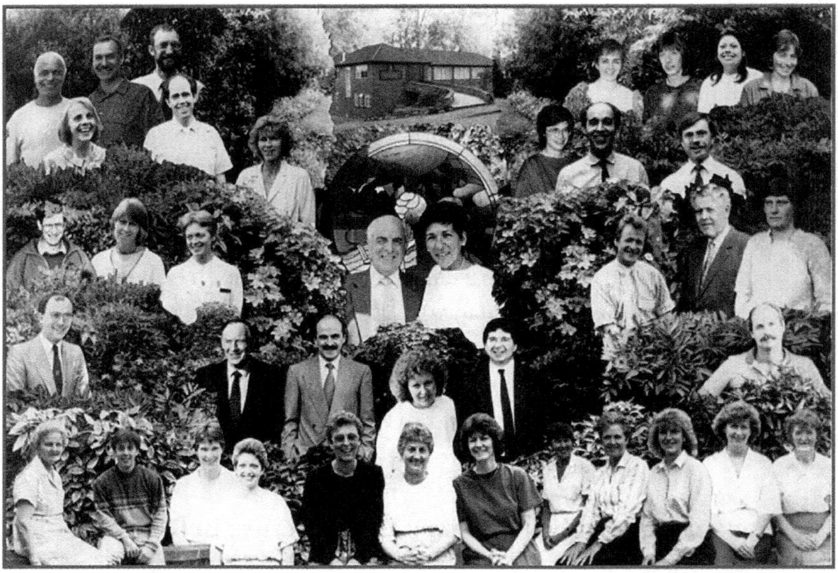

Figure 4.1. CTA and a collage of its faculty in the 1980s (Worsley in the centre left). Permission of reproduction kindly granted by Dr Martin Allbright (https://www.doctoracupuncture.co.uk/drmartinallbright.html).

its emphasis on the universal *qi* 氣 (typically translated as 'energy' or 'vital force'; cf. Chapter 1) and various therapies such as massage, moxibustion, and the use of inexpensive steel needles, Chinese medicine was collectively considered an appealing, cost-effective, and potent alternative to modern biomedicine. Based on the interconnectedness of body-mind-spirit, its holistic approach to health was highly valued by those seeking a more comprehensive form of care.

Wuxing and the Law of the Five Elements

Inspired by his travels across Asia, Worsley embraced the *wuxing* theory from Chinese medical tradition as the theoretical foundation for his own style of acupuncture. Founding his acupuncture college and naming it the College of Traditional Acupuncture, the ancient roots of the Five Elements theory became a powerful tool and evidence to serve FEA's legitimacy as a form of authentic Chinese acupuncture. Thereafter, during the following decade, Worsley and his CCM students also gave this tradition the countercultural gloss in their construction of the knowledge and professional identity of FEA as an alternative medicine in the UK.

In the FEA community, theoretical principles for clinical work are referred to as 'laws' (Eckman 2007, 216–18; Connelly 1976, 23–24, 92). This method corresponds to homoeopaths naming their theoretical doctrine the 'law of Similars' (meaning 'treating like with like'), with an implication of having its root in nature and the reliability of such doctrine as truth that 'will never alter' in time (Coulter 1984; Worsley 1984, 37). The laws in FEA's cosmology include the 'Law of Husband and Wife' for pulse taking, the 'Law of Midday-Midnight' – referring to a daily horary rule about when 'each of the organs within the Element is functioning at its peak of energy' – and the 'Law of Cure' – again borrowed from homoeopathy – pointing to the notion that symptoms can sometimes get worse before getting better (Coulter 1977, 362).

Among those laws, the 'Law of the Five Elements' has always enjoyed a fundamental role in the FEA system. A comparison between Worsley's law and the textual explanations of *wuxing* in foundational Chinese medical classics – such as the *Inner Canon of the Yellow Emperor* (*Huangdi neijing* 黃帝內經, commonly referred to as *Neijing*) and the *Canon of the Yellow Emperor's Eighty-One Difficult Issues* (*Huangdi bashiyi nanjing* 黃帝八十一難經, commonly referred to as *Nanjing* 難經), both of which were originally compiled around the first century CE – shows both consistencies and discrepancies.

As far as the discrepancies are concerned, the changes that occurred were partly due to practical concerns. In the Traditional Chinese Medicine (TCM) style I learnt in a five-year university programme in Beijing, concepts underlying clinical diagnosis and treatment consisted of *yin-yang* and *wuxing* paradigms (cf. Chapter 3). Without the former, I argue, *wuxing* is less an independent diagnostic system by nature as it is essentially a description of the physiological phenomena and functions of the human body rather than the causes and pathological processes of malfunction or imbalance. How was one to fill the gap between physiological teachings and the practical therapeutic requirements of seeing patients? In the absence of knowledge of other paradigms in Chinese medicine, Worsley had to extend and innovate the original *wuxing* theory into a Five Elements theory that was both the theoretical basis for explaining health and disease and a tool for making clinical diagnoses. To provide such a model for his Euro-American students, Worsley constructed his Law of the Five Elements with some basic categories from the ancient *wuxing* correspondence system (Table 4.1) and proposed an innovative concept which he called 'CF' (Causative Factor) (Connelly 1976, 93; Eckman 2007, 95). This concept has never been a feature of classical Chinese medicine, nor is it a characteristic of the modern forms of differential diagnosis that emerged in contemporary Chinese medicine during the mid-20th century.

Table 4.1. The canonised system of correspondences of the *wuxing*/Five Elements schema[4]

	Wood	Fire	Earth	Metal	Water
Organs	Liver/Gall Bladder	Heart/Small Intestine	Spleen/ Stomach	Lung/Large Intestine	Kidney/ Bladder
Seasons	Spring	Summer	Late Summer	Autumn	Winter
Environmental Factors	Wind	Heat	Damp	Dry	Cold
Growth & Development	Birth/Infant	Growth/Young adult	Transformation/ Adult	Reaping, Harvest/Old Age	Storage/ Death
Directions / Stages of the Day	East Dawn	South Midday	Center Transition	West Dusk	North Midnight
Emotions	Anger	Joy	Worry	Grief/Sorrow	Fear
Tastes	Sour	Bitter	Sweet	Pungent	Salty
Colours	Green	Red	Yellow	White	Blue
Sounds	Shout	Laughing	Singing	Crying	Groaning
Odours	Rancid	Acrid/Burnt	Fragrant	Rotten	Putrid

Worsley's method was much simpler than a typical Chinese medicine diagnosis. According to his law, a CF diagnosis means a determination of which one of the five Elements (Wood, Fire, Earth, Metal, or Water) is 'most seriously imbalanced' by observing 'the presence or absence of subtle colours, odours, vocal qualities and emotional tendencies' that correlate with the Five Elements correspondence system (Eckman 2007, 19). Ideally, the information from these categories would point to the same Element. For example, if a patient has 'a yellowish complexion, singing voice, fragrant odour and craving for attention and sympathy', then he or she would be diagnosed as having their CF in the element Earth (Eckman 2007; see Table 1).

As Vivienne Lo and Michael Stanley-Baker have observed, for declared living traditions such as Chinese medicine, a particular language and nomenclature (in the case of Chinese medicine, such terms include *yin-yang, wuxing*, and *qi*) act as the glue that provides a sense of continuity between the ancient and the contemporary (Stanley-Baker and Lo 2022). In the case of FEA, a comparison between those Chinese medical classics and Worsley's teachings (recorded in later published textbooks, journal articles, as well as video recording clips) indicates that Worsley adopted from his transnational learning experience some basic characteristics and framework for *wuxing*: the designation and characters of the five *xing* ('Elements' in FEA language), the relations between each Element, and some categories included in the

4 The author made this table based on the texts of *wuxing* in *Neijing* and *Nanjing*.

corresponding system of *wuxing* (as shown in Table 1). These preserved elements served as the scaffolding for Worsley's construction of his Law of the Five Elements, and, meanwhile, as the 'linguistic glue' that legitimised his claim to the authenticity of FEA as a traditional Chinese practice.

Worsley did not disclose any information regarding his decision to develop these four diagnostic categories over other alternatives. They are loosely based on the ancient Chinese diagnostic categories of *wang* 望 (to observe), *wen* 聞 (to smell), *wen* 問 (to ask), and *qie* 切 (to touch). But without access to classical texts, language training, or a proper translator for his studies in Asia, Worsley creatively used the limited knowledge he had gleaned from his masters and adapted it to the interests and passions of his young CCM audience. Despite all four categories being represented in premodern texts, his reinterpretations of them are idiosyncratic. The category of 'odour', for example, is read in modern Chinese medicine as the smell of a patient's urine and faeces and is less a feature of a person's more generalised odour. In Worsley's reinvention of CF diagnosis, he simplified the categories and resettled them in a daily life setting, assigning each patient a body odour related to their weak 'Element' according to the traditional *wuxing* correspondences. Thus, a patient who was weak in the Earth Element would smell fragrant, in the Fire Element would smell scorched, in the Wood Element would smell rancid, and in the Water Element, putrid. These were nature- and sensation-based associations that emphasised a person's connection to the environment (on nature and environment, cf. Chapter 3). When introducing his theory, Worsley always started with its links with nature, which he portrayed as something each of us could know innately.

> When we go into this system of medicine, we find it [...] is wholly based on natural laws. Man cannot pollute it; man cannot change it; man cannot improve upon it. [...] Do you know, a child of seven can understand the wisdom of traditional Chinese medicine? *It is so simple; it is so basic*; it is so natural. [...] The great tragedy is that we neglect the natural gifts we are given when we were first born. I firmly believe that no man nor woman can be your teacher. I do not believe in gurus, at least not in the form of human beings. I feel that our teacher is nature itself. Everything we want to know is out there in nature. (Worsley 1980, my emphasis)

Worsley's emphasis on the observation of the natural world was constructed to help students develop a better understanding of the Elements in order to diagnose CFs in patients and proved to be a very successful pedagogy. On the one hand, it reflects the aforementioned ecological and environmentalist concerns that CCMers were endorsing, where nature was seen as an essential source of healing (cf. Chapter 5). Only through 'direct contact with nature' can one channel this healing power and attain an authentic way of being and living (Umbach and Humphrey 2018, 30). In Worsley's teaching, nature rather than modern civilisation was presented as the primary source of healing, which he and his students could access through direct contact, observation, and learning. On the other hand, Worsley's teaching method for the CF is a sensation-based practice that prioritises individual experience, empowering each student with their own unique source of expertise. Thus, soon after the beginning of their course, students were asked to go and sensitise themselves to the world around them, starting with developing their personal sensory experiences of each season (cf. Chapter 3). As Janie recalled,

> He (Worsley) just said, 'It's not in the book. [...] You have to be in nature, you have to experience how the Elements work in nature. [...] [T]he only way you're gonna do it is *being in tune with nature*'. [...] And living in London was very frustrating in the winter. Because it was never cold enough. It wasn't proper cold, ever, to really know what winter does. So I used to go out to the country to see what winter was like. What happened – when it was icy – what happened to the ground, what happened to the plants. (Janie 2019, my emphasis)

The subsequent step required students to refine their experiences for clinical diagnosis. My interviewees recall being instructed by their teachers to visit a busy street or train station and observe the auras and odours of passersby. They were to listen to the sound of their voices and determine the CFs of the people they observed: identifying whether they were Earth, Water, Wood, Fire, or Metal individuals (Eckman 2007, 95):

> I love to be able to just sit here in a cafe and look across and think 'Oh yeah, they are a bit green'. I listen to the voice, 'Yeah, there's a bit of a shout in there'. And sometimes you know, I'll just be walking on the street, and I'll just see somebody walking towards me. I could see elementary what's going off with them. (Anna 2019)

In retrospect, Worsley's method of linking the source of healthcare knowledge to nature and individual senses was seen as authentic by his CCM students. This perception stemmed from its role as a form of rebellion and an alternative to the modern mainstream lifestyle and the orthodox biomedical system. The use of the five senses in the Law of the Five Elements provided an alternative way of knowledge production and formed a challenge to the exclusiveness of the professional biomedical establishment. When reviewing the reliability of conventional empirical knowledge of medicine in recent centuries, Coulter (1984) concludes that '[w]hen all can perceive, discuss, make comparisons, and draw conclusions, the resulting knowledge is reliable'. According to Coulter's analysis, Worsley's teachings earned certain legitimacy through the endorsement of collective experience while enhancing the sense of connection and devotion from his students through training the sensory acuity of their whole bodies 'as an instrument' for diagnosis (Baker 2016, 1521; cf. Chapter 3).

The Emphasis on the Emotions and Spirits of Points

There was a vital weakness in Worsley's 'Traditional Acupuncture'. The simplistic synthesis of an Element theory from the vast corpus of Chinese medical writing and experience barely provided any practical model for dealing with physical symptoms. My respondents remembered that in the first three-year programme, they spent most of the time learning the Five Elements theory and trying to identify the characteristics of each Element both in nature and in individual patients. There were also practical classes teaching pulse-taking and the location of acupuncture channels and points. However, the curriculum provided little training on the recognition, analysis, and treatment of illnesses as one would usually expect in medical education.

In claiming to identify the root cause of a person's illness, FEA took a fierce stance against conventional medicine as 'allopathic' – the therapeutic principle dedicated to attacking and reversing physical symptoms through the doctrine of opposites (cf. Chapter 8). This claim, again, was of its time. In the 1960s, Euro-American societies witnessed the most notorious scandal in the field of modern medicine: the Thalidomide crisis.[5] This disaster heralded a radical shift in public attitudes against science-based medicine. In the following decades, a growing 'disenchantment with modern science' and public disillusionment with conventional medicine spread to segments of

5 Thalidomide, (UK trade name Distaval), developed by the West German pharmaceuticals company Chemie Grünenthal in the 1950s, was marketed as a mild sedative and prescribed as safe for pregnant women. After being prescribed to relieve morning sickness, it was later recognised as having 'harmful effects on the foetus in early pregnancy'. The scale of the disaster remains unknown, but in 1979 knowledge of the 8,000 surviving thalidomide children in 46 affected countries heralded a public questioning toward science-based medicine. See Hayman (1961) and The Insight team of the *Sunday Times* (1979) for details.

the population in Europe and North America (Avina and Schneiderman 1978; Holden 1978). And since allopathy – the attack on physical symptoms – was an essential feature of the biomedical system (particularly its pharmaceutical arm), FEA's weakness in symptomatic treatment was perceived and legitimised as an advantage by its CCM followers. For example, John and David explained to me their concern with symptomatic healthcare and how this concern motivated their pursuit of FEA:

> When you're brought up in a country where Western medicine is the predominant thing, you go to the doctor and say, 'I'm feeling upset', he says, 'What else have you got?' He ignores, you know, personal distress things, which may be the key thing. And he deals with something else or gives people a tranquillizer, which isn't [...] always the best medicine. It does do a lot of magical things, surgery and so on are extremely effective. Just to be clear, [there are] a lot of people with physical problems. Sometimes the origin of it is mental anyway. (John 2020)

> The Oriental School of Medicine. Uh, I signed on for a year there [...]. [W]e weren't completely convinced by what we were being taught. It was *symptomatic*. And the registrar at that college saw that we were unhappy. And she was a patient of Worsley and also quite a powerful person. And she negotiated with him to come back to the UK to finish our training. And the whole group of 10 or 12 people moved to Worsley's for finishing our training. [...] It [van Buren's teaching] was syndromes. It was a, I can't remember the words, but it was very much learning facts, a bit like a medical doctor [...] *the whole group rebelled against.* (David 2018)

During the CCM period, the symptom-oriented approach to medical diagnosis and intervention faced significant criticism within British society, particularly from proponents of alternative medicines. For members of the FEA community, the prevailing negative sentiment towards symptomatic medicine served as a catalyst, bolstering their professional identity and sense of camaraderie. The limitation of FEA to treating physical ailments not only strengthened their bond but also authenticated their practice as the 'real' traditional Chinese acupuncture, setting it apart from symptomatic modern medicine. Meanwhile, the critique of modern medicine was instrumental in the rise of FEA among the UK public in the late 20th century. Just as Ludwik Fleck puts it, the prevalence of any medical thoughts in a society would occur 'only if they have a seminal effect by being performed at a time when the social conditions are right' (Fleck 1979, 45).

John's comment highlights a major critique of orthodox medicine by advocates of holistic medicine: the division of body and mind, both philosophically and clinically. Worsley constructed FEA with the same conviction, introducing his acupuncture with a tripartite focus on body, mind, and spirit. In FEA, the 'spirit' level was not limited to the 'spiritual and religious sides of a person' but rather to the sum of one's sensory perceptions and feelings, one's ability to 'be moved by fine music or art', or 'a feeling of God in their lives' (Mole 1985). Any malfunction on this level meant a loss of 'some feeling of closeness to nature', 'as if their spirit had no eyes through which to take in that beauty [of nature]' (Mole 1985). The 'mind' level referred to the 'cognitive faculty' as one's 'ability to think', instead of the psychological sense of one's personality or behaviour. Then, Worsley took a further step, stating that the spirit and mind were the deeper *roots* of the body and that any physical illness would be spontaneously healed by transforming a patient's *emotions*.

With this principle of seeing the mind and spirit as the root of physical disorders, FEA practitioners tend to prioritise emotional diagnostic questions over allopathic and physically oriented ones. Peter Mole, a student at the College who graduated in 1978, wrote in the group newsletter of 1985 the following: 'Profound change only comes about with a fundamental change in the emotions. Just as they produce the most destructive forces in the body, mind, and spirit, so the emotions can also provide the most constructive' (Mole 1985). Dianne Connelly, Worsley's student in the 1970s and author of the first unofficial FEA textbook, published her second book in 1987, *All Sickness is Homesickness*, in which she promoted the idea that all illness and symptoms are a way for us to come 'home' to our authentic selves, in the sense of knowing, healing, and fulfilling who we are physically, mentally, and spiritually (Connelly 1994).

In the Han dynasty (202 BCE–220 CE), emotions had already been included in the corresponding categories of the *wuxing* system, and it is certainly true that emotions have always been integral to the Chinese diagnostic process (Zhang 2007). Nevertheless, in building the FEA system, Worsley's focus on the emotional aspect of the diagnostic process to determine patients' CF was clearly shaped by the development of psychotherapy in 20th century Europe (cf. Chapter 6). The early FEA textbook (Connelly 1976, 90–100) provided FEA practitioners with a set of questions to ask patients during their initial session:

1. What is your age, date, time and place of birth?
2. With whom do you live?

3. Why are you coming to the clinic?
4. Any other problems or complaints? Are there things you might not ordinarily go to a doctor for? (e.g., 'I have difficulty in making decisions, I am angry a lot, I feel like moaning all the time.')
5. You and your family's medical history?
6. What is your emotional history? How were you as a child? Did you have any difficulties that can be remembered? Any strong features? How did you get along with others, how did you feel growing up? Was there any trauma in childhood, like moving or a family death, that was terribly upsetting?
7. How would you describe yourself emotionally?
8. What is your favourite colour?
9. What season/climate do you like or not like particularly?
10. What time of day do you feel better or worse?
11. What is your favourite taste?
12. How is your head? Do you wear spectacles? How are your ears, nose, mouth, skin, hair and scalp, nail, bones, muscles? Urination? Perspiration? Bowel movement?
13. How do you sleep? Do you dream? Is there any recurrent theme?
14. Smoke, drink and diet?
15. Are you taking any medications?
16. What is your menstrual cycle like?
17. How is your general energy level?

As this list shows, FEA practitioners were trained to spend a long time taking down a personal history, with a focus on feelings and emotions, as the key evidence to validate the CF diagnosis. 'What we are trying to do', Worsley explains, 'is to get right within you [the patient], so we can see you as a unique individual from all three levels (of body, mind, and spirit)' (Worsley 1984, 21). One FEA periodical in 1983 recorded a patient's perspective on his first FEA session for prostate dysfunction: 'The first appointment consisted of talking about myself for two hours: childhood and relationships with my parents; medical background; daily pattern of life – how I ate, slept and so on; my reactions to the seasons; emotional disposition – did I have "up" days and "down" days?' (Silverlight 1983).

In addition to the explicit answers to these questions, FEA practitioners were also encouraged to pay attention to more implicit messages through the patients' behaviour: the expression of emotions when speaking, the quality of their voice and the terminology they used would all give away their CF. These techniques had a clear resonance with the psychoanalysis used by psychologists, whose community was active and influential in the psychosomatic movement. With the rise of individualism in Euro-American societies in the last century, Bellah and colleagues (1985, 47–48) observed a parallel development of psychotherapy among the middle classes as a means of 'liberat(ing) and fulfil(ling) the self' and 'empowering the self'. The lay practice of acupuncture and Chinese medicine, practised in the same social groups and with the same concern for a holistic approach to the psychological and the somatic, underwent a process of 'psychologising' by members of the counterculture and New Age movements in the last decades of the 20th century (Barnes, 1998). It is not surprising, therefore, when Janie's patient commented that his FEA session was 'more like a therapy' (Janie 2019). Of the articles published in the Society's periodical in 1983, one-third are related to the application of psychological knowledge for FEA's clinical practice.

Drawing on the Word Association technique of psychoanalysis, in the FEA practice the 'exact words' used by patients not only contributed to the aforementioned diagnosis of CF, but in some cases could also direct the treatment plan by prescribing which acupuncture points to use. For example, a patient who repeatedly used the word 'weary' to describe her feelings led Janie to treat her with the point 'Palace of Weariness' (Janie 2019). Commonly, non-Chinese practitioners use a standardised alphabetical-numerical method to refer to acupuncture points, combining the channel to which a point belongs with an ordinal number for that specific point on the channel. In this system, the point mentioned in Janie's case is designated as Pericardium 8 (or PC8 for short). However, when first discovered and documented in China, each point originally had a lyrical name in Chinese. Drawing on this tradition, Worsley invented the concept of 'spirit of point', endowing each point with a spiritual healing effect based on his English translation of their Chinese names. In Worsley's view, the name of the acupoint implied its specific therapeutic effect – hence 'Palace of Weariness' for a patient feeling 'weary':

> He [Worsley] puts a lot of emphasis on the name of the point. He has names of the points. Some kind of translation of the points. To give you an example, like Liver 13, it's called *zhangmen* 章門. This was translated as Chapter Gate. So *men* 門 as Gate, and *zhang* 章 translated as Chapter. And then he would put his interpretation on this. So, it's a chapter, so you can open up a new chapter in a person's life. [...] Then you know a lot about the Liver. And Liver is a Wood Element. So it does planning and decision-making. Therefore it has got to do with chapters of your life. It's a plan for your life. (Volker 2018)

Indeed, acupuncture points were named and associated with healing effects in accordance with the classical philosophy of Chinese medicine, which lyrically describes the human body as a microcosm of the universe (Lo 2001; Lo and Stanley-Baker 2012). However, the FEA community's interpretation of this practice was more of a CCM unfolding, delivered without knowledge of or reference to the cultural context that had given rise to the point names in the first place. After all, as Worsley repeatedly assured his students, the essence of becoming a proficient FEA practitioner lies not in studying Chinese classics or other textbooks. Instead, it is found in gaining sensory experience in nature, engaging in psychoanalytic practice with patients, and harnessing intuition in the application of the spirit of acupuncture points, all of which are fundamental for providing holistic therapy to patients.

Conclusion

This chapter contextualises the cognition and recognition of knowledge within the FEA community, using Worsley's Law of the Five Elements as a case study, during the latter half of the 20th century. It is worth noting that Worsley's approach to the *wuxing* theory to accommodate the sociocultural context of his time is not an isolated historical occurrence. Since the Song dynasty (960–1279), Chinese physicians have applied *wuxing* as a canonical foundation for innovative medical theories stimulated by personal interpretations of classical texts and clinical experience (for *wuyun liuqi* 五運六氣, see Woolf 2022). In 1970s Britain, the Law of the Five Elements was recognised by Worsley and his students more in a British cultural sense – such as to use the law of nature and to combine contemporary spiritual and psychological trends – and less about its Chinese origin due to the lack of classical medical books translated into English at the time. Nevertheless, through transnational transmission, the skeleton of the *wuxing* theory was there to legitimate the identity of FEA as a 'traditional acupuncture' embraced by a CCM audience who espoused an alternative approach to the orthodox medical establishment. The FEA's approach was thus validated by its practitioners because it presented alternatives to the aspects for which modern society and orthodox medicine faced criticism: the alienation from and disregard of nature and subjective sensory experiences, along with the absence of a holistic perspective on the physical and mental dimensions in medical practice.

In this chapter, I argued that there was a 'counterculture Orientalism' embodied by the British FEA community of Worsley and his CCM generation of students. In Worsley's teaching and the shared discourse of his CCM followers, Chinese medicine and acupuncture were still considered an inert, traditional entity and a cultural Other, while their 'undeveloped' nature became the source of appeal as strategies for challenging the social and medical establishment (cf. Chapter 5). The Law of the Five Elements encapsulated an essentialist and romanticised collective imagination of 'traditional Chinese acupuncture', characterised by features that offered, to borrow Edward Said's words (1979, 2), a 'contrasting image, idea, personality, experience' in comparison to the Western, modern, orthodox medicine prevalent in their society. Formed and developed amidst the counterculture and New Age movements, the FEA theory assimilated and reflected the antiestablishment sociocultural traits of that era. On the one hand, within a context where the safety of pharmaceutical drugs was under fierce dispute, acupuncture's evident contrast with orthodox medicine – an external intervention focused on emotions instead of physical symptoms – legitimated it as a credible alternative therapy. On the other hand, an apparently ancient Chinese theory (the *wuxing* theory, through the lens provided by Worsley as the Law of the Five Elements), with its substratum focus on nature and sensory experience, provided an alternative knowledge source to interpret the body in simple terms and without recourse to the monopoly and authority of modern science.

In the first decade of the 21st century, the economic crisis, alongside shifts in the sociocultural and professional landscape in the UK, resulted in the shutdown of nearly all the major FEA colleges in the country, including Worsley's College of Traditional Acupuncture in Leamington Spa. Contrary to expectations, in the decade following its decline in the UK, FEA not only persevered but thrived in China, where it has undergone a reverse process of transmission. In 2012, the first FEA course was held in Nanning, Guangxi province. Since then, seven private training societies have emerged, along with a newly established professional body for FEA, uniting hundreds of practitioners across 18 Chinese provinces. This recent history of FEA's introduction and proliferation in China serves as a reflective lens, capturing intriguing trends and thought currents within the evolving Chinese TCM community. These dynamics, central to my doctoral dissertation (Yang 2023), warrant further scholarly attention and exploration.

Bibliography

Avina, Robert L., and Lawrence J. Schneiderman. 1978. 'Why Patients Choose Homeopathy'. *The Western Journal of Medicine* 128, no. 4: 366–69.

Baker, Michael. 2016. *A Chronological Journey Through Chinese Medical History on the Causes of Disease*. Bath and United Kingdon: Brown Dog Books.

Ballah, Robert N., Richard Madsen, William M. Sullivan, and Steven M. Tipton. *Habits of the Heart*. Berkeley: University of California Press, 1985.

Barnes, Linda L. 1998. 'The Psychologizing of Chinese Healing Practices in the United States'. *Culture, Medicine, and Psychiatry*, no. 22: 413–43.

Barnes, Linda L. 2005. *Needles, Herbs, Gods, and Ghosts: China, Healing, and the West to 1848*. Cambridge, Mass: Harvard University Press.

Berke, Joseph H., ed. 1969. *Counter Culture*. London: Owen.

Bivins, Roberta E. 2000. *Acupuncture, Expertise and Cross-Cultural Medicine*. London: Palgrave Macmillan. https://doi.org/10.1057/9780230287518.

Brink, Serena. 1992. 'The New Age: A Modern Synthesis of Mysticism'. *Agenda*, no. 15: 7–11. https://doi.org/10.2307/4065577.

Bull, G.M. 1973. 'Acupuncture Anaesthesia'. *The Lancet*. Originally published as Volume 2, no. 7826: 417–18. https://doi.org/10.1016/S0140-6736(73)92276-9.

Campion, Nicholas. 2015. *The New Age in the Modern West: Counterculture, Utopia and Prophecy from the Late Eighteenth Century to the Present Day*. London: Bloomsbury Publishing.

Chen, Yun-Ju. 2022. 'Yin, Yang, and Five Agents (Wuxing) in the Basic Questions and Early Han (202 BCE–220 CE) Medical Manuscripts'. In *Routledge Handbook of Chinese Medicine*, edited by Vivienne Lo, Michael Stanley-Baker, and Dolly Yang, 13–22. Routledge. https://doi.org/10.4324/9780203740262-3.

Cheng, Tsung O. 1973. 'Acupuncture Anesthesia'. *Science* 179, no. 4073: 521–21. https://doi.org/10.1126/science.179.4073.521.a.

Connelly, Dianne M. 1979. *Traditional Acupuncture: The Law of the Five Elements*. Columbia: Wisdomwell Press.

Coulter, Harris L. 1977. *Divided Legacy: A History of the Schism in Medical Thought*. Vol. 2. Progress and Regress: J.B. Van Helmont to Claude Bernard. Washington DC: Wehawken.

Coulter, Harris L. 1984. 'Homoeopathy'. In *Alternative Medicines: Popular and Policy Perspectives*, edited by J. Warren Salmon, 57–80. New York: Tavistock.

Daston, Lorraine, and Peter Galison. 2007. *Objectivity*. New York: Cambridge, Mass: Zone Books.

Eckman, Peter. 2007. *In the Footsteps of the Yellow Emperor: Tracing the History of Traditional Acupuncture*. California: Long River Press.

Fleck, Ludwik. 1979. *Genesis and Development of a Scientific Fact*. Translated by Thaddeus J. Trenn and Fred Bradley. Chicago: University of Chicago Press.

Foucault, Michel. 1972. *The Archaeology of Knowledge*. Translated by Alan Sheridan. London: Tavistock Publications.

Hamilton, Sidney, Percy Brown, Mary Hollington, and Kathleen Rutherford. 1972. 'Anaesthesia by Acupuncture'. *The British Medical Journal* 3, no. 5822: 352–52. http://doi.org/10.1136/bmj.3.5822.352-b.

Hayman, D. J. 1961. 'Withdrawal of Thalidomide ("Distaval")'. *The British Medical Journal* 2, no. 5265: 1499.

Heelas, Paul. 1996. *The New Age Movement: The Celebration of the Self and the Sacralization of Modernity*. Oxford: Blackwell.

Holden, Constance. 1978. 'Holistic Health Concepts Gaining Momentum'. *Science* 200, no. 4345: 1029. http://doi.org/10.1126/science.200.4345.1029.

Hollingworth, Clare. 1972. 'China's Faith in Acupuncture'. *Daily Telegraph*, 20 June: 13. The Telegraph Historical Archive, https://link.gale.com/apps/doc/IO0703673495/TGRH?u=ucl_ttda&sid= TGRH&xid=d01fc1b6. Accessed on 28 April 2020.

Hopton, A.K., S. Curnoe, M. Kanaan, and H. MacPherson. 2012. 'Acupuncture in Practice: Mapping the Providers, the Patients and the Settings in a National Cross-Sectional Survey'. *BMJ Open* 2, no. 1: e000456. https://doi.org/10.1136/bmjopen-2011-000456.

Leech, Kenneth. 1973. *Youthquake: The Growth of a Counter-Culture through Two Decades*. London: Sheldon Press.

Lo, Vivienne. 2001. 'Huangdi Hama Jing (Yellow Emperor's Toad Canon)'. *Asia Major* 14, no. 2: 61–99.

Lo, Vivienne, and Michael Stanley-Baker. 2012. 'Chinese Medicine'. In *The Oxford Handbook of the History of Medicine*, edited by Mark Jackson, 150–69. Oxford: Oxford University Press. https://doi.org/10.1093/oxfordhb/9780199546497.013.0009.

Melville, Keith. 1972. *Communes in the Counter Culture: Origins, Theories, Styles of Life*. New York: Morrow.

Mole, Peter. 1985. 'The Role of the Emotions in Body, Mind and Spirit'. *TAS Newsletter*, no. 18 (October): 4–6.

Musgrove, Frank. 1974. *Ecstasy and Holiness: Counter Culture and the Open Society*. London: Methuen.

Nelson, Elizabeth. 1989. *The British Counter-Culture, 1966–73*. London: Palgrave Macmillan.

Oliver, Paul. 2014. *Hinduism and the 1960s: The Rise of a Counter Culture*. London: Bloomsbury Academic. https://doi.org/10.5040/9781472594600.

Reston, James. 1971. 'Now, about My Operation in Peking'. *New York Times*, 26 July.

Roszak, Theodore. 1970. *The Making of a Counter Culture: Reflections on the Technocratic Society and Its Youthful Opposition*. London: Faber.

Said, Edward W. 1979. *Orientalism*. 1st Vintage Books ed. New York: Vintage Books.

Salmon, J. Warren, ed. 1984. *Alternative Medicines: Popular and Policy Perspectives*. New York: Tavistock.

Schumacher, E.F. 1999. *Small Is Beautiful: Economics as If People Mattered: 25 Years Later ... with Commentaries*. Point Roberts: Hartley & Marks Publishers.
Silverlight, John. 1983. 'The Point of It All'. *Traditional Acupuncture College* (*TAS*) *Newsletter*, no. 11: 7.
Sivin, Nathan. 2011. *Kexueshi fangfalun jiangyan lu* 科学史方法论讲演录 (Methodology of the History of Science). Beijing: Peking University Press.
Stanley-Baker, Michael, and Vivienne Lo. 'An Introduction'. In *Routledge Handbook of Chinese Medicine*, edited by edited by Vivienne Lo, Michael Stanley-Baker, and Dolly Yang, 1–10. London: Routledge. https://doi.org/10.4324/9780203740262-1.
Sunday Times of London Insight Team. 1979. *Suffer the Children: The Story of Thalidomide*. London: Deutsch.
Thomas, K.J., J.P. Nicholl, and P. Coleman. 2001. 'Use and Expenditure on Complementary Medicine in England: A Population Based Survey'. *Complementary Therapies in Medicine* 9, no. 1: 2–11. https://doi.org/10.1054/ctim.2000.0407.
Woolf, Deborah. 2022. 'The Importance of Numerology, Part 2 Medicine'. In *Routledge Handbook of Chinese Medicine*, edited by Vivienne Lo, Michael Stanley-Baker, and Dolly Yang, 91–108. London: Routledge. https://doi.org/10.4324/9780203740262-7.
Worsley, J.R. 1984. *Talking About Acupuncture in New York*. 2nd ed. Warwickshire: The College of Traditional Chinese Acupuncture.
Worsley, J.R. 1990. *Traditional Acupuncture Vol.II: Traditional Diagnosis*. Warwickshire: College of Traditional Acupuncture.
Yang, Yi. 2023. 'Constructing Authenticity and Embodying Tradition in a Globalising Medicine: A History of Five-Element Acupuncture (五行针灸, Wuxing Zhenjiu) from 1970s to Present'. PhD thesis, University College London.
Yinger, J. Milton. 1960. 'Contraculture and Subculture'. *American Sociological Review* 25, no. 5: 625–35. https://doi.org/10.2307/2090136.
Zhang, Yanhua. 2007. *Transforming Emotions with Chinese Medicine: An Ethnographic Account from Contemporary China*. Albany: SUNY Press.

Biography

Yang Yi's (PhD History, UCL) work is informed by her previous training in the field of biomedicine and Traditional Chinese Medicine. From 2006 to 2017, she was trained as a medical science researcher of TCM and acupuncture and practised as an acupuncturist in Beijing. Drawing on this experience, since 2017, she has turned to studying the modern history of Chinese medicine, specifically the crosscultural transmission of Chinese medicine in the 20th and 21st centuries.

5 From Eden to Aquarius

'Oriental Medicine', Natural Healing, and the Market of Self-Care Books in Brazil in the 1970s

Luis Fernando Bernardi Junqueira and Renata Palandri Sigolo[1]

Abstract: This chapter investigates the formation of a self-care and alternative healing book market in Brazil during the 1970s, a period characterised by the peak of the counterculture and the rise of the New Age movement within the country. As disillusionment with the materialistic foundations of biomedicine and its pervasive impact on notions of health and illness grew, a burgeoning community of Brazilian authors, translators, editors, publishers, and readers – all deeply interested in natural healing – sought an alternative in the 'Orient'. This imagined sphere was perceived as a source to complement, if not potentially supplant the perceived reductionist approaches to body, health, and life associated with biomedicine. In tandem with patterns observed in Europe and the United States, a rapidly expanding community of Brazilian enthusiasts invoked the concept of 'oriental medicine' ('medicina oriental' in Portuguese) as an antidote to what they identified as the 'Western materialistic malaise'.

Keywords: Oriental medicine, self-care, natural healing, New Age, Brazil

During the 1970s, Brazil was in the midst of a radicalisation phase within the US-backed civil-military dictatorship that had been established in 1964, an oppressive regime that would last until 1985. Despite this conservative political context, a wave of counterculture-inspired movements proliferated across the country in various fields such as the arts, literature, and healthcare

1 This work was supported by the Wellcome Trust [Reference: 217661/Z/19/Z]. Both authors have contributed equally to the research, writing, and revisions of this chapter.

Gaitanidis, Ioannis, Luis Fernando Bernardi Junqueira, Avery Morrow, and Sangyun Han (eds), *Therapy, Spirituality, and East Asian Imaginaries*. Taylor & Francis Group 2025
DOI: 10.5117/9789048559015_CH05

(Dunn 2016; on counterculture, cf. Chapter 4). Much has been written about the history of the counterculture and its aftermath in Europe and North America; English scholarship has, however, largely failed to appreciate the critical role played by the counterculture – and the subsequent New Age movement – in the diffusion of alternative therapies in Latin America, particularly in Brazil. This paper aims thus to analyse the Brazilian appropriation of ideas and practices originating from a loosely-defined 'Orient' within the transnational circulation of therapeutic knowledge between the late 1960s and early '80s. In tandem with the United States and Western Europe, the rise of upper-middle and upper-class movements such as the counterculture and New Age occurred within a search for new paradigms in body care, illness, and well-being. These new paradigms, positioned as alternatives to biomedicine, found in the Far East a powerful source of inspiration. Between the 1960s and '80s, Brazilians didn't need to journey to East Asia to encounter a plethora of representations of China, Japan, and India; these were already widely accessible in the public sphere. These references entered the country through a wave of translations from English, French, and Spanish into Portuguese, proliferating rapidly in the Brazilian press and popular culture. Their widespread impact on the Brazilian 'therapeutic landscape' – a term borrowed from Allison Williams (1998) – has persisted to this day.

The manual *From Eden to Aquarius: The Book of Natural Healing* (1974), translated from English into Portuguese as *Do Jardim do Éden à Era de Aquarius: O Livro da Cura Natural* in 1977, will serve as a case study to illustrate the formation of an 'orientally-inspired' market of alternative books in Brazil during the 1970s and '80s. The reason we chose this particular book is threefold. Firstly, *From Eden to Aquarius* was amongst the earliest titles published by Ground, a leading Brazilian publisher dedicated to promoting alternative therapies, spiritualities, and lifestyles associated with 'oriental culture'. Secondly, the book represents the expanding influence of American counterculture and the New Age in shaping new perspectives on health and illness within the middle and upper-class echelons of Brazilian society. Thirdly, *From Eden to Aquarius* demonstrates a creative interpretation of traditional East Asian ideas about the body through the lens of modern science, showcasing the broader New Age effort to appropriate 'oriental' concepts and practices and translate them for Western audiences (Hanegraaff 1996; Borup and Fibiger 2017).

Inspired by Sita Reddy's (2004) study of 'New Age Ayurveda' in the United States – where the author investigates how Ayurveda was portrayed and advertised in the American New Age market – our chapter delves into the surge of alternative medical literature in the 1970s and '80s in Brazil. We will pay particular attention to how this booming bookselling market played a pivotal role in popularising lifestyles, therapies, and concepts of the body that were purportedly derived from a distant Far East. More specifically, we will examine popular Brazilian representations of 'oriental medicine' and how these have transformed local perceptions of alternative health from the 1970s. Our purpose is not to criticise the widespread use of the term 'oriental medicine' – or 'medicina oriental' in Portuguese – but rather comprehend how, why, and what type of 'Orient' was being constructed and invoked in New Age publications aimed at spreading alternative views of body, health, and illness (cf. Chapter 4).

Since the 1960s, the Brazilian therapeutic landscape has featured a variety of ever-expanding therapies associated with 'oriental medicine' – including acupuncture, martial arts, *daoyin*, *reiki*, yoga, and macrobiotics – with numerous actors and organisations involved in their promotion and consumption. Elsewhere, we have analysed the popularisation of Chinese medicine in Brazil, arguing that whilst therapies such as acupuncture and martial arts had been introduced into the country through Japanese immigration around the mid-20th century, these practices garnered unprecedented attention in the 1970s thanks primarily to individuals associated with the emerging New Age world (Sigolo and Junqueira 2021). This chapter will build on our previous research by exploring the representations of oriental medicine through the new conceptions of the body presented in *From Eden to Aquarius*. How to cultivate health? What causes illness? How to heal oneself and others? We will conclude by arguing that the Orient depicted in *From Eden to Aquarius* – which, we should remember, is merely an example of a much vaster corpus of texts – tends to reveal much more about the concerns and self-representations of Americans and Brazilians around the 1970s rather than providing a comprehensive picture of East Asian cultures. In other words, the Orient introduced in alternative medical literature largely symbolises 'the other as the inversion of the self' (Burke 2001, 139).

Microcosm-Macrocosm

Biomedicine has been a major proponent of the mechanical concept of the body that has come to dominate modern societies. Based on Andreas Vesalius (1514–1564) and his anatomical studies in the 16th century, the body turned into an object that could be fragmented and separated from the cosmos (Le Breton 2013, 72). This view would develop over the next century with René Descartes (1596–1650) and the 'body-as-machine' metaphor, a lifeless body made of constituent parts that present themselves to the scientist's dispassionate gaze. Pushing imagination and the subjective away, the rise of such a 'sense of reason' championed mathematics as the only legitimate instrument for explaining nature and bodily experiences (Le Breton 2013, 91). The biochemical interpretation of the human frame thus rejected the prevailing Hippocratic principle that attributed health and disease to the balance of the humours. Like Hippocratic medicine, the healing traditions of China and India similarly embraced the perspective that the human body is a microcosm, mirroring and responding dynamically to changes in its environment (macrocosm) (Kuriyama 2002; Detrez 2002) – a perspective that would be often invoked by New Agers during the second half of the 20th century.

As the concept of the body as a machine gained increasing momentum in the European medical landscape (Detrez 2022, 45–47) from the 17th century onwards, spiritual or ostensibly subjective elements were sidelined as irrelevant. Concurrently, the focus on cadaveric studies accentuated the disease rather than the patient. As such, biomedicine gradually moved away from questions about what life is or what makes a body alive – questions that remained nevertheless central to the vitalist ethos underpinning various alternative healing modalities (Porter 2002). Meanwhile, the burgeoning interest in alternative medicine during the 1970s was also fuelled by a decline in the quality of the doctor-patient relationship (Queiroz 2003) – a concern already expressed in the 19th century's global rise of mind-cure and holistic movements (Harrington 2008; Whorton 2002). This decline was characterised by medical practitioners' reluctance to acknowledge their patients' own interpretations of their bodily functions and their relationships with other entities, both human and nonhuman.

According to Bernard Andrieu (1999, 10–11), the 1970s marked the heyday for the 'promotion of the individual body', wherein individuals were encouraged to appropriate medical knowledge in order to become doctors of their own bodies. The rise of alternative medicine was a direct consequence of this new paradigm: rather than dichotomising body, mind, and spirit, the 'doctor-of-my-own-body' endeavours to embody both physician and patient, symptom and cure, subject and object. Health restoration transcended the mere negation of illness, prioritising a holistic sense of well-being and personal cultivation (Moulin 2006). Within the dynamics of the doctor-patient relationship, alternative medicine purportedly focuses more on the individual experiencing illness than on the illness itself, founding its approach on the patient's narrative of suffering, thereby empowering them to become the protagonists in their healing journey (Le Breton 2013, 143).

Whether through a therapist or the individual itself, the 'doctor-of-my-own-body' often turns to 'natural remedies' existing in the potentiality of their own body as a means for self-healing (Andrieu 1999; Vrignon 2017). These intertwined facets are represented in the work we will examine below.

The term 'alternative medicine', however, is not so easily defined. According to Andrade (2006, 25–45), the WHO does not draw a clear line between 'complementary medicine' and 'alternative medicine', for example. Andrade argues that the term may imply a political position in favour of a less materialistic worldview, a movement closer to nature and free from the mechanistic conventions associated with biomedicine. Similarly, it could indicate opposition to biomedicine, as enshrined in the contesting universe of the 1960s and '70s (Barros 2008, 134). Critiquing the term 'parallel medicine' proposed by François Laplantine and Paul-Louis Rabeyron (1987), Olivier Faure and Hervé Guillemain (2018) contend that 'alternative' or 'heterodox' medical systems such as homoeopathy, mesmerism, and acupuncture were in fact integral to the sociopolitical milieu wherein they flourished. Far from walking parallel to biomedicine, such 'heterodox systems' were closely intertwined within the same healthcare universe and must thus be understood in their interconnections. Likewise, Roberta Bivins (2011) proposes viewing heterodox medicine as 'cross-cultural medicine', highlighting the transnational circulation of therapeutic practices as well as their local appropriations around the globe. Bivins astutely notes that such transcultural exchanges were not confined to the 1960s and '70s but became increasingly pronounced with the surge of globalisation in the latter half of the 20th century.

The United States, the Counterculture, and the Rise of New Age in Brazil

To fully understand the influence of American alternative medical literature on the emergence of the New Age movement in Brazil, it is essential to consider the complex interactions between the United States and Brazil over the past century. It is safe to say that no other country has had such a profound and lasting impact on the course of Brazil's economy, politics, and culture as the United States. The second half of the 20th century witnessed a series of military coups in Latin America, directly orchestrated or backed by the US government (Serrano 2010; Coggiola 2001; Rosenmann 2013). Given Brazil's strategic significance in the Latin American region and its wealth of natural resources, the United States intensified its engagement with the country, especially during the Cold War era (Braga 2002). In the 1960s, the American government aimed to secure control over the Brazilian political sphere, fearing the spread of communism, especially after the triumph of the Cuban Revolution in 1959, which served as an inspiration for local peasant leagues, students, labour, and leftist intellectual movements critical of American imperialism. The resignation of conservative President Jânio Quadros in 1961, followed by the ascension of the leftist João Goulart from the Brazilian Labour Party (PTB) to the presidency, alarmed the Brazilian military and the conservative and right-wing elites. In response, the US government did not hesitate to foster and support the military coup of 1 April 1964, initiating a dictatorship that would persist until 1985 (Green 2009, 25–26).

The United States' endeavour to control Latin America also fuelled the dissemination of the 'American way of life' through vigorous soft power initiatives. Cultural production – especially Hollywood cinema – and the introduction of American goods in the Brazilian market stimulated the insertion of values such as consumption, capital accumulation, and the ethos of the 'self-made man' as quintessential components of a developed nation (Ouriveis 2013). However, an unintended consequence of American cultural hegemony was the global exportation of counterculture, which found a receptive environment in Brazil. As Christopher Dunn has observed, in the mid-1960s, slogans like 'Make love, not war' served as a dual protest against both the atrocities of the Vietnam War and the oppression by the Brazilian authoritarian regime. Thus, while counterculture represented a transnational movement, it resonated particularly well within Brazil as a response to specific local conflicts and societal crises (Dunn 2016, 13–26).

Despite escalating political suppression, the late 1960s in Brazil were characterised by a tremendous cultural vibrancy. Movements challenging the ultranationalistic, puritanical, and antidemocratic values endorsed by the military dictatorship and its adherents surged across the nation. In this milieu, non-Christian spirituality and therapies, seen as alternatives to biomedicine and its mechanistic view of the body, health, and disease, emerged as potent means of subverting the Brazilian conservative establishment from within.

As a response to the disillusionment with a world marked by Cold War divisions, the looming threat of nuclear annihilation and the rampant capitalist consumerism emblematic of the American way of life, the counterculture movement emerged as a transnational phenomenon (Roszak 1969; Martins 2011; cf. Chapter 4). It presented itself as an antidote to the 'modernity malaise', advocating for the revitalisation of subjectivity through avenues such as psychedelic art, the consumption of psychoactive substances, and the pursuit of mystical experiences, with indigenous and Eastern religions playing a crucial role as sources of inspiration (Monneyron and Xiberras 2008). Counterculture adherents also redefined the relationship between humans and the nonhuman world (or 'nature), leading to a heightened awareness of environmental degradation. This shift precipitated the rise of other global movements like environmentalism and ecologism, alongside a resurgence of interest in 'natural diets' and 'holistic therapies' across Europe, the United States, and South America (Lowenberg 1989; Sigolo 2020). Additionally, this critical stance towards Western modernity catalysed the establishment of various intentional communities, including ecovillages and hippie communes, and fostered alternative networks within urban settings, often anchored by bookstores and publishing houses (Tavares 1985).

The 1960s marked a turning point in the history of alternative medicine. Drawing on lasting objections to orthodox medicine (Vrignon 2017), the counterculture's rebellion against authority and technocracy revived a search for alternative methods of healing based on subjectivity and self-care (Lowenberg 1989; Whorton 2002). At the individual level, adherents eschewed the reduction of the body into compartmentalised medical specialities, while on a broader scale, they envisioned humans as integral to their ecosystems (Queiroz 2003). Illness was perceived as the result of a dystopian industrial society that debilitated our bodies through estrangement from nature. Conversely, health was equated with a 'return to nature', embracing 'natural lifestyles' such as vegetarianism, physical exercise, sunbathing and a wholesome diet (Vrignon 2017). These alternative perspectives on healthcare would be instrumental in shaping the subsequent New Age movement. As Wouter J. Hanegraaff (1996) observed, the New Age resists easy categorisation, incorporating a range of beliefs and practices originating from 19th-century esoteric traditions, rejuvenated by the (predominantly) American countercultural experience.

Whereas acupuncture and martial arts had been known in Brazil for some time – mainly due to the efforts of Japanese immigrants – it was not until the late 1960s that these therapies began to garner broader interest, especially amongst the middle and upper classes (Sigolo and Junqueira 2021). The New Age's pursuit of physical, mental, and spiritual health was embraced by individuals and groups united by the conviction that health transcends the mere absence of disease, encompassing instead the achievement of overall well-being and a sense of wholeness. Although not every practitioner of alternative medicine identifies with or should be categorised as 'new agers' (Toniol 2016; Sigolo 2019), the influence of the New Age movement in enhancing the visibility of alternative therapies within the Brazilian public domain is unmistakable (cf. Chapter 8). Moreover, the movement has introduced an even broader array of heterodox cosmologies and healing practices, as will be detailed in the analysis to follow.

Publishing 'New Age' in Brazil

From Eden to Aquarius is situated within a period marked by the flourishing of the Brazilian editorial market. The ratio of books per inhabitant increased notably during the 1960s and '70s (Reimão 1996, 58), and with a growing number of university students, the period experienced a steady decline in illiteracy, broadening the base of potential readers (Hallewell 2017, 56, 797). Meanwhile, the trade of books received a significant boost in the late 1970s following the promulgation of a law that permitted more diverse distribution. Beyond traditional bookshops, books began to be sold in pharmacies, petrol stations, stationery stores, and via mail order, enhancing their accessibility and availability to the public (Reimão 1996, 62).

Founded in 1972, Ground, the publisher in charge of the Portuguese translation of *From Eden to Aquarius*, was part of a specific editorial universe built throughout the 20th century. Alongside other publishers such as O Pensamento and Cultrix[2] – established in 1907 and 1955, respectively – Ground catered for a readership avid for self-knowledge, spirituality, and the occult sciences, including 'oriental wisdom' (Hallewell 2017, 370–71). By the 1970s, the magazine *Planeta* – originated from the French magazine *Planète* – as well as the Palas Athena Association, the Horus and the Zipak bookstores also became important venues associated with this flourishing alternative readership (Cosson 2007, 31). José Magnani (1999) observes that publications promoting alternative lifestyles pertained to a dynamically evolving network, with members sharing beliefs and concerns that were seldom rooted in formal institutions but primarily in voluntary engagements.

The inception of Ground was the result of a collaboration between Marcio de Castro and Juracy Cançado in 1968, a partnership formed as both sought refuge in the United States to evade the repression of the Brazilian civil-military dictatorship. In an interview published in 1978, Castro and Cançado explained the purpose of establishing Ground: 'We can say

2 A loose English translation for O Pensamento would be 'The Thought'. Cultrix, on the other hand, is a Latin word meaning 'she who labours at or cares for a thing', a 'female inhabitant', or 'female worshipper' (Lewis and Short 1962, 488).

that we would like to publish books of a practical nature, to modify life habits, customs, diet, introducing new philosophical currents, if possible to improve humanity. [...] In short, Ground is concerned with presenting alternatives for survival in today's world' (Schild 1978). Castro and Cançado also operated a bookstore in a shopping centre in Rio de Janeiro – one of Brazil's largest and most influential cultural hubs. By the early 1980s, this bookstore boasted a collection of over 500 titles from various Brazilian publishers, covering a range of topics such as acupuncture, *daoyin*, massage, macrobiotics, natural diet, medicinal plants, energy healing, occult sciences, and spirituality – many of which were categorised as 'medicina oriental' (oriental medicine).[3] Ground's title catalogues and in-book advertisements reflect the plural and dynamic New Age market thriving in Brazil around the late 1970s. Notably, the back cover of the 1977 Portuguese edition of *From Eden to Aquarius* highlights Ground's commitment to publishing the 'finest works in Portuguese on subjects like medicine and natural diet, yoga, meditation, orientalism, astrology, education, counterculture, philosophy, religion, ecology, natural farming, martial arts, psychology, parapsychology, fantastic realism, scientific fiction and the occult sciences' (Brodsky 1977).

Indeed, Ground edited some of the most successful manuals of alternative lifestyles of the time, spearheading the category 'oriental medicine' in Brazil. Its debut publication, *Do-In: Técnica oriental de auto-massagem* (Do-In: Oriental Technique for Self-Massage)[4], first released in 1973, became a real bestseller: by 2006, it had already reached its 36th edition, with the first edition alone selling over 12,000 copies. Authored by a renowned proponent of macrobiotics and other 'oriental healing sciences', the Belgian-American Jacques de Langre (1925–1993), the manual's remarkable success prompted its translator, Ground's cofounder Juracy Cançado, to edit his own manual on the subject, *Do-In: Livro dos primeiros socorros* (Do-In: A First Aid Book), first published in 1976. Combining a variety of pressing, kneading, tapping, and stretching techniques of self-massage, Cançado's manual was heralded in newspapers and courses as an 'essential practical manual' whose knowledge offered a 'natural alternative to the aspirin, analgesics and other intoxicating drugs' ('Bases da medicina' 1978). By 2017, the manual was already enjoying its 50th edition.[5] A prolific author, Cançado remains

3 For an overview of Ground's vast catalogue, visit https://www.ground.com.br/historico.php.

4 This manual is still in print. Its alternative title is *Do-In: Guia prático de auto massagem* (Do-In: A Practice Guide for Self-Massage).

5 From 2017, it has been published under the title *Do-In: A milenar arte chinesa de acupuntura com os dedos* (Do-In: The Ancient Chinese Art of Acupuncture with Fingers).

a well-known name amongst practitioners of Chinese medicine in Brazil, being equally influential in promoting oriental medicine in Portugal and Spanish-speaking countries in Latin America (Sigolo and Junqueira 2021).

Apart from de Langre and Cançado's *Do-In*, other acclaimed manuals and resources published by Ground during the 1970s included *Mapa dos meridianos chineses* (Map of Chinese Meridians; 1975), *Liberdade através da alimentação* (Freedom through Food; 1977), *Prontuário de svásthya yoga* (Svasthya Yoga Handbook; 1977), *From Eden to Aquarius* (1977), and *Sugar Blues* (1978). These works, whether translated from American bestsellers or inspired by them, collectively sold well over 100,000 copies within six years of Ground's establishment, with each title seeing at least five editions within a decade of their initial release ('Os novos' 1979; Schild 1978).

Greg Brodsky and His From Eden to Aquarius

From Eden to Aquarius: The Book of Natural Healing was originally published in New York in 1974, making its way into Brazil in 1977, where it was rendered as *Do Jardim do Éden à Era de Aquarius: O Livro da Cura Natural* (henceforth: *Do Jardim do Éden*).[6] Authored by Greg Brodsky and illustrated by Maureen O'Brien, the manual offers a vast repertoire of alternative methods for self-care. In a review from an excited reader of *Correio Braziliense* – one of the oldest and most influential newspapers in Brazil at the time – alongside acupuncture and Reich bioenergetics, the manual also 'addresses other precious subjects, such as various methods of oriental and occidental massage, hydrotherapy, the therapeutic use of meditation, yoga and breathing exercises; the medicinal properties of foods and herbs, the oriental arts of Aikido and T'ai Chi Chuan; fasting and seasonal diet appropriate to the needs of each organism' (Borja 1978). Readers also praised Brodsky's insightful perspectives on the body and its role in humanity's 'physical and spiritual evolution' as 'profound', 'mind-blowing', and 'fascinating' (Borja 1978; Pires 1978).

Born on the East Coast of the United States in 1942, Brodsky relocated to New York City at the age of 18. During an interview with the authors in January 2023, Brodsky recounted that he first encountered his spiritual mentor and began studying *aikido*, *taiji*, and *karate* in New York. Indeed, his journey into the healing arts commenced following a shoulder injury

6 When referring to the Portuguese edition, we will use the Portuguese title *Do Jardim do Éden*. As for the English edition, we will adopt *From Eden to Aquarius*.

sustained during aikido practice.[7] Brodsky's short biography in *Do Jardim do Éden* introduces him as a practitioner of acupuncture, *daoyin*, medicinal herbs, *aikido*, *taiji*, hata, and kundalini yoga. His career spanned roles as a teacher in various American and European universities and as an instructor of natural healing in a community in Big Indian, New York (Brodsky 1977, 7). Together with his wife, Brodsky established the Santa Cruz T'ai Chi Chuan in Santa Cruz, California, in the early 1980s. This group remains active, focusing on the therapeutic aspects of Chinese and Japanese martial arts.

Brodsky's engagement with Chinese and Japanese cultures, along with alternative therapies, has been well documented through newspaper advertisements, articles in *T'ai Chi Magazine*, and the Santa Cruz T'ai Chi Chuan official website. It is said that Brodsky started to learn a variety of martial arts and healing techniques from Chinese and Japanese martial artists who moved to the United States in the 1960s and '70s, such as Cheng Man-ch'ing (1902–1975), William C.C. Chen (1933–), and Mikoto Masahilo Nakazono (1918–1994) ('Lineage' n.d.). This trend of learning from Chinese and Japanese immigrants was prevalent amongst self-care book authors not only in the US but also in Europe and Brazil during that period (Costa 2016; Sigolo and Junqueira 2021; cf. Chapters 2 and 4).

Following its first publication in the United States, *From Eden to Aquarius* would also be printed in the United Kingdom, Canada, and Spain, from where it spread to various Spanish-speaking countries in Latin America. The manual's wide circulation neatly illustrates the booming transnational market of self-care books catalysed by the counterculture and New Age movements. Indeed, between the 1960s and '80s, an unprecedented number of titles on alternative forms of healing would be translated into Portuguese from English, French, and Spanish, feeding Brazilians' growing interest in 'oriental wisdom' and thereby giving rise to the earliest Brazilian groups devoted to the study and practice of 'oriental medicine' and 'oriental spirituality' (Sigolo and Junqueira 2021; Magnani 1999; Nascimento, 2006). More broadly, this trend underscores the significant role that transnational cultural exchanges played in shaping Brazil's engagement with alternative medical practices and spiritualities.

By 1994, *Do Jardim do Éden* had reached its sixth edition, with sales surpassing 10,000 copies as early as 1978. It was promoted in the prominent daily *Jornal do Brasil* as 'a mind-blowing book that is stirring up all those who are beginners in the path of oriental healing methods and natural diet' ('Misticismo' 1979). The preface of *Do Jardim do Éden* and reviews published in

7 Interview conducted on 8 January 2023.

general-interest newspapers lauded Brodsky's skilful fusion of the 'traditional therapies of the ancients' and 'avant-garde medical research' (Borja 1978). In the words of Ground's editors, *Do Jardim do Éden* represented the 'perfect integration of modern technology and empirical knowledge derived from the traditional culture of the ancients', making the book 'particularly valuable to the challenges of current times' (Brodsky 1977, 8). In an early catalogue, Ground hailed it as 'a modern treatise of traditional medicine – certainly the most comprehensive book, in Portuguese language, dedicated to the methods of natural and spiritual healing', and advertised *Do Jardim do Éden* in its series of manuals heralding the 'dawn of a new consciousness' arising in Brazil and beyond (Catálogo 1978, 1).

The book's popularity was also expressed in Brazilian popular culture. In 1981, the title *Do Jardim do Éden à Era de Aquarius* became the parade theme of Unidos da Vila Isabel, one of the most traditional samba schools of Rio de Janeiro. Bringing together 'dragons, Buddhas, pharaohs', and other 'oriental elements', a reporter explained, the parade aimed to 'search for humanity's identity within time, as manifested in Brazil' (Paz 1981). In short, whilst rooted in 'traditional oriental wisdom', *Do Jardim do Éden* was portrayed as firmly supported by the latest discoveries in Western science, emblematic of the 'new cultural renaissance' of the 1970s (Brodsky 1977, 7).

From Eden to Aquarius: A Plurality of Bodies

Do Jardim do Éden presents a multifaceted representation of the body that intertwines with its conceptions of health, illness, and well-being. From its very cover, we already learn that there is a body to be transformed. Unlike the American and Spanish editions, the cover of the Portuguese translation features the central part of the painting *Unio Mystica*, by the Dutch surrealist painter Johfra Bosschart (1919–1998). The artwork portrays the divine transformation of a human being and her ascent to a higher plane of existence (Figure 5.1). This imagery aligns with the book's broader narrative, suggesting that the human body is not static but a site of profound spiritual and physical metamorphosis.

The book's title, extended in the Portuguese edition to *Do Jardim do Éden à Era de Aquarius: O Livro da Cura Natural*, situates the body within a vast temporal and spatial continuum. This continuum stretches from the Christian mythical past of the Garden of Eden to the prophesied future of the Age of Aquarius, implying that individuals in the contemporary era – more specifically the 1970s – are charged with the task of self-transformation.

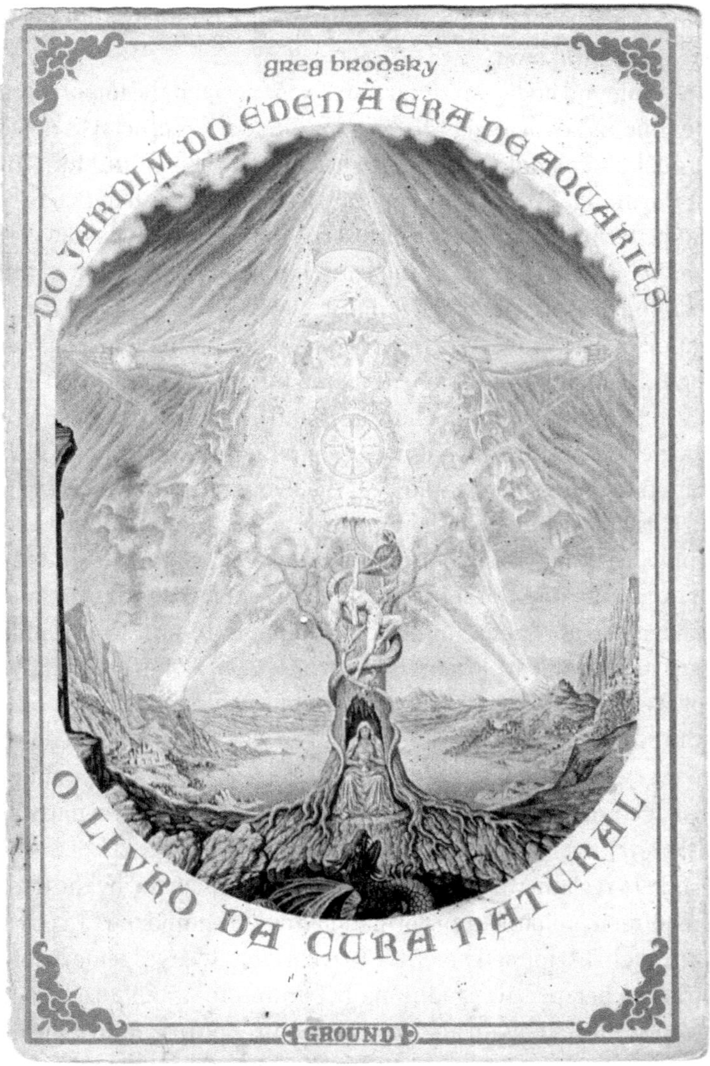

Figure 5.1. Front cover of *Do Jardim do Éden* (1977). Reproduced with the kind permission of Ground.

This transformative process is depicted as both a personal and collective journey towards achieving a state of holistic well-being, symbolised by the alchemical body. The incorporation of Leonardo da Vinci's *Vitruvian Man* right before the manual's introductory section further emphasises the ideal of the human body in balance and harmony, resonating with the manual's thematic focus on the integration of subjective bodily experience (cf. Chapters 2 and 3). The *Vitruvian Man*, representing the principles of proportion and symmetry, serves as an iconographic reminder of the pursuit of a 'perfect' body – perfect not just in physical health but in its alignment with cosmic and natural laws.

To grasp the profound bodily-spiritual transformation and the importance of 'natural healing' as advocated in *Do Jardim do Éden*, it is crucial to delve into Greg Brodsky's cosmological perspective on the body and human evolution. In the manual's opening chapter, 'The Garden of Eden', Brodsky outlines what he terms the 'growth cycles of the human race'. These cycles were projected to peak in the Age of Aquarius, marked by the advent of the 'Third Civilisation' in 2011. According to this view, the 'First Civilisation' reached its apex of spiritual evolution in Eden, where it lived for 100,000 years. During this era, humans, unencumbered by the constraints of time and space, lived in a state of perfect harmony and unity with the cosmos.

This idyllic period of spiritual abundance gradually gave way to a new cycle dominated by materialism, marking the evolution into the 'Second Civilisation'. This era is characterised by significant strides in science and technology, but also by an increase in conflicts and violence and a growing rift between humanity and the spiritual domain. The transition from one civilisational cycle to another, as Brodsky articulates, requires conscious intent. It suggests that the evolution toward the 'Age of Aquarius' and the emergence of the 'Third Civilisation' is contingent upon a deliberate choice by humanity to embrace a more spiritually attuned way of living. This choice involves moving beyond the materialistic predilections of the current era to re-establish a connection with a lost spiritual essence and the natural world (Brodsky 1977, 17).

The aspiration to reclaim the paradisiacal state once inhabited by the First Civilisation requires a profound transformation from the mundane to a pure, divine body through disciplined practice. This concept diverges remarkably from the Christian perspective traditionally familiar to Brazilians, where the body is seen as marred by sin and thereby requires purification (Detrez 2002, 31). Brodsky's approach instead posits the material body as a vessel for achieving spiritual enlightenment, offering a foundation for restoring the unity once experienced in Eden. This process of 'returning to the divine within ourselves' aligns well with the religiosity articulated by the New Age movement and, whether consciously or not, seems to resonate with the Daoist pursuit of self-cultivation and immortality.

Moving away from a patriarchal, distant, monotheistic god, the New Age hailed the divine as a 'perfect self'. This internal divine essence can be unveiled through the transformation of the material body, suggesting a path to spiritual awakening that is both personal and internal (D'Andrea 2018). Such a view is reaffirmed in a reader's annotation on a blank page of the first Portuguese edition: 'God is not the well-known Western God who is conceived of as an arbitrary God and who fights demons that cannot be vanquished'.

Brodsky delineates the metamorphosis of the body as based on five distinct states of being or levels of consciousness: U-O-A-E-I (1977, 17–27). Humans are born in the state of U-level, which includes basic needs. The development of memory, experience, and intellect corresponds to the O-level. The emergence of the A-state signifies the nurturing of spirituality, enhancing an individual's awareness of the divine presence within. If the person advances, they attain the E-level, whereby they understand the cycles of life and the importance of searching for order and harmony. According to Brodsky, this state enables one to lead a life of sanity and health, transcending competition, philosophy, or religion – a level attained by historical figures such as Jesus, Gautama Buddha, Moses, and Mohammed (1977, 24–25). The final phase, the I-level, represents the realisation of the divine and grants ultimate access to the Age of Aquarius.

At the core of Brodsky's theory of human evolution, as introduced in *Do Jardim do Éden*, is the profound influence of his master, Nakazono Mutsurō 中園睦郎 (1918–1994), a 'teacher of natural medicine [...] [who] brought me the secrets of an ancient and nearly forgotten philosophy which explained everything from the nature of the DNA molecule to the evolutionary patterns of life itself' (Brodsky 1977, 12). Later known as Mikoto Masahilo Nakazono, Nakazono was a healer and martial artist who moved from Japan to France in 1961 and then to Santa Fé, New Mexico, in 1972, where he established the Kototama Institute and lived until his death.

In an interview with the authors in January 2023, Brodsky reminisces about meeting 'Nakazono-sensei' in Paris in 1965 and how he became his student. 'Mr. Nakazono was very kind to me. He believed that a coming Age of Enlightenment would begin in the U.S. when enough people would have attained the consciousness of the fifth level according to the Kotodama teachings. He came to the U.S. and taught me there'.[8] Nakazono is introduced in Brodsky's book as a master of *kendo, judo, karate, aikido*, acupuncture, macrobiotics, and the Kototama Principle. Kototama or Kotodama 言霊 – variously translated as 'the power of words' or 'the spirit of language' – is an old Japanese concept that explains that 'sounds placed in a certain order each carry a particular quality of energy' (Vergonjeanne 2012, 3). Kotodama is considered the spiritual foundation of *aikido* (Kaku, Machin, and Nakamura 2000), whose founder, Ueshiba Morihei 植芝盛平 (1883–1969),

8 Interview conducted on 8 January 2023.

was Nakazono's master. Nakazono's emphasis on Kotodama goes beyond its martial applications, viewing it as a pathway to physical, mental, and spiritual realisation – 'the final truth of human life and the universe as one' (Nakazono 1984, 4). Borrowed from Nakazono, the U-O-A-E-I vowel system introduced in *Do Jardim do Éden* comprise the five stages of human development through the vibration of sounds.

In Brodsky's framework, health is achieved through the realisation of the divine within ourselves, a process that paves the way to entering the Age of Aquarius, facilitated by our transformed bodies. This transformation emphasises the interplay between the visible/physical body and an 'invisible body' imbued with energy (cf. Chapter 1). Here, the mind emerges as a critical connection agent, acting as the conduit through which the physical body is transformed by the energy body (Brodsky 1977, 34). To explain the behaviour of the energy body, Brodsky resorts to 'oriental' concepts, notably from Indian tantra and Chinese and Japanese medicine. He delves into the anatomy of the chakras or 'energy centres', illustrating how energy circulates throughout the body:

> The entire body works as a spiritual and physical whole. [...] All the chakras will eventually be opened if you can allow your energy to flow through them and awaken them. It is a simple process to begin to 'work' with them, but it requires considerable sensitivity and perseverance. Using the chakras also helps absorb life energy – *Ki*, to use the Japanese term (*ch'i* in Chinese, *Prana* in India; the Western term is 'bioenergy'. (Brodsky 1977, 58; on *qi*/*ki*, cf. Chapters 1, 2, and 3)

A map of this energy body appears prominently in the richly illustrated chapter on acupuncture. There, Brodsky explains that inserting needles into the physical body and stimulating them can activate energy flow within the meridians, thereby restoring the unity between the material and spiritual worlds within us. Whether from the Indian or Chinese point of view, this invisible anatomy cannot be properly appreciated without understanding the flow of energy throughout the physical body. Brodsky then bridges spiritualist notions with scientific concepts, drawing parallels between 'Western science' and 'Eastern metaphysics'. He posits energy as the foundational element of the material world, manifesting within our bodies as 'energy spirals', analogous to the DNA molecule (Brodsky 1977, 33–38). Further, Brodsky compares the spiral of the DNA to the Japanese deities Izanagi and Izanami, depicted in his manual as a *yin-yang* symbol intertwined as a vortex (Brodsky 1977, 66–69).

Do Jardim do Éden equips readers with a diverse array of methods to unlock the mind's latent capabilities, from meditation, hypnosis, and Kotodama-inspired techniques to breathing exercises, martial arts, and massages. These techniques are unified by their potential to unblock and enhance the flow of stagnant energy, thereby fostering health and well-being. The physical body is portrayed as both a conduit for energy flow and a barrier to it. To address this, Brodsky extensively details, both textually and visually, various yoga poses and *taiji* and *aikido* movements (1977, 159–67). Moving bodies exhibit the possibilities of energy mobilisation – with the caveat that these are not 'ordinary physical exercises'. Interestingly, the only visibly 'Western' therapy in Brodsky's manual is Swedish massage, whose human bodies are illustrated at rest, receiving massage stimuli from another person (Brodsky 1977, 179). The reader is warned that this technique should nonetheless be done by someone capable of holding their 'inner self' (Brodsky 1977, 174) – a reminder that whatever the therapy adopted, it acts not only on the physical but primarily on the energetic body.

The focus on physical exercises in *Do Jardim do Éden* also underscores the importance of maintaining good health by eliminating toxins from the body through specific physical movements. The notion of detoxification as a way to restore health is given particular attention in the chapter 'Food as Natural Medicine' – one of the highlights in Brazilian reviews of the manual. Here, Brodsky states that the search for 'complete realisation' must be underpinned by daily care with what nourishes the body, namely 'good food, whole food, live food. [...] When given live energy to use as fuel, [the body] can carry out all its functions with a minimum of waste while providing you with a maximum of energy' (Brodsky 1977, 90). The author devotes several pages to the properties of various foods, explained in terms of both *ch'i* [qi] and vitamins – another example of what the Brazilian editors declared to be 'the perfect integration' of traditional (Orient) and modern (Occident) knowledge. The ultimate goal, according to Brodsky, is to select foods that support the body's 'constant renewal' by enhancing the dynamic flow of energy while simultaneously purging toxins.

Final Remarks: The Age of Aquarius as the Resumption of Eden

Brodsky's view of body care transcends the idea of health as the mere absence of disease. Instead, health is attained by transforming the physical body into a divine body through a variety of alternative methods of health promotion, such as natural diet, acupuncture, yoga, *aikido*, *taiji*, and meditation.

This metamorphosis does not involve the creation of a new body; rather, it entails the return to a primordial state – by regaining the essence of the Garden of Eden, the individual enters the Age of Aquarius. Interestingly, while the concepts of the Garden of Eden and the Age of Aquarius originate from Western traditions, their realisation is facilitated through 'oriental' practices. The pursuit of a primordial paradise, a notion often associated with Christian theology, is sought through the adoption of Japanese and Chinese spiritual and medical frameworks.

The fusion of 'East-West' and 'traditional-modern' also sought to reconcile religion and science, allowing the author to reinterpret organic structures such as the DNA molecule in terms of Eastern mythologies. Indeed, the Brazilian editors of *Do Jardim do Éden* hailed this manual as illustrative of the 'new paradigm in healthcare' that was awakening throughout the Western world during the 1970s. This paradigm, though contemporary in its manifestation, found potent inspiration from imagined traditional and Eastern cultures, noted for their 'greater intimacy with nature and with our own bodies':

> Ancestral Natural Medicine is now abandoning its marginal condition to be gradually assimilated by sophisticated modern therapies – digital acupuncture, the oriental methods of massage which are now integrated into the current techniques of relaxing and bioenergy, the oriental thought merging with the elements of bold forms of psychotherapy – all these are but a few signs of this tendency. This encounter between the ancient and the new, the Orient and the Occident, the 'esoteric' and the 'scientific' constitute the foundation of integral medicine: the Medicine of Man. (Brodsky 1977, 8–9)

The concept of 'energy' was instrumental in Brodsky's view of the human body, establishing a powerful link between what the Brazilian editors of his manual called the 'ancient and the new, the Orient and the Occident'. Whilst energy has become a shared vocabulary amongst most alternative medical systems today (Oschman 1996; Stein 2021), this relatively modern Western concept is not as universal as it might initially appear (cf. Chapter 1). Homoeopathy, Chinese medicine, and Ayurveda, for instance, all underline the nonmaterial elements of the body as key to understanding health and disease (Wunenburguer 2008; Stanley-Baker 2022). However, in efforts to popularise these 'alternative' medical systems, native terms such as vital force, *qi*, and prana often end up being used interchangeably with the loosely defined 'energy'. This process of cultural translation aims to assimilate into and gain legitimacy from scientific discourse, particularly quantum physics, which has become a prominent trend in New Age literature (Burwell 2013; Hanegraaff 1996, 62–63, 398, 407, 421–23, 517).

The circulation of a book like *From Eden to Aquarius* in Brazil became possible due to the rising awareness of health as an individual responsibility as well as a growing interest in self-care and alternative healing from the late 1960s – primarily driven by the spread of counterculture and New Age amongst the Brazilian middle and upper classes. The concept of the individual as a 'doctor-of-oneself' (Andrieu 2001) was fuelled by what Anthony Giddens (1991) calls 'reflexivity', a characteristic of the second half of the 20th century. Reflexivity is characterised by an attitude wherein institutional certainties are replaced by personal and fragmented choices, exemplified by the 'reflexive project of the Self'. In this new paradigm, people tend to eschew rigid, predefined behavioural models in favour of constructing their lifestyles around personal choices. These choices are informed by both local and global factors, with individuals assessing the potential risks associated with their decisions. In this regard, individuals are viewed not as passive recipients of social structures but as active participants, influencing these structures through their personal actions and decisions. This approach underscores the notion that our individual choices heavily affect our physical and mental well-being, positioning the management of these choices as a key objective in our lives.

The Brazilian 'doctor-of-oneself' could count on a plethora of publications offering guidance on how to achieve a healthy state through natural methods. Their many suggestions were greatly influenced by the United States, where the New Age movement was born. As a result, the 'oriental philosophies' underpinning many alternative therapies in Brazil can be seen as Brazilian appropriations of American reinterpretations of what 'oriental wisdom' is or ought to be. Indeed, these therapies are typical examples of 'cross-cultural medicine' (Bivins 2011; 2007), an appropriation process that, in our case, must take into account both the American and Brazilian historical contexts. *Do Jardim do Éden* was but one within a wave of lay-oriented manuals published from the 1970s dedicated to the then nascent field of 'oriental medicine'. Over time, such publications fostered the creation of dedicated spaces for oriental therapies and reflected their growing popularity amongst the Brazilian middle and upper classes. This movement culminated with the insertion of many such therapies – including Chinese medicine, Ayurveda, and *reiki* – in Brazil's Public Health System (Sistema Único de Saúde, or SUS) in 2006, thereby extending their accessibility to a wider spectrum of Brazilian society.

How, then, was the term 'Orient' invoked in New Age Brazilian publications of alternative medicine between the late 1960s and early '80s?

Examining the process that led Brazilian biomedical doctors to study Chinese medicine in the 1980s and '90s, Maria Nogueira and Kenneth de Camargo Jr. (2007) observed that the Orient sought by these professionals was not limited to a specific geographic location but rather comprised an 'imagined world' roughly associated with China, Japan, and India. Their view of the Orient fed the stereotypes of the Western imagination, which found, in this imagined space, the opposition of what it considers itself to be – a process famously defined by Edward Said (1979) as 'Orientalism' (cf. Chapters 6 and 8). In this context, the Brazilian interpretation of the Orient aligns closely with the perceptions held by American and European New Agers of their time. Publications by Ground, for example, have often depicted the Orient as a repository of tradition, natural wisdom, mysticism, exoticism, and femininity – characteristics lauded as being of equal, if not greater, value compared to Western virtues and ideals (for a similar view, cf. Chapter 4). Such glorification of the Orient reveals the enduring impact of cultural representations and the imaginative force in moulding Western, including Brazilian, perceptions of the Far East. It highlights a collective yearning for therapeutic and spiritual alternatives perceived to be lacking in Western traditions, thereby reinforcing the complex interplay between cultural fantasy and the search for authenticity and self-realisation in alternative medicine.

Bibliography

Andrade, João Tadeu. 2006. *Medicina alternativa e complementar: Experiência, corporeidade e transformação.* Salvador: EDUPBA, 2006.

Andrieu, Bernard. 1999. *Médecin de son corps.* Paris: PUF. https://doi.org/10.3917/puf.andri.1999.01.

Andrieu, Bernard. 2001. 'Médecin de soi-même'. In *Michel Foucault et la médecine. Lectures et usages*, edited by Philippe Artières. Paris: Éditions Kimé. https://doi.org/10.3917/kime.artie.2001.01.0084.

Barros, Nelson F. 2008. *A construção da medicina integrativa.* São Paulo: Hucitec.

Bases da medicina chinesa em curto intensivo de Do-In. *Diário de Pernambuco,* 21 October 1978: C-2.

Bivins, Roberta. 2007. *Alternative medicine? A History.* New York: Oxford University Press.

Bivins, Roberta. 2011. 'Histories of Heterodoxy'. In *The Oxford Handbook of the History of Medicine*, edited by Mark Jackson, 579–598. New York: Oxford University Press. https://doi.org/10.1093/oxfordhb/9780199546497.013.0032.

Borja, Wagner. 1978. 'Livros'. *Correio Braziliense*, segundo caderno, 10 August: 3.

Borup, Jørn, and Marianne Q. Fibiger, eds. 2017. *Eastspirit: Transnational Spirituality and Religious Circulation in East and West*. Leiden: Brill.

Braga, Paulo R. 2002. 'Os interesses econômicos dos Estados Unidos e a segurança interna no Brasil entre 1946 e 1964: Uma análise sobre os limites entre diplomacia coercitiva e operações encobertas'. *Rotas de Interesse* 45, no. 2: 46–65. https://doi.org/10.1590/s0034-73292002000200003.

Brasil. 1986. *Relatório da 8ª Conferência Nacional de Saúde*. 17–21 March. https://bvsms.saude.gov.br/bvs/publicacoes/8_conferencia_nacional_saude_relatorio_final.pdf. Accessed on 29 October 2022.

Brodsky, Greg. 1974. *From Eden to Aquarius: The Book of Natural Healing*. New York: Bantam.

Brodsky, Greg. 1977. *Do jardim do Éden à era de Aquarius: Livro da cura natural*. 1st ed. Rio de Janeiro: Ground.

Burke, Peter. 2001. *Eyewitnessing: The Uses of Images as Historical Evidence*. London: Reaktion Books.

Burwell, Jennifer. 2013. 'Figuring Matter: Quantum Physics as a New Age Rhetoric'. *Science as Culture* 22, no. 3: 344–366. https://doi.org/10.1080/09505431.2013.768222.

Coggiola, Osvaldo. 2001. *Governos militares na América Latina*. São Paulo: Contexto.

Cosson, Rildo. 2007. *Fronteiras contaminadas, literatura como jornalismo e jornalismo como literatura no Brasil dos anos 1970*. Brasília: UNB.

Costa, Matheus O. da. 2016. *Daoismo Tropical: A transplantação do Daoismo ao Brasil*. São Paulo: Fonte Editorial.

D'Andrea, Anthony. 2018. *Reflexive Religion: The New Age in Brazil and Beyond*. Leiden: Brill. https://doi.org/10.1163/9789004380110.

Descola, Philippe. 2021. *Les formes du visible: Une anthropologie de la figuration*. Paris: Éditions du Seuil.

Detrez, Christine. 2002. *La construction sociale du corps*. Paris: Éditions du Seuil.

Dunn, Christopher. 2016. *Contracultura: Alternative Arts and Social Transformation in Authoritarian Brazil*. Chapel Hill: University of North Carolina Press. https://doi.org/10.5149/northcarolina/9781469628516.001.0001.

Faure, Olivier, and Guillemain Hervé. 2019. 'Pour une autre histoire des pratiques médicales alternatives'. *Histoire, médecine et santé* 14: 9–28. https://doi.org/10.4000/hms.1656.

Giddens, Anthony. 1991. *Modernity and Self-identity: Self and Society in the Late Modern Age*. Redwood: Stanford University Press.

Green, James N. 2009. *Apesar de vocês*. São Paulo: Cia das Letras.

Ground. 1978. *Catálogo: Livros para uma nova consciência*. Rio de Janeiro: Ground.

Hallewell, Laurence. 2017. *O livro no Brasil*. São Paulo: EDUSP.

Hanegraaff, Wouter J. 1996. *New Age Religion and Western Culture: Esotericism in the Mirror of Secular Thought.* Leiden: Brill. https://doi.org/10.1163/9789004378933.

Harrington, Anne. 2008. *The Cure Within: A History of Mind-Body Medicine.* New York: W.W. Norton.

Kaku, Kouzo, Roger Machin, and Mami Nakamura (2000). 'Ki in Shinto and Aikido'. In *The Mysterious Power of Ki: The Force Within*, edited by Kouzo Kaku, 73–86. Leiden: Brill.

Kaminski, Leon, ed. 2019. *Contracultura no Brasil, anos 70.* Curitiba: CRV. https://doi.org/10.24824/978854443212.9.

Kuriyama, Shigehisa. 2002. *The Expressiveness of the Body and the Divergence of Greek and Chinese Medicine.* New York: Zone Books.

Laplantine, François, and Paul-Louis Rabeyron. 1987. *Les médecines parallèles.* Paris: PUC.

Le Breton, David. 2013. *Anthropologie du corps et modernité.* Paris: PUF. https://doi.org/10.3917/puf.lebre.2011.01.

Lewis, Charlton T., and Charles Short. *A Latin Dictionary. Founded on Andrews' Edition of Freund's Latin Dictionary.* Oxford: Clarendon Press, 1879.

Lineage. *Santa Cruz Tai Chi.* http://santacruztaichi.com/?page_id=19. Accessed on 5 December 2022.

Lowenberg, Jones S. 1989. *Caring and Responsibility: The Crossroads Between Holistic Practice and Traditional Medicine.* Pennsylvania: University of Pennsylvania Press.

Magnani, José Guilherme C. 1999. *Mystica urbe.* São Paulo: Nobel.

Martins, Marcos L. 2011. 'Utopias na Era de Aquário'. In *Histórias de países imaginários, variedades dos lugares utópicos*, edited by Marcos Antonio and Renato Moscateli, 143–166. Londrina: Eduel.

Misticismo e ciência unidos. 1979. *Jornal do Brasil*, 10 August, caderno B: 4.

Monneyron, Frédéric, and Martine Xiberras. 2008. *Le monde hippie: De l'imaginaire psychédélique à la révolution informatique.* Paris: Imago.

Moulin, Anne Marie. 2006. 'Le corps face à la médecine'. In *Histoire du corps. 3. Les mutations du regard, le XXe siècle*, edited by Jean-Marie Jacques Courtine, 15–71. Paris: Éditions du Seuil.

Nakazono, Mikoto Masahilo. 1979. *Inochi: The Book of Life.* Santa Fé: Kototama Institute.

Nascimento, Marilene Cabral do. 2006. 'Acupuntura, medicina e interculturalidade'. In *As duas faces da montanha: estudos sobre medicina chinesa e acupuntura*, edited by Marilene Cabral do Nascimento. São Paulo: Hucitec.

Nogueira, Maria Inês, and Kenneth R. de Camargo Jr. 2007. 'A orientalização do Ocidente como superfície de emergência de novos paradigmas em saúde'. *História, Ciências, Saúde – Manguinhos* 14, no. 3: 841–861. https://doi.org/10.1590/s0104-59702007000300009.

Os novos camponeses: Misticismo e ciência Unidos. 1979. *Jornal do Brasil*, 19 August, caderno B: 4.

Oschman, James L. 1996. 'Healing Energy Part 1: Historical Background'. *Journal of Bodywork and Movement Therapies* 1, no. 1: 34–39. https://doi.org/10.1016/s1360-8592(96)80013-1.

Ouriveis, Maíra. 2013. 'Soft Power and Cultural Industry: US Foreign Policy Present in the Daily Life of the Individual'. *Academic Journal of International Relations* 2, no. 4: 168–196.

Paz, Arnaldo. 1981. 'Imperatriz: Favorita num desfile de atrasos'. *Correio Braziliense*, 4 March, nacional: 3.

Pires, Ézio. 1978. 'Livros'. *Correio Braziliense*, 6 July, segundo caderno: 3.

Porter, Roy. 2002. *Blood & Guts.* London: Penguin.

Queiroz, Marcos de Souza. 2003. *Saúde e doença: Um enfoque antropológico.* Bauru: EDUSC.

Reddy, Sita. 2004. 'The Politics and Poetics of "Magazine Medicine": New Age Ayurveda in the Print Media'. In *The Politics of Healing: Histories of Alternative Medicine in Twentieth-Century North America*, edited by Robert D. Johnston, 196–217. New York: Routledge.

Reimão, Sandra. 1996. *Mercado editorial brasileiro.* São Paulo: FAPESP.

Rosenmann, Marcos R. 2013. *Tiempos de oscuridad: Historia de los golpes de Estado en América Latina*. Tres Cantos: Ediciones Akal.

Roszak, Theodore. 1969. *The Making of a Counter Culture.* Oakland: University of California Press.

Said, Edward. 1979. *Orientalism.* New York: Vintage Books.

Schild, Susana. 1978. 'Editora Ground: Os bons negócios do do-in, ioga, macrobiótica e meditação transcendental'. *Jornal do Brasil*, 10 June: 6.

Serrano, Felipe V. 2010. 'Estado, golpes de Estado y militarización en América Latina: Una reflexión histórico política'. *Argumentos* 23, no. 64: 175–193.

Sigolo, Renata P. 2019. 'Homeopatia, medicina alternativa: Entre contracultura, Nova Era e oficialização (Brasil, década de 1970)'. *História, Ciências, Saúde – Manguinhos* 26, no. 4: 1317–1335. https://doi.org/10.1590/s0104-59702019000400017.

Sigolo, Renata P. 2020. 'O alimento como remédio natural: Saúde e estilo de vida alternativo no Brasil na década de 1970'. *Revista Hydra* 4, no. 8: 6–33. https://doi.org/10.34024/hydra.2020.v4.10675.

Sigolo, Renata P., and Luis Fernando B. Junqueira. 2021. 'Entre agulhas e mãos: A medicina chinesa no Brasil da década de 1970'. *Locus* 27, no. 1: 122–151. https://doi.org/10.34019/2594-8296.2021.v27.32716.

Stanley-Baker, Michael. 2022. 'Qi 氣'. In *Routledge Handbook of Chinese Medicine*, edited by Vivienne Lo and Michael Stanley-Baker, 23–50. London: Routledge. https://doi.org/10.4324/9780203740262-4.

Stein, Justin B. 2021. 'Energy Healing: Reiki, Therapeutic Touch, and Healing Touch in the United States and Beyond'. In *The Routledge Handbook of Religion, Medicine, and Health*, edited by Dorothea Lüddeckens, Philipp Hetmanczyk, Pamela E. Klassen and Justin B. Stein, 229–243. London: Routledge. https://doi.org/10.4324/9781315207964-19.

Tavares, Carlos A. P. 1985. *O que são comunidades alternativas*. São Paulo: Brasiliense.

Toniol, Rodrigo. 2016. Cortina de fumaça: Terapias alternativas/complementares além da Nova Era. *Rever* 16, no. 2: 31–54. https://doi.org/10.21724/rever.v16i2.29281.

Vergonjeanne, François. 2012. 'Le Kotodama'. *Actualités en analyse transactionnelle* 143: 1–17. https://doi.org/10.3917/aatc.143.0001.

Vrignon, Alexis. 2017. *La naissance de l'écologie politique en France. Une nébuleuse au cœur des années 68*. Rennes: Presses Universitaires de Rennes. https://doi.org/10.4000/books.pur.154722.

Whorton, James C. 2002. *Nature Cures: The History of Alternative Medicine in America*. New York: Oxford University Press.

Williams, Allison. 1998. 'Therapeutic Landscapes in Holistic Medicine'. *Social Science & Medicine* 46, no. 9: 1193–1203. https://doi.org/10.1016/s0277-9536(97)10048-x.

Wunenburguer, Jean-Jacques. 2008. *Imaginaires et rationalité des médecines alternatives*. Paris: Les Belles Lettres.

Biography

Luis Fernando Bernardi Junqueira (PhD History, UCL) is a D. Kim Foundation Postdoctoral Fellow at the Department of History and Philosophy of Science, University of Cambridge. He is a global historian specialising in the intersections of science, medicine and religion in 19th- and 20th-century China, with extended interests in the histories of esotericism, psychology and mental health in modern East Asia and the history of alternative medicine in South America (https://luisfbj.com/).

Renata Palandri Sigolo is an Associate Professor and head of the Center for History, Health, and Society in the Department of History at the Federal University of Santa Catarina, Brazil. Her academic interests include the history of alternative medicine, health, and the environment, as well as the formation of intentional communities in Brazil and France during the second half of the 20th century. Additionally, she is a leading public historian known for her educative outreach initiatives pertaining to the global history of medicinal plants.

6 Buddhist Self-Help Healing Narratives and the Meditative Turn

Christina Lee

Abstract: The rise in popularity of mindfulness between the late 20th and early 21st centuries has led to a meditative turn in global self-help culture. Using personal experiences of transformation through meditation and neuroplasticity, authors claim to demystify mindfulness and meditation as a form of brain training without the cultural baggage of religious doctrines. This chapter explores the role of mindfulness self-help literature in shaping mindfulness into a transnational cultural product not only in Europe and America but also in East Asia. It critiques neuro-orientalist approaches to meditation in mainstream discourses of mindfulness and examines the ways in which healing narratives by Asian-American Buddhist writers challenge binary constructs of East/West, tradition/modern, spirituality/science.

Keywords: Buddhism, East/West, healing, meditation, orientalism, self-help

According to the ISBN database, in 1999, only six English-language books were published with the word 'mindfulness' in the title. By 2019, however, this number had risen significantly to 680 (ISBNdb 2024).[1] These titles include mindfulness-based therapy handbooks like Zindel Seagl, Mark Williams, and John Teasdale's *Mindfulness-Based Cognitive Therapy for Depression* (2001) and mindfulness self-help guides for everyday practice like Andy Puddicombe's *The Headspace Guide to Mindfulness & Meditation* (2011). This 'meditative turn' to mindfulness in self-help literature is part of what *Time* magazine

1 Results generated by entering 'mindfulness' as search term for English language books in 1999 and 2019 on ISBN Database.

Gaitanidis, Ioannis, Luis Fernando Bernardi Junqueira, Avery Morrow, and Sangyun Han (eds), *Therapy, Spirituality, and East Asian Imaginaries.* Taylor & Francis Group 2025
DOI: 10.5117/9789048559015_CH06

has called the 'Mindful Revolution' (Pickert 2014). An emergent subgenre of mindfulness self-help literature is what I call the mindfulness healing narrative. Examples include Ruby Wax's *Sane New World* (2013), Dan Harris's *10% Happier* (2014), and Ed Halliwell's *Into the Heart of Mindfulness* (2016), which relate how meditation and mindfulness-based cognitive therapy helped them recover from depression. As religious studies scholar Jeff Wilson observes, the abundance of accessible books, articles and materials on mindfulness means that it is 'no longer necessary even to have a Buddhist or meditation instructor' as anyone can take up meditation at any time at their own ease (Wilson 2014, 52). In its ubiquity, mindfulness has become a spiritual idiom so commonplace and recognisable that it is 'barely distinguishable from any number of other self-help programs' (Wilson 2014, 53).

While many scholars have commented on the commodification of mindfulness in the mainstream self-help industry, few have noted the role of personal self-help narratives in shaping transnational and transcultural discourses of mindfulness. Although these mindfulness self-help books are principally intended for a white, middle-class, Euro-American readership, they are increasingly finding a receptive audience in East Asia where the mindfulness market is rapidly expanding (Data Bridge Market Research 2022). Since its transmission by Buddhists from Asia to North America in the 1970s, mindfulness is now being retransmitted from North America back to Asia as a form of therapeutic self-help (for a similar movement, cf. Chapter 4). As Hendriks and Nehring et al. have shown, American and American-style self-help literature have a strong transnational reach and exert considerable influence on therapeutic culture in countries like China (Hendriks 2017; Nehring et al. 2016).[2] Though the number of people with depression and anxiety in China continues to rise, the majority of people choose self-treatment. Asian patients remain wary of the side effects of pharmaceutical interventions and mindfulness is seen as a cheaper, more accessible, less stigmatising alternative to conventional psychiatric treatment (Yang 2017). At the same time, despite its positive reception in Asia, mainstream American mindfulness has been criticised for its role in the erasure of Asian American experiences of meditation and of undermining the efforts of local Buddhist communities.

This chapter discusses how self-help literature between the late 20th and early 21st centuries helped construct the 'Mindful Revolution' and

2 While it is true that the Chinese self-help book market is full of translated American books, it is fundamentally 'glocal', as Chinese self-help entrepreneurs actively appropriate and blend American therapeutic discourses into local conditions and concerns (Nehring et al. 2016, 73).

shape mindfulness therapeutic discourse in the Global North and East Asia. It explores how American authors mobilised personal experiences to authenticate mindfulness's therapeutic efficacies (on personal experience, cf. Chapters 2, 3, and 4) and demystify mindfulness for the average non-Buddhist reader. I broadly define self-help literature as books that offer advice, guidance, and instructions on a variety of topics with the intention of directing readers towards certain goals, such as better health, change in life attitudes, or new skills. I include in this definition guidebooks, manuals, popular psychology books, and memoirs of recovery from illness that aim at inspiring others to follow their lead. I approach mindfulness from a literary perspective and use narrative analysis to show how mindfulness self-help writers embody cultural authority by presenting themselves as pastors and mediators of both ancient Asian Buddhist traditions and modern Western science. I examine the discursive strategies through which mindfulness self-help writers rehabilitated Buddhist concepts through the lenses of Western neuropsychology to present mindfulness as a value-neutral, culturally unmarked product of scientific modernity. I call this endeavour 'neuro-orientalism'.[3] As I show, neuro-orientalism not only works to reinscribe mindfulness as a Western scientific discovery but serves to flatten sectarian and cultural differences in its construction of the universal cerebral therapeutic subject. I show how attempts to demystify meditation fall back on familiar tropes of Asian culture as 'Other' and invalidate local Asian and Asian American experiences of Buddhism. In the last sections, I turn to alternative healing narratives by Buddhist writers to explore how they deployed Buddhist ethics to rescript the neuro-orientalist narrative.

Remaking *Dharma*

In 1979, molecular biologist and long-term meditator Jon Kabat-Zinn developed the stress reduction and relaxation programme (SR&RP) for patients with chronic pain at the University of Massachusetts Medical

3 Dylan T. Lott (2016) has previously used 'neuro-Orientalism' in a similar context to describe the effects produced in dialogues between neuroscience and Buddhism of framing a people as 'the (projected) locus of an exotic, esoteric otherness, made answerable to a representation which is valued and coveted within a technological framework thought to be free of biasing effects' (242). In my usage, I employ neuro-orientalism specifically in the context of transnational self-help therapeutic culture as a discursive technique that frames Buddhist meditation as a distant and exclusive religious practice made universally accessible and relevant to modern urban readers through neuroscience.

Centre. As characterised by Kabat-Zinn in his book *Full Catastrophe Living,* the SR&RP is 'a systematic approach to developing new kinds of control and wisdom in our lives, based on our capacities for relaxation, paying attention, awareness, and insight' (Kabat-Zinn 1990, 2). SR&RP is rooted in diverse Buddhist and yogic traditions including Theravada, Zen, and Vedanta and incorporates meditative techniques like sitting meditation and hatha yoga. In the eight-week SR&RP, delivered as a complement to existing treatments, patients were taught to observe sensations in their bodies, including unpleasant and painful ones, without identifying with or reacting to them. Jon Kabat-Zinn calls this *mindfulness*, namely 'the awareness that emerges through paying attention on purpose, in the present moment, and nonjudgmentally to the unfolding of experience moment by moment' (Kabat-Zinn 2003, 145). This definition was inspired by the Pali word *sati,* meaning 'memory', and carries the notion of 'attention' or 'awareness' (Thera 1962). Kabat-Zinn intentionally uses the term 'mindfulness' to differentiate Mindfulness-Based Stress Reduction from other nonmeditative stress management therapies and to make it into a 'place-holder' for *Dharma,* the Buddha's teachings on 'the nature of mind, emotion, and suffering and its potential release' (Kabat-Zinn 2003, 145). In the sermon on the Four Noble Truths and the origin and cessation of suffering, Buddha taught that life, with its cycles of birth, sickness, old age, and death, is full of suffering and dissatisfactions (*dukkha*). *Dukkha* is generated by craving (*tanha*) for pleasure and permanence. To liberate oneself from suffering (*nibbana*) and leave the cycle of rebirth (*samsara*), one must eradicate cravings and attachments. This can be achieved through meditating on the impermanence of the body and following the Eightfold Path.

Findings from the SR&RP showed that patients experienced significant reductions in pain and distress as well as positive changes in self-perception (Kabat-Zinn 1991, xxxi). The study not only confirmed meditation's effectiveness in altering autonomic stress responses as suggested in Herbert Benson's *The Relaxation* Response (1975) but demonstrated how Buddhist concepts like mindfulness could be integrated into existing clinical frameworks as a therapeutic intervention. The SR&RP was later renamed Mindfulness-Based Stress Reduction (MBSR). The successes of MBSR saw the emergence of other mindfulness-based interventions (MBIs), such as Mindfulness-Based Cognitive Therapy (MBCT) and Dialectical Behaviour Therapy (DBT). In the late 1990s and early 2000s, researchers used neuroimaging technologies like fMRI (functional Magnetic Resonance Imaging) to study the effects of mindfulness on neuroplasticity, the brain's capacity to adjust its structures and function in response to changes in behaviour or the environment. The studies found evidence that meditation can thicken the neural tissues in the prefrontal cortex and strengthen the anterior cingulate cortex (Davidson and Lutz 2008). These findings suggested that meditation can enhance emotional regulation, memory, and concentration (Hanson 2009). Today, MBSR and MBCT are delivered in mainstream healthcare for a range of conditions and used in schools and workplaces for mental health support across the UK and the US. The Global Mindfulness Collaborative, run by Brown University's Mindfulness Center, also has partner institutions offering MBSR and MBCT in China, Korea, Japan, and Taiwan (Global Mindfulness Collaborative 2024).

The Mindful Self-Help Pastor

In *Mindful America,* Jeff Wilson describes six kinds of processes involved in the mindful movement: (1) 'mediation', the historical translation and development of Buddhism and of meditation from Asia to America by Asian Buddhist monks and lay Western teachers who travelled to Asia in the 1970s; (2) 'mystification', the process of deemphasising traditional religious Buddhist concepts like karma and reincarnation to accommodate American culture and values; (3) 'medicalisation', the process of modifying mindfulness into a therapeutic intervention for secular healthcare settings through mindfulness-based interventions like MBSR in the 1980s and '90s; (4) 'mainstreaming', the assimilation of mindfulness into the everyday life of average middle-class Americans; (5) 'marketing', where mindfulness is turned into a consumer commodity; and (6) 'moralising', the process of bringing mindfulness into education and the workplace to make America a more compassionate and productive society (Wilson 2014). Since Wilson's study principally focuses on mindfulness's expansion in America after its transmission from Asia and transformation into MBSR, he does not consider mindfulness's development outside the US. Yet self-help books have been instrumental in marketing mindfulness as a universally accessible therapeutic practice in East Asia. Although countries like China and Japan have a rich history of Buddhism, meditation was largely practised in Buddhist monasteries. As the founder of the Xi'an Jiaotong Liverpool University Mindfulness Center, Pan Li, writes, compared to ancient texts on meditation, translated foreign mindfulness books were much more accessible and practical for lay Chinese people (Li 2023; cf. Chapter 9).

Despite assumptions about their supposed lack of literary merit, self-help books are important, as they 'constitute an interface between psychological, medical and religious forms of expert knowledge and public narratives of the self, self-development, and the relationships between self and society' (Nehring, et al. 2016, 8). With rising medical costs and growing distrust towards mainstream media, individuals are becoming increasingly reliant on self-help writers and health experts who lie 'outside the traditional confines or intuitional parameters of the doctor-patient relationship' (Barker 2014, 175). Michel Foucault called this form of government of individuals' conduct 'pastoral power'. In Foucault's usage, government refers not only to 'political structures or to the management of states' but also to 'the way in which the conduct of individuals or of groups might be directed' (Foucault 1982, 789). In this sense, government is the 'direction (*conduit*) of souls' to control others' possible fields of voluntary actions and delineate their subjectivity. According to Foucault, pastoral power was a form of religious power aimed at ensuring individuals' salvation in the next world. In its ancient Hebraic religious sense, 'Pastorship is a fundamental type of relationship between God and men [...] a religious type of power that God exercises over his people' (Foucault 2009, 125). After the decline of the Christian Church, the pastoral function was transferred from religious institutions to the state and other political institutions. The aim of pastoral power today is 'no longer to lead people to salvation in the next world but rather ensuring it in *this* world' (Foucault 1982, 784). In contemporary neoliberal Western societies, salvation now means stability of income, personal security, material comfort, and physical and mental well-being. Pastoral power was relocated from parish pastors to experts like doctors and counsellors, who provide guidance and practical advice to individuals on how to be healthier, wealthier, and happier.

In addition to playing a 'translational and mediational role' and relaying medical information advice to the public, self-help authors have also become important sources of pastoral care (Rose 2007, 41). These narratives sell mindfulness as 'a lifestyle product embodied in the iconic form of the expert self-help author' (Wilson 2014, 142). The pastoral authority of self-help writers lies in their lived experiences of personal transformation and their capacities for identification with readers of all backgrounds. Positioning themselves as rational sceptics-turned-believers, they present their own experiences of recovery through mindfulness meditation as readily accessible 'maps' available to anyone in need of relief from suffering. In the translator's preface for the Chinese edition of Kirk Strosahl and Patricia Robinson's *The Mindfulness and Acceptance Workbook for Depression*, Xu Shousen argues that in addition to the strategies described in the book, what makes the book appealing is Strosahl's 'unique experiences' (*dute jingli* 独特经历) of mental illness. Despite cultural differences, Strosahl's depression allies him with the millions of Chinese people who struggle with depression and this makes the book much more persuasive (*geng ju shuofuli* 更具说服力) and practical (*geng ju shixiaoxing*更具实效性) (Xu 2021, foreword).

Demystifying Mindfulness

According to Wilson, a key strategy for mainstreaming and marketing mindfulness in America is mystification, the process of obscuring mindfulness's Buddhist roots by repackaging Buddhist concepts in modern American terms (Wilson 2014, 44). Mystification often simultaneously involves demystification, the removal of 'bewilderment' and 'irrational beliefs' around meditation through the affirmation of secular mindfulness's this-ageliness (*saeculum*, age), its relevance to people in contemporary society facing everyday problems of suffering (OED 2023; Batchelor 2017, 3). In mindfulness healing narratives like Dan Harris's bestselling *10% Happier* (2014) and Ruby Wax's *A Mindfulness Guide for the Frazzled* (2016), mystification and demystification are mediated by the sceptical mindful pastor, who 'road-tests' meditation to show that mindfulness is wholly compatible with modern life and accessible to average Americans: 'if it can work for me, it can probably work for you, too' (Harris 2014, Preface).[4] In *10% Happier*, Harris grants readers 'exclusive access' to the 'voice in his head' so they can witness the difficulties he encountered in meditation and avoid the pitfalls in their practices (Harris 2014, Preface). Harris experienced a drug-induced panic attack while presenting on live television in 2004, caused by the cocaine he was using to control the symptoms of post-traumatic stress disorder (PTSD) and depression he had developed since his return from war zones. After the panic attack, he was reassigned to report on faith and spirituality, where he interviewed New Age gurus and exposed religious cults. A self-professed agnostic sceptic rationalist, Harris had thought of meditation as 'ringing bells, ogling crystals, intoning *om* and attempting

4 *10% Happier* was published in China by China Youth Press as *Yige mingxiangzhe de juezhishu Gaobie jiaozao miming yali de ziwo xunlianfa* 一个冥想者的觉知书：告别焦躁、迷茫、压力的自我训练法 [*A Meditator's Book of Awareness: Self-Training to Get Rid of Anxiety, Confusion, and Stress*] (2015). *Mindfulness for the Frazzled* was published in Taiwan by Times Culture Press as *Quanxin liuzhou zhengnian lianxifa Quanqiu zuire chaoliu renren dou zai zhuiqiu de neizai zhengli rangni jinru zuijia gongzuo zhuangtai huochu yuyue rensheng* 全新6週正念練習法：全球最熱潮流，人人都在追求的內在整理，讓你進入最佳工作狀態，活出逾悅人生！[*All New 6 week Mindfulness Training: The Hottest Trend in the World, the Inner Reorganisation Everyone is Looking For, So You Can Work in Your Best Form, and Live a Joyful Life!*] (2016).

to float off into some sort of cosmic goo' (Harris 2014, 97, 87). It was only after interviews with Buddhist psychiatrist Mark Epstein, neuroscientist Jud Brewer, and the Dalai Lama that he realised that he had been 'blinded by his own scepticism' and had 'closed his mind prematurely' to meditation (Harris 2014, 218).

As Harris argues, mindfulness and Buddhism are not inherently difficult or irrational; it is the cultural baggage around meditation and 'false advertising' in American culture that mystifies mindfulness (Harris 2014, 102). Contrary to his earlier beliefs about the Buddha, Harris learned that the Buddha was not a god but an 'original psychoanalyst' who discovered the nature of the mind and its suffering and invented mindfulness to change the mind (Harris 2014, 88). Understanding *dukkha* as the mental suffering and anxieties generated by the 'inner chatter' in his head, he learned to use mindfulness to 'short-circuit' the 'habitual, mindless chain reactions' that usually follow such chatter. Rather than being 'a recipe for passivity', Harris found that mindfulness made him more productive and '10% happier than before' (Harris 2014, 154).

Ruby Wax, an American-British comedian and mental health advocate with recurrent depression, describes a similar conversion to mindfulness. After other psychotherapeutic interventions failed, she decided to try meditation and then undertook a master's degree in MBCT at Oxford under the supervision of Mark Williams, the founder of MBCT. In *A Mindfulness Guide for the Frazzled*, Wax describes suffering as being 'frazzled', constantly burnt-out and stressed. Having spent years in the 'Land of Frazzledom', Wax decided to become an 'expert tourist guide' for readers with depression by sharing her own journey to the 'exit route' through meditation (Wax 2016, Foreword). Wax had previously thought meditation was a Buddhist practice involving chanting 'long meaningless mantras' and worshipping 'some elephant with a thousand arms or a smiling fat man' (Wax 2013). Yet, as she learned in her MBCT course, mindfulness did not involve humming mantras but was, in fact, a mental fitness regime that trains the mind to notice mind-wandering and can be practised at any time during any activity, including when showering or making tea. Through narrating her experiences of depression and meditation with light-hearted humour and demonstrating how mindfulness transformed her response to mental suffering, Wax shows that liberation from suffering is not something to be attained in the next life but is possible in *this* life right now.

Although Harris and Wax primarily wrote for a white, European-American audience, it is also easy to see why they would equally appeal to Asian readers. Harris's and Wax's concerns about career advancement and the stresses of working in hypercompetitive environments are highly relatable to overworked urban Asian readers. While there are positive signs of changing attitudes towards depression in East Asia, public disclosures of mental illness (especially when combined with substance abuse) still incur shame (Zhang 2020, 9). Few Asian writers have the licence to write about depression with the same frankness and explicit humour as Harris and Wax. This ability to write about the difficult and unseemly aspects of depression bolsters their authority as a guide not just for Americans but for anyone struggling with depression.

Neuro-Orientalism and Cerebral Self-help

As well as showing how mindfulness both emerges from and responds to everyday experiences of suffering, the convinced sceptic of mindfulness healing narratives also plays a key role in demystifying and translating the science of mindfulness into plain, nonspecialist language to create a common-sensical 'American vocabulary' of mindfulness (Kabat-Zinn 2011, 288). In his mindfulness self-help guide *Meditation for Fidgety Skeptics* (2017), Harris dismisses traditional art depicting meditators on a misty mountain with 'beatific looks on their faces' as misleading and unreflective of the actual experience of meditation (Harris 2017, Ch. 1). The actual experience of meditation is much closer to taming a beast, which he illustrates with the drawing of a man with a whip, holding a chair in front of him, against a large brain on a stool. Rather than a serene, tranquil experience, mindfulness is 'a rigorous brain exercise' of 'trying to tame the runaway train of the mind' (Harris 2014, 101). Pointing to neuroscience research on neuroplasticity, Harris claims that traits and attributes like resilience and kindness are skills that can be 'trained the same way you build your body in the gym' (Harris 2014, Preface). As Harris suggests, it is possible to 'sculpt your brain through meditation' and 'grow' the grey matter' that controls emotion and resilience 'the way doing curls grows your biceps' (Harris 2014, 168). In *A Mindfulness Guide,* Wax writes that since taking up meditation, she has become more focused and less self-centred than before such that she could actually 'feel the muscle of attention growing from a puny little bump to a something quite powerful' (Wax 2016, Ch. 9). These metaphors of mindfulness as brain-training exemplify what Audun Roald calls 'cerebral self-help', where individuals seek to optimise or change their lives by manipulating neuroactivities (Roald 2012, 770). Transposing the language of neuroplasticity onto discourses of personal development and self-optimisation, cerebral self-help frames mental exercises like mindfulness as 'a means of taking responsibility for our brains' that 'gives the subject direct access to his or her brain' (Madsen 2014, 66).

By reframing spiritual cultivation as 'brain gym', the rhetoric of cerebral self-help renders 'innocuous the less familiar or palatable elements of Buddhist mindfulness' and transforms mindfulness into a uniquely modern enterprise (Wilson 2014, 44). I call this discursive technique of repackaging Asian contemplative traditions in neuroscience 'neuro-orientalism'. For Edward Said, the Orient is 'an idea that has a history and a tradition of thought, imagery, and vocabulary that have given it reality and presence in and for the West' (Said 2003, 5; cf. Chapters 4 and 5). The relationship between the Oriental East and the Occidental West is essentially a relationship of domination and power, sustained by a system of knowledge production about the Orient that enables the positional superiority of Western identity. In Orientalist discourses, the Orient is a 'symbol of true spirituality and a repository of exotic terminology' from which a new, healthier, purer and more peaceful world order may evolve (Hanegraaf 1996, 517). The Far East is imagined as a wellspring of forgotten ancient wisdom preserved by a few elect Buddhist masters (represented by the iconic male Asian 'Oriental monk') whose unparalleled insight into the human condition provides moral guidance to the civilised but spiritually lost Christian West (Iwamura 2010, 6). In neuro-orientalist discourses, the otherworldly mystical aesthetics that once characterised Eastern wisdom is rejected and instead the Orient is actively reimagined as a site of scientific excavation. The very brain of the Oriental Monk himself is an object of curiosity whose knowledge can only be accessed through Western science and brain scanners (Waldron 2017, 84). The tale of the Oriental monk who travels to the West to find a spiritual successor in the spirited white male is here rehearsed in the narrative of the determined Western scientist who assists the master in spreading the essence of Buddhism to benefit humanity. Though benign and wise, the Asian Buddhist monk's ties to religious tradition and detachment from worldly affairs make him impenetrable to the average non-Buddhist. It is the Western expert who can translate religious notions like enlightenment (*nibbana*) in scientific terms and 'speak' to the concerns of ordinary people dealing with the stresses of living in a cosmopolitan world.

Neuro-orientalist discourses present mindfulness as both 'confirmed by ancient wisdom' and grounded in scientific empirical evidence, its universal applicability proven by the longevity of the thousand-year-old practice and the biological sameness of the human brain (Nehring and Frawley 2020, 1186). This is readily seen in neuropsychologist Rick Hanson and neurologist Richard Mendius's bestselling book *The Buddha's Brain*, in which they propose that 'an awakening mind means an awakening brain' and that 'if the brain is the cause of suffering, it can also be its cure' (Hanson and Mendius 2009, 11–12). Extending their argument, science journalist Donna Jackson Nakazawa suggests that it is possible to use meditation to 'reverse engineer' the neural circuitry that causes unhappiness and disease (Nakazawa 2013, 10). According to Nakazawa, early childhood traumatic events like the death of a parent and continuous exposure to stress in later life can alter genetic expressions that activate autoimmune conditions like Guillain-Barré syndrome, where myelin sheaths of the nerves become inflamed and cause numbness (Nakazawa 2013, 13). As Nakazawa suggests, by interrupting the cycles of stress that trigger the condition, meditation can promote the healing of the myelin sheaths and deactivate the gene that causes disease. Here, the Buddhist concept of *samsara*, the cycle of death and rebirth that causes endless suffering, is translated into neurophysiological terms as chronic hyperarousal and negative feedback cycle, while healing is reconceptualised as the neurobiological healing of the myelin sheaths of the nerves. In this way, the awakened mind becomes the awakened brain, and the path to awakening is the neural pathways to happiness and a healthy brain.

Though featured most prominently in American self-help, neuro-orientalism also appears in meditation books by East Asian authors. Kabat-Zinn, in his foreword for Taiwanese mindfulness teacher Chen Te-Chung's *Training in Mindfulness and Stress Reduction* [*Zhengnnian jianya de xunlian* 正念減壓的訓練], writes that mindfulness 'comes from deep inside Chinese culture and civilisation' and that MBSR is 'far more Eastern in both origin and essence than it is Western' (Kabat-Zinn 2017, Foreword). This framing of mindfulness as a modern, scientifically proven derivative of Asian meditation being returned to its place of origin by the Western scientist de-emphasises its foreignness, with local authors in Asia adopting this narrative to appeal to younger cosmopolitan readers. In *If You Feel Tired, Meditate* [*Ganjue lei le jiu mingxiang ba* 感觉累了，就冥想吧], Li Shangqing李上卿 writes that although meditation is ancient (*gulao* 古老), it is not mysterious (*shenmi* 神秘). Stressing that meditation is neither a religion (*zongjiao* 宗教) nor a philosophy (*zhexue* 哲学), she argues that meditation is popular today because it has been scientifically explained and proven to benefit health and to remake (*gaizao* 改造) our brains (Li 2014, Foreword, 3). By interlacing descriptions of traditional arts and monastic living with scientific studies about the positive neurophysiological benefits of meditation, Li reconstructs mindfulness into a pragmatic modernised form of *xiushen yangxing* 修身养性, the Chinese philosophy of self-cultivation. The subtitle for Li's book, *10 Minutes of Meditation Equals 2 Hours of Deep Sleep*[5] echoes *5 Minutes of Meditation Equals 1 Hour of Deep Sleep,*[6] the title for the 2011 Chinese edition of *The Buddha's Brain*. This association through mimicry further enhances Li's cultural authority as she installs herself as Hanson and Mendius's unofficial interlocutor who mediates mindfulness's return to the East from the West.

The Limits of Mindful Salvation

In Kabat-Zinn's reflections on his initial vision for MBSR, he states that he did not intend to decontextualise mindfulness from its Buddhist roots but recontextualise *dharma* within the frameworks of science, medicine, psychology and healthcare so that it would be 'maximally useful' to people who would not otherwise have interest in or access to mindfulness (Kabat-Zinn 2011, 288). Although mindfulness self-help pastors have helped increase public knowledge about mental health, they have also eroded the role of mindfulness as a practice for gaining insight into suffering as a conditioned experience. In their discursive self-fashioning as wounded pastors, mindfulness writers adopt a survivalist mentality that presents mindful resilience as part of the 'protective cocoon' that insulates the individual from the anxieties generated by illness and enables the individual to 'carry on' with day-to-day life (Giddens 1990, 3). Cerebral self-help localises suffering as a neurophysiological and psychological problem inside the individual and instead of challenging the social conditions that generate stress, the rhetoric of mindful resilience encourages readers to become self-sufficient entrepreneurial therapeutic subjects and overcome stress in a hypercompetitive environment (Cook 2016). This is particularly problematic in China where mindfulness self-help is operationalised as therapeutic governance to direct unhappy individuals to question their own competencies rather than government policies (J. Yang 2017). Rather than leading readers to salvation, mindfulness pastors become complicit in perpetuating suffering by concealing the causes of suffering.

Neuro-orientalist discourses of mindfulness have also had a significant impact on Buddhist communities in both East Asia and North America. Although Buddhism is a major religion in China, there are concerns that it

5 *Mingxiang 10 fenzhong dengyu shushui erxiaoshi* 冥想10分钟等于熟睡二小时.

6 *Mingxiang 5 fenzhong dengyu shushui yixiaoshi* 冥想5分钟，等于熟睡一小时.

remains associated with superstition; neuro-orientalism, on the other hand, promises to provide a safe, depoliticised way to promote meditation (Zhang 2020, 183). However, mindfulness self-help downplays the importance of spiritual communities and Buddhist leaders have objected to the dilution of Buddhist ethical frameworks which misleads people to view relaxation as the goal of mindfulness rather than the cultivation of righteous intention for the sake of the world and other people (Hendriks 2017, 206; Matsuyama and Shimada 2018).

Asian writers' adoption of the neuro-orientalist narrative of mindfulness is troubling because neuro-orientalism essentially grew out of a 'racialised dynamic of power' that marginalises Asians as the exotic Other (Hsu 2016, 373). The celebration of mindfulness as revived by Western scientists invalidates both the cultural work done by local Buddhist communities in Asia and the achievements of Buddhism-inspired culturally specific psychotherapies like Morita therapy and *naikan* therapy, which Asian psychologists have been doing since the early 20th century (Zhang 2020, 143). Despite claiming to demystify meditation, writers do not interrogate the role of popular culture in the production of religious stereotypes. Harris's uncritical evocations of stereotypes like 'bearded swarmis' to juxtapose well-dressed Harvard scientists demonstrate how Western mindfulness accentuates and grounds its authoritative modernity by establishing it in opposition to a 'racial otherness' (Hsu 2016, 374). The term 'cultural baggage', originally used to categorise the religion and customs imported by Asian American immigrants, not only renders the contributions of Asian American Buddhists to the mindfulness movement invisible but also exacerbates anti-Asian and anti-Buddhist sentiments amid an increase in anti-Asian racism in the Global North (Hsu 2016; Fleming, Womack, and Proulx 2022). For Asian Americans, as ethnic minorities in a white Christian-majority society, the devotional Mahayana Buddhist practices and beliefs that white Theravada practitioners dismiss as superstitious provide a deep connection to ancestral families integral to their formation of self-identities (Han 2021, 80). When dominant cultures exercise the power to 'pick and choose what cultural forms to absorb or discard, and what is regarded as worthy or unworthy of consideration in defining Buddhist practice for Western communities', they extend legacies of 'oppressive sociopolitical histories' (L. Yang 2017, 47).

The Art of Being Sick

Notwithstanding the cultural dominance of neuro-orientalism, some nonmainstream Asian-American writers have pushed back by centring

Buddhist ethics in their mindfulness healing narratives. In *The Embodied Mind,* neuroscientist and cofounder of the Mind and Life Institute Francisco Varela, philosopher Evan Thompson, and psychologist Eleanor Rosch argue that while it is important to understand the neurobiological mechanisms of meditation, we must also recognise the significance of meditation as an integrated experience and exercise that involves the application of bodily and cognitive skills in 'situated and ethically directed action' (Varela, Thompson and Rosch 2016, xxv). As they observe, mindfulness is not simply about the inner observation of mental activities instantiated in neural networks and the acquisition of cognitive skills through individual mental training but primarily the application of skilful embodied action in interactions between individuals. As such, it is better to compare meditation to 'the ongoing practice of an art' like painting rather than to the 'development of a technical ability' as implied in metaphors of brain gym (Batchelor 2015, 257).

In *Mindfulness as Medicine,* Vietnamese American Buddhist nun and former doctor Sister Dang Nghiem writes that although she was trained in biomedicine, it was not her medical knowledge but the practice of mindfulness she learned at the monastery that taught her the 'art of being sick' (Nghiem 2015, 229). In 2011, Nghiem contracted Lyme disease, a tick-borne disease caused by the bacterium *Borrelia burgdorferi.* In the late stages of Lyme disease, the bacteria infect the nervous system and lead to neuropsychiatric symptoms such as neuropathic pain and cognitive dysfunction (Dumes 2020, 2). Instead of isolating and distracting herself with busyness like she used to when she was a doctor, Nghiem practised Touching the Earth meditation. In this meditation, the practitioner prostrates and sends gratitude to the Earth and her biological and spiritual ancestors. When Nghiem practised Touching the Earth, she realised that she and the tick that bit her are interrelated and share Buddha nature. Therefore, rather than rejecting Lyme disease, she could live in harmony with the tick in her body as it was. This insight brought 'a moment of deep healing' because it removed feelings of fear and aversion towards her body and changed the dynamics of her interactions with others (Nghiem 2015, 249).

In the framework of interbeing, 'the healing of one person can heal many because we inter-are' (342). As Nghiem became at peace with her ill body, she could transmit peace rather than pain to the people around her. According to the Buddhist principle of dependent origination (*paticcasamuppada*), all actions arise from previous actions, and each person's present thoughts and actions will impact the behaviour of others. Thich Nhat Hanh calls this 'interbeing' (Hanh 1996, 88). Nghiem remaps interbeing in neuropsychological terms and compares it to the mirror neuron theory. Mirror neuron theory is the idea that mirror neurons enable human self-awareness and empathy (Ramachandran and Oberman 2009). Mirror neurons are neurons found in the premotor cortex. When observing a person, mirror neurons are activated to allow the observer to imitate the person's actions and feel the other person's emotions in themselves. Using this model of neuropsychological interbeing, Nghiem rejects individualistic readings of mindfulness by insisting that caring for one's own suffering is always connected to caring for others' suffering. In showing her experiences of suffering and healing, Nghiem's narrative also becomes a textual mirror that reflects readers' suffering and makes the 'healing of many others possible' (Ngheim 2015, 342).

In *Occupy This Body* (2019), Korean American Buddhist scholar Sharon Suh extends the notion of dependent origination to examine how the voice in her head does not simply generate mental suffering but is also conditioned by her social and cultural environment. Suh's mother, who had anorexia and bulimia, used to force-feed and body-shame Suh while she herself took laxatives to stay thin. As a result, Suh developed disordered eating habits and continued to experience body insecurities throughout her adult life. Determined not to transmit her suffering to her young daughters, Suh practised yoga and meditation to change her relationship with food and her body. As she meditated and tried to inhabit her body without judgement, she saw that much of her anxieties came from other people and external forces like social media and women's magazines. Just as Mara, the Buddhist demon of delusion, sent an army of monsters and his daughters (craving, desire, discontent) to tempt the Buddha away from the path of enlightenment, women are constantly subjected to the 'Mara of marketing and popular culture', deprecating comments about their bodies and pressured to conform to impossible beauty standards (Suh 2019, 181). This realisation that women across generations and cultures experience the same kind of suffering prompted her to focus on her body from the inside out through mindful awareness so she could develop an awareness of 'how it feels in the present moment without the external chatter' (183). Calling her readers to turn away from the false images in culture's mirrors, Suh encourages women to 'withdraw from the onslaught of socially constructed *dukkha* and outer harm' that tell women their bodies are less than ideal and 'tune out' external voices that govern what they eat and how they look (Suh 2019, 189). Using Buddhist mythology to remystify and defamiliarise suffering as conditioned by dependent origination, Suh reclaims Asian Buddhist 'cultural baggage' as cultural resources for resisting oppressive gender norms and directs women towards alternative ways of being with their bodies.

Being Refuge

> 'Be the refuge' has become my strategy for engaging Buddhist practice in my battle with cancer. I'm okay with not reaching the fully liberating refuge of enlightenment in this lifetime. It would be enough if I could have somewhat of a refuge for myself from pain and anxiety, and then to try to be a refuge for those around me. (Arunlikhati 2016)

In 2016, Aaron J. Lee posted on his blog under the pseudonym 'arunlikhati' that he was dying from cancer. He was diagnosed with a metastatic non-Hodgkin lymphoma that affected his bone marrow, kidneys, and central nervous system. Being of mixed Asian descent meant that his chances of finding a stem cell donor were extremely slim. As he struggled with the gruelling chemotherapy regimes, he recalled the Buddha's teachings on the Four Noble Truths and resolved to create a refuge for himself. For Aaron, a refuge is a space where someone can feel safe, comforted, and nurtured. Meditation was a refuge as focusing on his breath allowed his mind to 'dwell in a comfortable space during some rather uncomfortable procedures' (Arunlikhati 2016). In turn, cultivating tranquillity of mind enabled him to use mindful speech and action to become a refuge for others around him. Accepting help from friends and family with gratitude was his way of relieving their feelings of helplessness and making them less uneasy about his illness. Before his diagnosis, Aaron previously kept a blog called Angry Asian Buddhist, in which he criticised the whiteness of American Buddhism and worked to expand the representation of Asians and Asian-American Buddhists. His final message to readers to 'be the refuge you wish to see in this world' was a continuation of that work to create refuges where marginalised people can find 'true comfort and wellbeing'.

As Aaron's realisation shows, though disease causes suffering, it can also be a 'catalytic factor' for new insight since illness inspires meditation on the body's impermanence. The knowledge one gains from experiencing illness can bring the sick person in communion with the suffering of other sentient beings and inspire action for change (Birnbaum 1979, 3). Meditative experiences expose the 'inherent impermanence' of ability-based identities, and 'when linked to a socially engaged Buddhism [meditation] can also support work to eradicate the social and political oppression (Squier 2004, 50). In mainstream self-help culture, the goal of healing is emphatically individualistic; it can be achieved through perseverance and determination. The psychologisation of mindfulness as a mental attention-training exercise constructs meditation as a personal, solitary practice that 'overlook[s] the value of togetherness'. When the Buddha told his followers to bring his teachings into their direct experience, he was inviting them to draw on their collective experience of community to explore 'what it means to awaken together' (L. Yang 2017, 48).

In the Pali canon, the Buddha is named the Supreme Physician, Dharma is likened to a medicine, and members of the *sangha* are compared to attendants of the sick (Birnbaum 1979, 3). In *How to Be Sick*, Buddhist teacher and former law professor Toni Bernhard describes how she healed through *sangha*. As a chronically ill person living with Myalgic Encephalomyelitis (ME) and chronic fatigue, Bernhard is frequently unable to participate in social gatherings. Over time, she lost contact with friends and even her local Buddhist group. As she looked for support outside face-to-face contact, she turned to online support groups for disabled and chronically ill people, whom she calls 'the culture of the sick' (Bernhard 2010, 155). Even though they are not Buddhists and do not use the term *dukkha*, Bernhard considered them part of her *sangha* because they taught her how to see suffering differently, as something that connects her to the world rather than separating her from it. Just as Nghiem and Suh use the Buddhist notion of dependent origination to show how our suffering is interrelated to the suffering of people around us by reframing the diseased body as a vehicle for awakening and communion, Bernhard maintains that healing is not an individual enterprise but one that necessarily relies on the support of others. This rescripts modern culture's valorisation of independence and enables individuals to openly accept care from others without shame or humiliation as a practice of collective healing.

Conclusion: A Culture of Healing

Since the onset of the meditative turn at the turn of the 21st century, mindfulness has expanded rapidly and become normalised in many societies. Americans' relationships with meditation and Buddhism have changed drastically since the introduction of MBSR. As this chapter has shown, mindfulness self-help books and narratives have been instrumental in changing perceptions of Buddhism and meditation across North America and East Asia. In their ongoing dialogues with both science and Buddhism, mindfulness self-help writers have been crucial in breaking through the tired dichotomies such as traditional/modern, science/religion, East/West, sick/healthy to find new ways of living with bodily and cultural differences (cf. Chapter 9).

Though under-appreciated, mindfulness healing narratives added very important practical and personal dimensions to meditation that mainstream mindfulness self-help overlooks. Writing as fellow sufferers, they encouraged readers to reconceptualise what it means to be ill and to be healed outside a rigid biomedical paradigm. Just as there is no 'right' approach to meditation, there is no single way of healing. Healing can mean liberation from intergenerational trauma, racism, and social injustices. Healing is also a collective practice. Although illness can be isolating, it can also unite people through their shared suffering. More than a health fad, mindfulness has an enduring influence on modern society, because of its capacity to create a refuge from pain not only within oneself but also outside, in the community, and in doing so, transform the culture of the sick into a culture of healing.

Bibliography

Arunlikhati. 2016. 'Be the Refuge'. *Be the Refuge.* December 16. https://medium.com/be-the-refuge/be-the-refuge-289870435744.

Barker, Kristin K. 2014. 'Mindfulness Meditation: Do-It-Yourself Medicalization of Every Moment'. *Social Science & Medicine* 106: 168–76. https://doi.org/10.1016/j.socscimed.2014.01.024.

Batchelor, Stephen. 2015. *After Buddhism: Rethinking the Dharma for a Secular Age.* New Haven: Yale University Press. https://doi.org/10.12987/9780300216226.

Bernhard, Toni. 2010. *How to Be Sick: A Buddhist-Inspired Guide for the Chronically Ill and Their Caregivers.* Boston: Wisdom Publications.

Birnbaum, Raoul. 1979. *The Healing Buddha.* Boulder, Colorado: Shambhala.

Cook, Joanna. 2016. 'Mindful in Westminster: The Politics of Meditation and the Limits of Neoliberal Critique'. *HAU: Journal of Ethnographic Theory* 6, no. 1: 141–61. https://doi.org/10.14318/hau6.1.011.

Data Bridge Market Research. 2022. *Asia-Pacific Meditation Market – Industry Trends and Forecast to 2029.* https://www.databridgemarketresearch.com/reports/asia-pacific-meditation-market.

Davidson, Richard J., and Antoine Lutz. 2008. 'Buddha's Brain: Neuroplasticity and Meditation'. *IEEE Signal Process Mag.* 25, no. 1: 174–76. http://doi.org/10.1109/msp.2008.4431873.

Dumes, Abigail A. 2020. *Divided Bodies: Lyme Disease, Contested Illness, and Evidence-Based Medicine.* London: Duke University Press. https://doi.org/10.2307/j.ctv15kxg1w.

Fleming, Crystal M., Veronica Y. Womack, and Jeffrey Proulx, eds. 2022. *Beyond White Mindfulness: Critical Perspectives on Racism.* New York: Routledge. https://doi.org/10.4324/9781003090922.

Foucault, Michel. 1982. 'Subject and Power'. *Critical Inquiry* 8, no. 4: 777–95. https://www.jstor.org/stable/1343197.

Foucault, Michel. 2009. *Security, Territory, Population: Lectures at the Collège de France 1977-78.* Edited by Michel Senellart. Translated by Graham Burchell. Houndsmill: Palgrave Macmillan.

Giddens, Anthony. 1990. *Modernity and Self-Identity: Self and Society in the Late Modern Age.* Cambridge: Polity Press.

Global Mindfulness Collaborative. 2024. 'Global Mindfulness Collaborative'. https://www.brown.edu/public-health/mindfulness/global-collaborative.

Han, Chenxing. 2021. *Be the Refuge: Raising the Voices of Asian American Buddhists.* Berkeley: North Atlantic Books.

Hanegraaff, Wouter J. 1996. *New Age Religion and Western Culture: Esotericism in the Mirror of Secular Thought.* Leiden: E. J. Brill. https://doi.org/10.1163/9789004378933.

Hanh, Thich Nhat. 1996. *Being Peace*. Berkeley: Parallax Press.

Hanson, Rick, and Richard Mendius. 2009. *Buddha's Brain: The Practical Neuroscience of Happiness, Love, and Wisdom.* Oakland, CA: New Harbinger.

Harris, Dan. 2014. *10% Happier: How I Tamed the Voice in My Head, Reduced Stress Without Losing My Edge, and Found Self-Help That Actually Works.* London: Hodders & Stoughton.

Harris, Dan. 2017. *Meditation for Fidgety Skeptics: A 10% Happier How-To Book.* London: Hodder & Stoughton.

Hendriks, Eric. 2017. *Life Advice from Below: The Public Role of Self-Help Coaches in Germany and China.* Boston: Brill.

ISBN. 2024. *ISBN Database.* https://isbndb.com/search/books/mindfulness?column=title&edition=&year=1999&language=.

Iwamura, Jane. 2010. *Virtual Orientalism: Asian Religions and American Popular Culture.* Oxford: Oxford University Press. https://doi.org/10.1093/acprof:oso/9780199738601.001.0001.

Jackson Nakazawa, Donna. 2013. *The Last Best Cure: My Quest to Awaken the Healing Parts of My Brain and Get Back My Body, My Joy, and My Life.* London: Penguin Books.

Kabat-Zinn, Jon. 1990. *Full Catastrophe Living: Using the Wisdom of Your Body and Mind to Face Stress, Pain, and Illness.* New York: Delta Trade.

Kabat-Zinn, Jon. 2003. 'Mindfulness-Based Interventions in Context: Past, Present, and Future'. *Clinical Psychology Science and Practice* 10, no. 2: 144–56. http://doi.org/10.1093/clipsy.bpg016.

Kabat-Zinn, Jon. 2011. 'Some Reflections on the Origins of MBSR: Skilful Means and the Trouble with Maps'. *Contemporary Buddhism* 12, no. 1: 206–81. http://doi.org/10.1080/14639947.2011.56484410.

Kabat-Zinn, Jon. 2017. Foreword to *Zhengnian jianya de xunlian Fengxing quanqiu Hafo yixueyuan Google Maikengxi Pingguo dou zai yong* 正念減壓的訓練：風行

全球、哈佛醫學院、Google、麥肯錫、蘋果都在用 [Training in Mindfulness and Stress Reduction: Trending Around the World, Used by Harvard Medical School, Google, McKinsey and Apple], by Te Chung Chen. Taiwan: Fang Zhi Press.

Li, Pan. 2023. '*Cong dongfang chuandao xifang you huidao dongfang Xijiao-Liwupudaxue zhengnianzhong de dansheng* 从东方传到西方, 又回到东方: 西交利物浦大学正念中心的诞生' [From the East to the West, and back to the East: The Birth of the Xi'an Jiao-tong Liverpool University Mindfulness Centre]. In *Mindfulness-Based Stress Reduction Work Professionals' Experience* [*Zhengnian jianya kecheng congyezhe gongzuo xinde* 正念减压课程从业者工作心得], edited by Li Pan, Wang Susu, and Nie Chongbin. Shanghai: Shanghai Jiao Tong University Press. Kindle.

Li, Shangqing. 2014. *Ganjue leile jiu mingxiangba Mingxiang shifenzhong dengyu shushui liangxiaoshi* 感觉累了, 就冥想吧: 冥想十分钟等于熟睡两小时 [If You Feel Tried, Meditate]. Harbin: Northern China Literature and Art Publishing House.

Lott, Dylan. 2016. 'From Interiority to Inner Territory: Tibetan Buddhism, Neuroscience, and the Politics of Representation'. PhD thesis, University of Illinois.

Madsen, Ole Jacob. 2014. *Optimizing the Self: Social Representations of Self-Help.* New York: Routledge. https://doi.org/10.4324/9781315693866.

Matsuyama, Daiko, and Yuka Shimada. 2018. '*Maindofurunesu wa seichō yokkyū o sageru no ka* マインドフルネスは成長欲求を下げるのか' [Does Mindfulness Reduce the Desire for Growth?]. *President Woman.* 23 February. https://president.jp/articles/-/24416?page=2.

Nehring, Daniel, Emmanuel Alvarado, Eric C. Hendriks, and Dylan Kerrigan. 2016. *Transnational Popular Psychology and the Global Self-Help Industry: The Politics of Contemporary Social Change.* New York: Palgrave Macmillan. https://doi.org/10.1057/9780230370869.

Nehring, Daniel, and Ashley Frawley. 2020. 'Mindfulness and the "Psychological Imagination"'. *Sociology of Health & Illness* 42, no. 5: 1184–201. http://doi.org/10.1111/1467-9566.13093.

Nghiem, Sister Dang. 2015. *Mindfulness as Medicine: A Story of Healing Body and Spirit.* Berkeley: Parallax.

Oxford English Dictionary. 2023. 'Demystify, v.'. *Oxford English Dictionary Online.* Oxford University Press. https://www.oed.com/view/Entry/49897?redirectedFrom=demystify&.

Pickert, Kate. 2014. 'The Mindful Revolution'. *Time*, February 3: 34–38.

Ramachandran, V.S., and L. Oberman. 2009. 'Reflections on the Mirror Neuron System: Their Evolutionary Functions Beyond Motor Representation'. In *Mirror Neuron Systems: The Role of Mirroring Processes in Social Cognition*, edited by Jaime A. Pineda, 39–62. Totowa: Humana Press. https://doi.org/10.1007/978-1-59745-479-7_2.

Roald, Audun E. 2012. 'Cerebral selvhjelp [Cerebral Self-Help]'. *Tidsskrift for Norsk Psykologforening* 49, no. 8: 766–70.
Rose, Nikolas. 2007. *The Politics of Life Itself: Biomedicine, Power, and Subjectivity in the Twenty-First Century.* New Jersey: Princeton University Press.
Said, Edward W. 2003. *Orientalism.* London: Penguin Books.
Squier, Susan M. 2004. 'Meditation, Disability, and Identity'. *Literature and Medicine* 23, no. 1: 23–45. https://doi.org/10.1353/lm.2004.0012.
Suh, Sharon. 2019. *Occupy This Body: A Buddhist Memoir.* Ottawa: Sumaru Press Inc.
Thera, Nyanaponika. 1962. *Heart of Buddhist Meditation.* London: Rider & Co.
Varela, Francisco J., Evan Thompson, and Eleanor Rosch. 2016. *The Embodied Mind: Cognitive Science and Human Experience.* Cambridge, MA: MIT Press. https://doi.org/10.7551/mitpress/6730.001.0001.
Waldron, William S. 2017. 'Reflections on Indian Buddhist Thought and the Scientific Study of Meditation, or: Why Scientists Should Talk More with Their Buddhist Subjects'. In *Meditation, Buddhism, and Science*, by David McMahan and Erik Braun, 84–113. Oxford: Oxford University Press.
Wax, Ruby. 2013. *Sane New World.* London: Penguin Books.
Wax, Ruby. 2016. *A Mindfulness Guide for the Frazzled.* London: Penguin Books.
Wilson, Jeff. 2014. *Mindful America: Meditation and the Mutual Transformation of Buddhism and American Culture.* Oxford: Oxford University Press. https://doi.org/10.1093/acprof:oso/9780199827817.001.0001.
Xu, Shousen. 2021. Foreword to *Yongbao nide yiyu qingxu Ziwo liaoyu de jiuda zhengnian jiqiao* 拥抱你的抑郁情绪：自我疗愈的九大正念技巧 [The Mindfulness and Acceptance Workbook for Depression: Using Acceptance and Commitment Therapy to Move Through Depression and Create a Life Worth Living (Embrace Your Depressive Emotions: Nine Mindfulness Self-healing Techniques)] by Kirk Strosahl and Patricia Robinson. Translated by Xu Shousen. Beijing: China Machine Press.
Yang, Larry. 2017. *Awakening Together: The Spiritual Practice of Inclusivity and Community.* Somerville, MA: Wisdom Publications.
Yang, Jie. 2017. *Mental Health in China: Psychologization and Therapeutic Governance.* Maiden, MA: Polity.
Zhang, Li. 2020. *Anxious China: Inner Revolution and Politics of Psychotherapy.* Oakland: University of California Press.

Biography

Christina Lee is a Research Associate for the 'Disability Matters' project at the University of Sheffield and an Honorary Research Fellow at University

College London. She completed her PhD in English and Medical Humanities at King's College London. Her research focuses on self-care, narratives of healing, and intersectional approaches to illness and disability.

Part 3

Alternative Therapies Across Epistemic Fields and Professions

When discussing the professionalisation, institutionalisation and other kinds of systematisation that allow the therapies analysed in this book to be taught and practised within established frameworks of care, the discursive alternativity of these therapies in comparison to other types of care tends to take centre stage. Indeed, while commentators often note how these therapies need to abide by wider standards of practice, they also frequently assume that their practice presents challenges to these standards, thus turning their alternative character into both a quality and a defect. Indeed, discussions about the systemisation of alternative therapies make at least two wrong assumptions: 1) they assume that the systems into which these therapies are implemented are devoid of controversies, and 2) they presume that this systemisation is uniform. It helps, however, to consider how more 'mainstream' fields of care, such as that of psychiatry, have had and continue to experience similar issues of systematisation that even lead them to question their very purpose.

In her detailed history of American psychiatry's efforts to define a biological mission for itself, Anne Harrington describes a variety of influential factors: the two world wars, idiosyncratic leaders, such as Adolph Meyer (1866–1950), and a stint of discriminatory ideologies that pervaded contemporaneous society and the pharmaceutical discoveries of the 1950s, from ableism and racism to sexism. By doing this, she demonstrates that there cannot be a linear understanding of how, time after time, psychiatry came to declare itself the new expert on every mental suffering (Harrington

2019, xvi). The three chapters in this section offer similar glimpses into the pluralistic and localised development of the therapies they respectively analyse. While the 'value' of these therapies as 'East Asian'-inspired or 'East Asian'-based may seem to define their entry into (or legitimisation among) specific systems of care, idiosyncratic practitioners, socio-legal contexts that often inadvertently work for or against them, and the quintessential strive of all therapies to be *particularly holistic* – namely to present a simple cure for as wide an array of ailments as possible – play an equally significant role. After all, alternative therapies are, first of all, therapies.

Harrington, Anne. 2019. *Mind Fixers: Psychiatry's Trouble Search for the Biology of Mental Illness*. New York: W.W. Norton.

7 A Collaboration Between Mother and Baby

Sophrology in a Japanese Maternity Clinic and the Making of Medical Knowledge

Pamela Runestad

Abstract: Sophrology has been conceptualised as a method to facilitate patient entry into a psychological state that would improve the efficacy of other health interventions. In this chapter, I describe how sophrology is used in a birth clinic in Japan as a case study. Additionally, I describe how sophrology is explained by three types of Anglophone writers. I argue that sophrology in these contexts is not different from the circulation of scholarly ideas and medical technologies in general, where ideas intermingle and are remade, but that the Anglophone publications on sophrology highlighted here provide clear examples of exotification of Asia. While the adoption of sophrology in Japan may suggest some level of occidentalism, it certainly leads to more questions about how various stakeholders value it. In exploring these points, I demonstrate the need for a critical-reflexive bricolage, whereby readers and writers consider not just who needs to be cited for their audiences but why and how, in order to avoid exoticism and appropriation.

Keywords: Japan, sophrology, maternity, transnational ideologies, exoticism, critical-reflexive bricolage

Scholars of health and medicine have long recognised movements and articulations of ideas about the body and theories of health and disease across space and time. Common examples include relationships between Islamic and Greek medical texts (Good and DelVecchio Good 1992), the prevalence and variety of humoral theories in medical knowledge around the world

Gaitanidis, Ioannis, Luis Fernando Bernardi Junqueira, Avery Morrow, and Sangyun Han (eds), *Therapy, Spirituality, and East Asian Imaginaries.* Taylor & Francis Group 2025
DOI: 10.5117/9789048559015_CH07

(Horden and Hsu 2013), and shifts in perceptions about human anatomy in Japan due to Chinese and Dutch influences at different times (Kuriyama 1992). Such examples demonstrate that the production of knowledge is social and dynamic: it is an ongoing, never-ending process that occurs through interactions and flows of people and ideas rather than something that is static. Knowledge production is also cultural: what is known and how it is shared or used is contextual, associative, and shaped by what is accepted by stakeholders at a given moment. But as critical theories have gained prominence, questions about intellectual property and the ownership of ideas have come into stark relief: the tendency for humans to be constant bricoleurs makes identifying who influenced whom a complicated endeavour that is bound up with power and essentialism that can take the forms of ethnocentrism and exoticism (such as orientalism and occidentalism). Classroom discussions, for example, may include attempts to parse appreciation (respectful use of the knowledge of others through citation or acknowledgement) from appropriation (which is often described as a form of neocolonialism, 'Columbusing', or outright theft) (Zhen 2019). While it is important to acknowledge contributions to knowledge production and the power relations in which they are made, dichotomisation runs the risk of oversimplification and directs attention away from questions about why particular ideas are attractive at particular times and among specific groups in the first place. In this chapter, I discuss the use of sophrology techniques in a Japanese maternity clinic, adopting it as a case study to illustrate how scholars might conceptualise transnational knowledge flows in the era of critical theories, critical pedagogies, and rapid digital flows by practising what I call critical-reflexive bricolage.

Ideas in Motion: Introducing Caycedo and Sophrology

Alfonso Caycedo (1932–2017) was a Colombian-born psychiatrist who earned his degrees and practised in Spain (Caycedo Institute, n.d.). Caycedo has gained acclaim, particularly in Europe, for developing sophrology in 1960 (Caycedo Institute, n.d.). In a seminal work, Caycedo (1964) described the need to engage in a type of psychosomatic medical practice that acknowledges connections between body and mind and retains a sceptical position towards pharmaceuticalisation. He explained sophrology with references to Greek roots: *Sos* (safety, tranquillity, security, serenity); *Phren* (mind); and *Logos* (treatise, study) (Caycedo 1964, 103). sophrology is now termed 'the study of consciousness in balance' by his legacy organisation, Sophrocay (which was previously the Caycedo Institute) (n.d.). Caycedo referenced European influences such as Husserl's phenomenology, ideas from Kraepelin's Munich School of psychiatry and hypnosis, and research by Swiss researcher Ludwig Binswanger (Caycedo 1964, 103), Additionally, Caycedo referenced influence from 'relaxation techniques and Oriental systems of concentrations such as yoga, Zen, and its derivatives which have been practised for millennia' (Caycedo 1964, 103). There are indications that Caycedo elaborated on how his experiences with yoga and Zen influenced particular steps or components of sophrologic processes in lectures or trainings, most notably captured in English explanations of sophrology applied to pedagogy by W. Jane Bancroft in 1982, who cites both scholarship in French and her notes from attending a four-day seminar by Caycedo in 1979. Caycedo's contemporary and collaborator, Isaac Gubel (1967), referred to sophrology as a method for encouraging patients to retreat into themselves into a trance-like or hypnotic-like state that allows them to change how they experience outside stimuli and bodily sensations, thereby enabling 're-education' or 're-orientation' through psychotherapy. In other words, sophrology, in its nascent form, was a means to put patients into a state in which they would be more likely to benefit from psychotherapy: it was a tool to facilitate psychotherapeutic outcomes. Caycedo founded the Caycedo Institute in 1991, where he continued to refine and utilise sophrology. More recently, Caycedo's daughter Natalia Caycedo, also a psychiatrist, assumed the primary role at the Caycedo Institute, now Sofrocay, in Spain, in 2010 (Caycedo Institute n.d.).

As will be described in detail below, various sources – lay publications, sophrology websites, and health science scholarship alike – describe Alfonso Caycedo's development of sophrology as a kind of East-meets-West philosophy that he developed through experiences traveling to India, Tibet, and Japan and engagement with yoga and Buddhist meditation. Notably, Sophrocay currently does not include this information on its website, nor does it refer explicitly to the practices above. Rather, Sophrocay seems to have shifted from such references and instead describes sophrology as 'personal training based on relaxation techniques and activation of the body and mind' with attention to consciousness, body perception, and the body-mind relationship (Caycedo Institute n.d.). Current practitioners state sophrology combines meditation, concentration, visualisation, breathing techniques, and movements into a 'discipline that reshapes techniques into a structured approach' to confront pain, stress, and anxiety and achieve a sense of relaxed alertness (Malina 2011).

Since its debut, sophrology has enjoyed popularity in Spain, France, and Switzerland in particular, where it has been used in settings ranging from education and sports to medicine since the 1970s (Moreau et al 2020; Romieu et al 2017; Caycedo Institute n.d.). It is considered a possible method to alleviate stress, anxiety, and pain that may improve general wellbeing and specific health outcomes. Sophrology practitioners credit Dorna Wilson-Revie for translating sophrology practices for an Anglophone audience in 2006 (Malina 2011), but as noted above, Bancroft has written about sophrology in scholarly publications in English since the 1980s. The emergence of sophrology websites in English seems to indicate that sophrology's presence is growing in the UK and making inroads in the United States as a professional qualification attained through courses, a technique to be used in daily life by everyday people and as a therapeutic element that can be incorporated into medical treatment plans. A PubMed search for 'sophrology' in English (one term only) yielded 113 sources, the vast majority of which are in French, Spanish, Italian, and German. Only 25 were in English and just six of those were focused on labour and childbirth. The majority of the English sources – regardless of where in the world the research was conducted – were written in the past decade.

Interestingly, a search of the Japanese database CiNii for sophrology (one term) yields 56 sources published between 1988 and 2020, the vast majority of which are about birth practices in Japan. Such investigations indicate that, in the past few years, sophrology has been taken up in the medical settings of Japan, South Korea, and China. To summarise, it appears that Caycedo, a Colombian-born psychiatrist trained in Spain, developed a philosophy and method of practice that grew out of his academic training in Europe and experiences in Asia that he termed sophrology (for a similar example of transnational flows, cf. Chapter 4). Sophrology was taken up in Europe first and has more recently been incorporated into medical research and practice in East Asia – and specifically for use during labour and delivery in Japan.

It is fairly common for Japanese medical practitioners to read medical literature in English, and sometimes in German or French. When I visited the hospital down the street from the maternity clinic, issues of *The New England Journal of Medicine* and *The Lancet* lined the bookshelf of the physicians' lounge. From 2003 to 2006, I worked with a group of Japanese physicians who employed me to revise English-language versions of articles they planned to submit for publication or present at conferences where the primary language was English, in addition to practising how to discuss case studies in English. Given that context, it is not surprising that obstetrician Matsunaga Akira (松永昭) thus learned about sophrology in Paris (where it had been applied to childbirth starting in 1972) in 1987 and started the Japan Sophrology Association shortly after (JSA n.d.). On the Association's website, the 'international' nature of sophrology – as something from Europe and circulating in America – is highlighted.

Drawing from ethnographic work conducted in 2013 and 2016 in a maternity clinic in central Japan where sophrology is practised and a review of English language literature in PubMed, I demonstrate that cases like the use of sophrology in a Japanese maternity clinic complicate simple dichotomies of appreciation and appropriation, orientalism and occidentalism, and professional epistemologies versus the lay public's ways of knowing. I argue that Caycedo's professional training in psychiatry and travel experiences in 'the East' are sometimes collapsed and uncritically circulated in the three Anglophone spheres where his work is most often used: in web publications by media influencers interested in wellness, in websites of practising sophrologists and in health science research. Moreover, sophrology becomes a mode of exoticism, depending on whether writers in Europe focus on its 'Asian' influences or writers in Asia focus on its European roots. Finally, I return to the case study of sophrology in a Japanese birth clinic (outlined below) to demonstrate how using a framework I call 'critical-reflexive bricolage' can help scholars and students discern how the tensions between these ideas can be usefully explored so that we can consider how and why particular ideas about health and wellbeing are circulated and rearticulated to fit evolving ways of being in an increasingly critically oriented transnational milieu. As the editors of this volume point out, perhaps it is not so much the origins of a practice or information themselves but the narration of origins as context-dependent associations that is more instructive about how people attempt to engage with and legitimise particular forms of knowledge. This has implications for research, teaching, and general media consumption.

Case Study: Labour in a Japanese Sophrology Clinic

'Call the clinic when you notice labour has begun', the midwives told a room of expectant parents during a parenting workshop. 'When contractions are five to ten minutes apart, you should come here for the next stages of labour'. This advice, and the first hours of labour at this Nagano clinic, are similar to medical practices elsewhere. Upon arrival, labouring women are checked in and examined. They labour – breathing strategically and with intention – supported by partners and nursing staff. In some ways, the breathing encouraged in early labour is akin to breathing techniques where rhythmic breathing is a mechanism to block out (Lamaze) or cope with (Bradley) the rhythmic pain of contractions (Tournaire and Theau-Yonneau 2007).

There are a number of differences that make labouring at this local clinic stand out, however. Labouring mothers often move through different spaces in the clinic as they progress through the stages of labour rather than stay in one place: they begin in the larger wardroom, move to a private room to labour with the midwife and finally move to the delivery room when delivery is imminent. The clinic offers no epidurals or other pharmaceutical means of pain relief. While in the ward, women may be treated with a leg or back massage with essential oils by the nursing staff to facilitate relaxation and alleviate pain. In private rooms, women may be encouraged to eat and drink in order to keep up their strength and hydration for the last stage of labour – something that is considered controversial in some settings due to a fear of aspiration should the woman need to undergo an emergency caesarean (Maharaj 2009). The midwives, who coach the labouring women through labour pains through controlled breathing, may also help alleviate pain with massage or show family members how to do it. Changing positions may also be part of the efforts to mitigate pain. Visualisation and music come into play in the delivery room.

There are also differences between the clinic delivery room and the bright, white, noisy hospital labour and delivery unit nearby: although the clinic's delivery room is equipped with a labouring bed and surgical instruments should such instruments be needed, it is darkened and soft music – just one song – plays on a loop. The music is from a sophrology CD that patients are given at the first of their 'parent workshops' (discussed below). By the time they arrive in the room, women have theoretically been listening to and completing visualisation and breathing exercises along with the music for months. Thus, playing this music in the background in the delivery room, in the relative dark, is a means to help the labouring woman achieve what sophrology practitioners call a state of 'relaxed alertness' in which they calmly focus and work with their baby through a midwife-assisted birth using the breathing and visualisation they have been practising. The physician generally only attends the birth and is present to 'catch' the baby, stitch up the mother if needed if she tears, or perform an emergency caesarean.

The brother-sister pair of physicians that owns and operates this clinic has been practising sophrology-informed obstetrics since the early 2000s. Their 17-bed practice has been in their family for three generations. They report that, to the best of their knowledge, theirs is the only clinic in the region that has taken up sophrology. The breathing and visualisation techniques taught to women in the childbirth workshops and used during births at this clinic are based on guided imagery paired with music, which was introduced to Japan by Dr Akira Matsunaga of the Japan Sophrology Association (Suzuki et al 2012). In a personal conversation, the clinic physicians explained to me that they chose to implement sophrology because of the female physician's personal experiences with the birth of her first child:

> As a new physician, I encouraged my patients to *gambare* [persevere] and work hard through their labours. After I had my first baby, I was so tired and sore from clenching my muscles I couldn't even hold my baby. And after that I felt bad for all my previous patients. I thought there had to be a better way. So, we looked and looked and we found sophrology and decided to try it. I had my next baby that way. And here we are.

An important point to make at this juncture is that the shift to sophrology is a shift from advising women what to expect during birth to teaching them how to train for it so that they would feel better during and after birth. This is slightly different from goals such as mitigating pain, reducing interventions, or improving maternal/neonatal outcomes that clinical researchers might have had in mind when investigating the merits of sophrology, as is discussed below. Additionally, birth is highlighted within pregnancy and motherhood and not necessarily treated as a discrete event; moreover, the primary focus is not necessarily on pain. Overall, sophrological training throughout pregnancy to improve labour and birth experiences (and not simply outcomes) is part of this clinic's theory, practice, and self-narrative.

Below, I elucidate other narratives circulating about sophrology, noting how they illustrate interest in the 'familiar-strange' by various stakeholders. At the end of the chapter, I return to this case study to demonstrate the importance of investigating how such narratives become social facts as opposed to simply accepting them as 'facts'.

Narrating Caycedo and Sophrology: Examples from 3 Genres in English

As noted above, sophrology is better known and more frequently practised in western Europe, particularly in Spain, France, and Switzerland, than in Asia and other parts of the world. This is likely due to Caycedo's location of practice, professional connections, and dominant languages of these places. To a lesser degree, mention of sophrology can be found in three distinct spheres in English with reference to practice around the world:

the general media, trade and lay publications, websites maintained by practising sophrologists, and health science research. When viewed side by side, it is clear that writers from all three spheres describe Caycedo's background and explanations of sophrology using similar phraseology in English that highlight its 'Asian' influences, regardless of writers' goals, disciplines or audiences; there are also obvious overlaps in these spheres that facilitate this. This complexity suggests that there is something about the associations these writers make about places that they hope provides legitimacy to Caycedo, sophrology, and their own endeavours (practice or research), even if those associations seem problematic, superficial, and/or appropriative from a humanities, social science, or area studies perspective. Although it would be fascinating to explore these associations in each of these languages, because of my own linguistic limitations and the limitations of this chapter, I explore only the English-language publications with regard to how Caycedo and sophrology are introduced and what its uses are.

Lay and Trade Publications

According to Michelle Botes of Switzerland-based Age-well.org (n.d.), 'Sophrology is a science that combines the Western philosophies of psychiatry and psychotherapy with Eastern philosophies of Yoga, Zen and Buddhism'. She states Caycedo was motivated to find better ways to treat war victims from World War II and highlights the work he did with Swiss psychiatrist Ludwig Binswanger and Swiss physician Raymond Abrezol. Botes also notes Wilson-Revie's efforts to bring sophrology to English speakers and that most English speakers do not know what sophrology is but asserts that most French and Swiss nationals do.

Emma Ledger (2017) of *The Guardian* offers a somewhat similar explication of sophrology, stating that it is a set of self-development techniques that use 'mental and physical exercises to try to achieve an alert mind in a relaxed body [that] combines mediation, breathing, relaxation [...] movement and visualization'. Like Botes, Ledger goes on to explain that Caycedo developed sophrology after 'he spent decades exploring yoga, Tibetan Buddhist meditation, hypnosis, and Japanese Zen [...] [and] the resulting philosophy sits at the crossroads between western relaxation and eastern meditation'.

Dancing Times writer Debbie Malina (2011, 34) states that sophrology encompasses 'yoga, hypnotherapy, and guided meditation' and therefore uses 'elements of both eastern and western traditions'. Like Botes, she also notes connections to Dr Abrezol and the plethora of French resources on sophrology compared to the dearth of those in English until Wilson-Revie translated sophrology methods.

All three writers attempt to associate the development of sophrology with Caycedo's travels to and experiences in Asia. One interpretation of these explanations is that associations with Asian countries (India, Tibet, and Japan) and bodily practices (breathing and meditation in yoga), and with religious frameworks (including Zen, which is separated from Buddhism by Botes), are all collapsed into a vague and exoticised set of 'Eastern traditions', an imagined Orientalist complement of spirituality to an equally ethnocentric 'West' grounded in science (cf. Chapters 5 and 8). Written this way, Caycedo's travels give him experiences that allow him to overcome Cartesian dualism which could not be done with European psychiatry and phenomenology alone. Sophrology becomes a method to treat modern European illness and rediscover a type of spirituality that Asians have been perceived to have had all along – while simultaneously ignoring scientific bodies of knowledge in Asia. The promise of something familiar with something 'new' may appeal to readers. When Botes indicates that the French and the Swiss know more about sophrology than English speakers, she plays on historic rivalries between Anglophones and Francophones that further complicate this collapse and fan the flames of competitive exoticism. Not only is it something familiar with something 'new'; there is an element of 'keeping up with' or being 'better than', with little attention to why such endeavours matter or what is at stake in engaging in them.

It is worth noting that although they use similar phrases and explanations, these writers' assessments of sophrology do differ. Botes (n.d.) seems convinced that sophrology is a 'natural way' to combat stress in general and that sophrology can 'train your mind to become happier and stronger'. Malina (2011, 35) advocates more specific uses, stating that dancers can use sophrology to deal with pain, overcome addiction, and cope with body image issues. Ledger (2017) is less convinced of the staying power of sophrology, calling it 'the new mindfulness' and 'the next buzzword answer to all our problems'. Regardless of these differences, the seeming need for these writers to associate Caycedo and sophrology with Asian places, practices, and traditions seems to indicate that for them the use of exotic references is an effective way to draw in readers. It could also be true that these associations were a draw for these writers, too.

As I show below, the writers highlighted in this section are likely not the origins of these associations; nor are they the only ones to employ them. While that does not nullify points of exoticism, it does complicate simple explanations and accusations of appropriation, raising questions about the responsibility of writers and readers and the uncritical consumption of information.

Practitioner Websites

The websites of sophrology institutes and practitioners typically include information about Caycedo and their versions of the history of sophrology. There are some recurring descriptions about origins on these websites and, as stated above, there are some direct connections between the three spheres I parse out here. Below, I describe three major websites, compare the phraseology, and indicate where their influence on writers like Ledger, Botes, and Malina appear. It is important to note that the purpose of these websites is to promote sophrology, but there is a proprietary framework employed because readers are potential patient-clients, or even future sophrology practitioners. Exact methods of sophrology remain opaque even when components such as meditation or visualisation are listed, for example. Some include testimonials like an everyday product.

The Sophrology Institute in the UK was founded by Philip Carr-Gomm, who trained with Dorna Revie – the woman credited by practitioners with introducing sophrology into English. He works with three other practitioners who offer courses and sell publications on sophrology. There are clear definitions of sophrology and a short bio of Caycedo on this website:

> Sophrology means, literally, "the study of Science of Harmonious Consciousness," and comes from three Greek words: *sos* (harmonious, serene), *phren* (consciousness) and *logos* (study, science). It's a fusion of techniques drawn from *modern western neuroscience and psychology* with methods used by the *ancient wisdom traditions of the east.* Sophrology uses visualization, simple postures and physical movement, combined with attention to breathing and awareness, to deeply relax the body and mind, while also introducing a sense of vitality and stimulating the cognitive functions, such as memory, imagination and concentration. *Inspired by Yoga, Buddhism, Zen, Neuroscience and Phenomenology, it offers a path of self-development as well as specific methods for improving the quality of life.* (The Sophrology Institute n.d., italics added)

Caycedo's travels to India and Japan (without reference to specialists there) and interests in hypnotism and yoga are highlighted along with his training in psychological phenomenology alongside Viktor Frankl, Ludwig Binswanger, and Sigmund Freud. There are no citations for these, but it seems likely that this information was drawn from Caycedo's publications (the definition is similar to that found in his 1964 publication) or transmitted from Caycedo to Revie to Carr-Gromm via training. Through the website, one can sign up for courses or purchase sophrology materials, and there are a number of exercises and videos. There are no testimonials.

Be-Sophro.com (n.d.) is a blog maintained by sophrology practitioner Dominique Antiglio in the UK. She states that she trained directly with Caycedo. Antiglio writes, 'created from *both Eastern practices and Western science,* sophrology uniquely combines breathing, dynamic relaxation, gentle movement, medication, and visualization techniques' (italics added). According to Antiglio, Caycedo studied Johannes Heinrich Schultz's work on autogenic training and researched alongside Ludwig Binswanger. She states that Caycedo travelled with his yoga-teacher wife to 'India, Japan and Nepal for 2 years to study how Yoga and its asanas, Yoga of sound, meditation and contemplation, Zen and Tibetan meditation, and some of the philosophies behind these practices were positively influencing consciousness'. On another page of this website, she states that 'Caycedo drew from his experience as a neuropsychiatrist, his studies in Greek philosophy, phenomenology and autogenic training, and his travels to India, Tibet and Japan to study yoga, Zen and Buddhism'. Online courses and Audio exercises are available, and there are a number of testimonials as well. Again, the sources of information are likely Caycedo's early articles and/or Antiglio's training.

There are some discrepancies between places Caycedo purportedly visited (even within the same site), and the two sites offer somewhat different information, but the overall message is very similar: sophrology is a combination of 'East' and 'West' that is a product of Caycedo's (Western) training and (Eastern) travels. The names of European scholars are highlighted, while the only reference to an actual yoga practitioner is Caycedo's own wife (who is also not named), which privileges Western epistemologies over Asian expertise. The associative currency of sophrology-Caycedo- 'Asia' seems operative: such combinations are not just interdisciplinary but also point to a 'worldliness' or 'international' perspective of health: Asian contributions (glossed as they are) provide a special draw. Questions arise about the need for practitioners to highlight such connections without giving a more nuanced explanation of sophrology or Caycedo's experiences. Did he train or study with practitioners during his travels? If so, with whom, and why are his scholarly engagements with European specialists highlighted, while Asian contributors are not? Is this a limitation in Caycedo's or sophrologists' transmission of such information, or is it more about perceptions about what Western audiences are familiar with and would care about? In what context would the intellectual contributions of specific Asian practitioners and traditions be considered important? Are the mere mention of the places and traditions all that is perceived to be important for practitioner audiences (for similar reflections, cf. Chapters 4 and 5)?

Some of the information Botes, Ledger, and Malina share about the origins of sophrology seems to have been drawn from these sophrology practitioner websites. Ledger explicitly mentions Dominique Antiglio of the UK-based Be-Sophro.com. Malina interviewed Florence Parot of the UK-based Sophrology Academy and includes information about the International Sophrology Federation in Geneva, where Wilson-Revie was associated. Malina (2011) refers to sophrology's incorporation of 'eastern and western traditions [to enable the] body and mind to operate in harmony', so it's likely that she is drawing directly from these sources. Botes offers no citations or sources, but the 'Zen and Buddhism' construct she uses suggests familiarity with sources such as these.

Interestingly, the Sophrocay website includes none of these explicit references to Asia. Instead of references to yoga and Buddhism similar to those that Caycedo himself used, the Sophrocay website (Caycedo Institute for the English site) highlights Natalia Caycedo's professional training in medicine and psychiatry, her ties to the founder (Alfonso Caycedo is her father), and their efforts to be scientific, international, and multidisciplinary – the 'authentic' version of sophrology. The Sophrocay definition removes place-based references: 'Sophrology is a personal training based on relaxation techniques and activation of the body and mind. It is based on the observation and study of consciousness, body perception, and the body-mind relationship, as well as their influence on lifestyle' (Caycedo Institute n.d.). The website contains testimonials, links to publications, and sign-ups for courses. Sofrocay, the Caycedo Method, and Caycedo Dynamic Relaxation are all trademarked. The website also includes the scientific articles that Sofrocay practitioners have published. Here, sophrology is a way of life, a therapeutic method, a topic of scientific research, and a family business.

One interpretation of the shift in emphases is that while Alfonso Caycedo (1964) wrote about his travels alongside his training, and seems to have described to his students how he was influenced by his travels (Bancroft 1982), Sophrocay under Natalia Caycedo has made efforts to de-emphasise past explanations that played up stereotyped dichotomies. And yet, the movement away from such characterisations is also complicated. It would be possible to argue that, rather than erase associations with Asian places, practices, and traditions that were once core to Caycedo's explanations, it would be better to explicate them in an effort to do justice to them. In other words, the erasure of the inspirations of sophrology could be interpreted as appropriation. Questions remain: which is more problematic, using thin references to inspirations that may be perceived as Columbusing or Orientalism, or not providing references for inspiration at all and risking accusations of appropriation – particularly when Alfonso Caycedo made such linkages so central to his work in the past? Is there an in-between? Does that depend on who the audience is perceived to be and the purposes or goals of the organisation?

Health Science Research

From an academic perspective, it is perhaps unsurprising that the associations with Asia would be made uncritically as described above; but similar associations show up in academic sources, particularly in the health sciences literature as well. In the sections below, I first review the uses of sophrology in the medical literature and then examine uncritical sourcing.

Recall that sophrology was originally conceptualised as a way to help patients enter a state that would facilitate their treatment in psychotherapy (Caycedo 1964, Gubels 1967). More recently, applications of sophrology include attempts to alleviate stress and anxiety, which could be an end in and of itself: less stressed, less anxious people may have a better quality of life (on similar health issues, cf. Chapter 6). Based on a study of 70 participants over a four-week intensive sophrology training period, Natalie Caycedo and colleagues argue that sophrology can be used to reduce anxiety and depression (van Rangelrooij et al 2020). Additionally, other teams have shown interest in examining whether sophrology, through various relaxation techniques, can lead to better patient outcomes, either because patients need fewer interventions or because patients report a reduction in perceptions of pain or improved experiences. This is very similar to the way it was leveraged to improve psychotherapy outcomes: sophrology becomes a tool to facilitate biomedical treatments. Research teams have explored using sophrology for asthma, cancer, cystic fibrosis, fibromyalgia, heart disease, and tinnitus in addition to applications for dentistry and childbirth. I discuss a select few of these publications below.

Bertrand et al. (2018, 6) report that patients who underwent sophrologic training before radiology procedures experienced decreased stress, anxiety, and pain compared to the control group. Moreover, the reduction in patient stress seemed to result in calmer breathing and fewer sudden movements during procedures, which made it easier for practitioners to access deep lesions and resulted in fewer complications. Romieu et al. (2017) applied sophrology to children with severe asthma and found that although there were no differences between the sophrology and test group with regard to hospitalisation time, medication requirements, or quality of life scores, shortness of breath improved with sophrologic training. Similarly, de Almeida Silva et al. (2019) found that sophrology contributed to improvements of patients with fibromyalgia in terms of their physical resistance, social aspects of health, general health, and pain, but that resistance training was more effective for improving strength and functional capacity than sophrology. Essentially, using sophrology in these settings functioned as an adjuvant: a strategy that could be used to support but not replace an evidence-based biomedical treatment for a specific physiological condition.

A number of studies report the benefits of sophrology in pregnancy, labour, and postpartum care. Betegon et al. (2017) report that sophrology reduced anxiety in a group of Spanish pregnant mothers with small-for-gestational-age foetuses and increased birth weights. Three teams based in East Asia sought to explore how sophrology could be used to ameliorate pain and improve birth outcomes for both mothers and infants. Labour contractions and pain can lead to hyperventilation and an increase in blood pH, which in turn could result in a reduced transfer of nutrients and oxygen to the foetus during labour (Kim et al 2008). In theory, breath control and anxiety control via sophrology could therefore improve birth outcomes both for mothers in terms of experience and for infants in terms of birth outcomes. Bonapace et al. (2018) acknowledge the connection between physical and psychological components of labour pains and advocate for a holistic approach to preventing the suffering of labouring women that includes nonpharmacological options such as sophrology.

In a study of 138 women split into a test and a control group, the researchers noted that there were no statistically significant differences between the groups because of the sample sizes, but women who underwent sophrology were less likely to require oxytocin and had lower blood pH levels; neonates had a lower level of acidaemia (Kim et al 2008). Liu and Hu (2019) found in their study of Chinese patients that a blend of sophrology-Lamaze-Kegel training improved delivery experiences and decreased haemorrhage volume at birth; improved pelvic floor function, decreased incidence of depression, and increased sexual function in mothers post-birth; neonates had both higher birth weights and higher Apgar scores. Suzuki et al. (2012) found that women in a sophrology-assisted group had lower amounts of biopyrrin in their urine, which the team was observing as a measure of stress. Overall, the application of sophrology to pregnancy and birth in the English literature indicates that sophrology may be used to support positive birth outcomes for women and infants in general.

As noted above, physicians in my field site chose sophrology to improve patients' experiences during and just after birth. But just what constitutes improved experiences and how such perceptions are related to clinical outcomes is murky and will be the subject of my next inquiries. Additionally, it will be interesting to see if clinical research conducted on this topic in East Asia continues to grow in English and Japanese: there have only been 10 publications in the past 10 years in Japanese. However, more careful review of these sources reveals that although biomedical researchers have worked hard to test whether their versions of sophrology are efficacious vis-à-vis other treatments, their adoption of narratives about sophrology has been uncritical and mirrors what is seen in lay and trade sources described above.

Making Sophrology Scientific

Prior to the publication of the studies discussed above, Pandey (2009) wrote a scathing review of scientific discussions of sophrology in the *Indian Journal of Social Science Researches* in which he lamented the lack of a clear definition of sophrology, the lack of proper authentication and referencing, and poor research design in scientific literature. Such literature often presents constructs and facts that lack adequate empirical support. Although the publications above seem to suggest that biomedical rationales for using sophrology and attempts to study its impacts through designs such as case-control studies have improved, issues Pandey described regarding definitions and histories remain in some publications.

For example, de Almeida Silva et al. (2019, 383) write that Caycedo created sophrology 'having spend [sic] a number of years studying meditation and yoga, notably in India and Japan' and after spending 'some years in Asia, immersed in Yoga, Tibetan Buddhism and Japanese Zen' – without citation. Some East Asian scientists follow this pattern as well. Kim et al. (2008, 18–19) write that sophrology is 'based on a combination of Western relaxation therapy and Eastern yoga and meditation' and includes 'exercises of oriental Yoga and Zen methods' without any citation, even though they note that there are 'questionable claims on Sophrology'. Suzuki et al. (2012) use this phrasing almost verbatim, citing Caycedo's 1964 work to explain its basis on 'Western relaxation therapy and Eastern yoga or meditation'. In other words, they sound a lot like publications in the general media and some practitioner websites (excluding Sophrocay) that all draw on the descriptions Caycedo started using in the 1960s – descriptions that were more accepted at the time.

Not all research teams use such references. Natalia Caycedo's team describes sophrology as based on Husserl's phenomenology and consisting of 'a structured training program using dynamic relaxation, contemplation, and meditation techniques', and compares sophrology to autogenic relaxation, yoga, meditation, and mindfulness, instead of explaining these as intellectual contributors to it (van Rangelrooj et al. 2020, 201). Liu and Hu (2017) explain sophrology as a guided relaxation and breathing exercise and do not discuss the origins or components of sophrology at all. Romieu et al. (2017) and Moreau et al. (2020) likewise avoid place and tradition-based descriptions of sophrology. Romieu et al (2017) state that it 'requires a structured method consisting in very practical physical and mental exercises, using techniques such as concentration, deep breathing, relaxation, visualization, and simple movements', which is repeated by Moreau (2020). There is no source indicated for this explanation in either publication, although the repetition is likely due to shared coauthors on the papers. Bertrand et al. (2018, 1–2) opt to summarise sophrology as Caycedo's method for studying 'consciousness and to control the body balance spirit' and allocate space to describe the actions of the sophrology-trained technician in clinical encounters. Even though de Almeida Silva et al. used the tradition and place-based explanation in their introduction, they provided a more complete explanation of the training of practitioners and patients alike than many studies do – and certainly more than can be found on sophrology websites. After all, methods must be articulated in scientific papers in order to test validity, reliability, and generalisability.

Particularly in recent publications, there is some variation in how sophrology and Caycedo are included (or not) in scientific articles that aim to examine sophrology's clinical uses. It may seem surprising that some of the explanations in the health science literature are not so different from the explanations that circulate on the internet. Back in 2009, Pandey, who is in psychology, noted it was difficult to find sources that could be authenticated. This may have to do with how sophrology has been taught and marketed to and by some of Caycedo's early students, and/or in what languages information was available. It's also possible that because methods can be considered proprietary for some practitioners, they may not want to publicise them lest the methods be used in ways they were not intended or they render the practitioner irrelevant to potential patient-clients or trainees. Not all practitioners are also researchers or psychiatrists or medical doctors like members of Caycedo's team are, although it is this team that blurs the lines of business-treatment-research the most.

Likewise, researchers are all trained in different ways. For example, training in power and hegemony is likely to be differently prioritised for medical researchers than it is for medical social scientists and medical humanities scholars, so it may not be surprising that the scientific rationale for testing sophrology in clinical settings and the methodologies for doing so are becoming robust even if explanations of what it is and how it came to be are less so. In her research on food safety, Heather Paxon (2016) demonstrates that the rationale for policy can be 'black-boxed': people forget the rationale for its creation and uncritically perpetuate the need to adhere to policy without knowing the underpinnings. In this case, it is taken for granted in some of the scientific literature – regardless of who is writing – that the East-West dichotomy that has been cultivated and maintained as a key aspect of sophrology is normal and natural. What would it look like to 'unbox' this assumption and still describe sophrology's components? What could be understood about applications of sophrology if this assumption were removed? And what are the ramifications for juxtaposing sophrology with yoga, as van Rangelrooij et al. do, when a direct connection was made previously by the founder?

Discussion: Associations and (Re-)Contextualisations

Of course, there is variation within and between the spheres I describe above, and there are also connections across the groups because neither people nor ideas fit neatly into boxes: they are in dialogue with one another. Journalists interview sophrologists and read their webpages. Some sophrologists are practitioners *and* researchers. All of these writers are professionals of some kind, with various obligations and frameworks that, depending on their discipline or field, shape not only how they write but how they view the world. These shape how and why they engage with sophrology in the first place. Untangling these is a challenge.

In the works described above, all the writers work to provide some sense of legitimacy to sophrology by describing its origins and associations, to legitimise their own work or conceptions of the world, or both. Lay authors unsurprisingly seem to pull from sources that are most accessible to them, and their tendencies to repeat details about sophrology's origins and Caycedo uncritically reinforces stereotyped ideas about the 'West' and the 'East' whereby Anglophone readers are enabled to view themselves and 'Asian' others in problematically flat and stereotyped ways – even if this is not done intentionally and is a function of implicit biases. In short, the commentary they contribute ensures some aspects of popular culture endure (stereotypes about self and other), while other aspects change ('sophrology is the new mindfulness').

The same types of things happen when practitioners of sophrology and health science researchers circulate such details uncritically. For some researchers, there are strong efforts to 'scientise' sophrology through clinical trials or studies. But while the science advances, some of the stereotypes remain: there is a tenacious tendency to draw connections between Caycedo's travels to Asian countries and engagement with Asian traditions. While the tendency to repeat information without much qualification or sourcing is less surprising in the general media, even if it is problematic, the same tendency in academic genres where sourcing is expected indicates the degree to which associations with place or traditions – where readers can imagine 'the other' in comparison to themselves – still have some currency. That currency should be cause for reflection and scholarly investigation. Are these details included because they are interesting to the writer, perceived as interesting to the reader, or because they seem necessary because they are what others have said? Is it because information on origins was generated by people in other disciplines so it is harder to critique or decide not to use?

For many practitioners, sophrology is their profession because it is a way of life that they themselves find appealing. Antiglio, for example, describes her own experiences as a means to convince readers of its efficacy. This is repeated by Niamh Lyons of American Sophrology, who includes her testimonial about being cured of her pain through sophrology along with other testimonials (American Sophrology n.d.). The philosophical connection between mind and body and the ability to take less medication – or none at all, in the case of Lyons – may appeal to those who want to take charge of their own health rather than rely on medical practitioners, who are sceptical of biomedicine and/or pharmaceuticalisation, and who are interested in holistic wellness practices that are purported to treat root causes of poor health (on similar views, cf. Chapters 4 and 5). Sophrology may play the conceptual role that practitioners and patients alike may have found to be deficient not just in medicine but in daily life where they reside. Thus, what happens 'over there' with regard to understanding health appeals. Moreover, with practitioners like Lyons and Antiglio, the line between practitioners and patient-clients is blurred; with both self-help materials, educational courses, and therapy as possible purchases on many sophrology websites, the line between wellness care and business is blurred as well.

Sofrocay is perhaps the most complicated of all because the people who comprise the group may be balancing the complexities of each of the spheres laid out above, but with the added pressure of enduring over time and being the 'authentic' authority on sophrology: 'Sophrology, for a serene, positive, and meaningful life at every age and stage of life' (Caycedo Institute n.d.). Sofrocay promotes the use of sophrology as developed by Caycedo (and trademarked by the company), trains professionals, organises courses and events, and spreads sophrology throughout the world – while also conducting research (parsed as qualitative and scientific). As Caycedo's methods have been trademarked and aspects of sophrology move throughout various networks, it is perhaps unsurprising that there has been a shift from emphasising origins other than Caycedo himself and increased interest in highlighted venues where his practices have been systematically used and validated.

Sophrology has been taken up by various health science researchers, with variation in whether it is considered a tool for general well-being or one that can replace or support biomedical treatments. It has circulated through various locations around the world, at different times and by different generations of people who speak different languages, are trained differently, and think differently about issues of citation/reference, appropriation, and essentialism. With regard to epistemologies and medicine, medical anthropologists have discussed medical syncretism (a synonym of bricolage) and medical pluralism (simultaneous use of different systems) with specific attention to Asia for decades (Lock and Nichter 2002). Common questions included, why did people use the tools or frameworks they did? What did it mean socially for someone to choose a specific treatment, a set of responses to illness, or even to choose responses from multiple medical systems at once (Crandon Malamud 1991)? The questions asked then influence the questions I have asked here: Why are people using these narrative frameworks for sophrology? How are they trying to use it as a tool? How does it legitimise them and the work they have been doing up to this point?

The Mama-Baby Collaboration

'Labour is a collaboration between mama and baby', the midwife told the group of expectant parents at one of the three workshops parents are required to attend. 'Baby is trying to come out and you are trying to help them come out. Breathing gives you the oxygen you need for your muscles, and your brain and your baby's brain. It helps labour progress. And having food and water, too. We are here to support you and help you'.

The midwife held up a CD. 'You will all get one of these to help you practice'. She put it into the CD player and played the song through until it started over. 'So it's up to you to think of an image you want to focus on while you listen and breathe. Practice this 20 minutes a day until the birth and it will be easier'. Women are encouraged to engage the pain, breathe with it, and view it as a means of collaborating with their baby to work through labour – so that they can meet their baby. This was followed by another possible exercise: 'Practice when you poop! Breathe when you poop and relax. Don't clench! Just let the poo out! It's like mini labour. Papas can practice this, too', she said with a laugh.

So why would a Japanese clinic adopt sophrology? How do visualisation, breathing practice, and guided meditation paired with music fit with other Japanese ideals? Why would a Japanese woman be interested in a sophrology-enhanced birth?

First, mama-baby (or mother-child) collaborations are common in family routines in Japan. Anne Allison's seminal 1991 article about how mothers and children collaborate through the production and consumption of school lunch boxes (*o-bentō*) is a useful example: mothers create *o-bentō* their children can and will eat according to the practical constraints of the school day (such as lunchtime duration), the tastes and capabilities of their children (what needs to be made bite-sized, for example), and in an enticing way where lunch box food becomes art that kids want to eat. Mothers find ways to encourage their children to learn how to eat a variety of healthy foods through this practice, steering them away from being picky eaters while also teaching them how to follow routines according to a timetable and rules. In the process of teaching children the rules and how to follow them through food, women reaffirm gendered rules about mothers as nurturers. Allison argues that lunch box production and consumption is a way that both parties enact their roles of being good Japanese citizens. With sophrology, mothers and children work together to birth the nation; according to Allison, they work together to grow the next generation, too. And that work is processual rather than discrete.

Second, Tsipy Ivry (2010) has elucidated the ways in which pregnant women's bodies are considered the healthy environment for the foetus in her ethnographic work on pregnancy in Japan. Ivry describes how prenatal care in Japan deemphasises genetic testing and instead emphasises health regimes of the mother such as eating a balanced diet, exercising, not smoking or drinking, and avoiding stress. All of these practices make the mother's body an ideal environment for the foetus. There are also examples that note Japanese preferences for 'natural' or herbal therapies in place of 'harsh' pharmaceuticals (Lock 1984), particularly in the case of women's health and reproduction (Sandberg 2019). In the case of the clinic in question, prenatal care that encourages visualisation and a form of guided meditation set to music is promoted alongside good nutrition; thus, the clinic promotes a particular version of a healthy pregnant woman whose everyday practices facilitate the growth of her baby and also facilitate the birth. A healthy mom who is sophrologically conscious and attuned to both her body-mind and her connection to her baby has a better chance for a 'good birth' that is unmedicated and requires no interventions and a healthy baby who scores high on Apgar tests at birth. In fact, the clinic's c-section rate is two per cent, although this is partial because complicated pregnancies are referred to the local hospital (for example, if a baby remains in the breech position as the 40-week mark approaches, patients are referred to a local hospital).

Third, the clinic's use of sophrology may be better understood within the local context. Like many places in Japan, one of the main attractions in town is a popular Buddhist temple famous for being a pilgrimage site. The temple is a main feature of local identity and a source of pride. Regardless of one's official religious affiliation, if they have one at all, participation in temple events is a popular everyday activity for many local people. Also, like other areas in Japan, Nagano is a site of intense internationalisation through Olympic, Special Olympic, and World Cup events. Investment in infrastructure for these events was accompanied by a rise in Western-style restaurants and coffee shops, as well as materials at government offices and private businesses in foreign languages. It is possible that sophrology techniques may have appeal because of both the vague familiarity of its supposedly Asian roots, as well as its status as a technique developed in Europe – the same familiar-exotic characteristics that make it popular in Europe. Recall the emphasis on the 'international' nature of sophrology and references to France, Europe, and America on the Japan Sophrology Association website. It is worth noting that meals at the clinic, which include Japanese, local, and non-Japanese themed dishes, operate in similar ways: as vehicles to both care for patients medically and by serving foods that are familiar and comforting or non-Japanese and therefore interesting, food production and consumption (like therapeutics) demonstrate ongoing negotiations about self, communities, and nations (Runestad 2023).

Further Questions

The work I have presented here documents steps in a research project on birth clinic practices and conceptualisations of citizenship and belonging through engagements with food and medical systems that I began several years ago and wrote about in 2016 and 2023. Many questions remain. Some of these include: How central is pain to the pregnancy, labour, and birth experience for patients and physicians compared to other concerns (as highlighted by the clinical research here)? How do stakeholders, patients, and clinic staff alike conceptualise pain and clinical concerns during labour and birth? Is pain something to prevent or to leverage, or something else? How do such conceptualisations shape pregnancy, labour, and birth experiences?

While some narratives about 'natural birth' describe unmedicated birth as important physiologically and morally, the avoidance of pain medication (epidurals) and the embrace of sophrology at this particular clinic does not appear to me to be a simple 1:1 relationship whereby the clinic physicians avoid pharmaceuticals because such pharmaceuticals would interfere with visualisation techniques. Rather, it seems more that the clinic physicians are utilising tools that they feel give women more agency and a sense of empowerment through systematic attention to their own bodies in pregnancy, labour, and birth – at least for uncomplicated pregnancies. An overarching question remains: what is the 'sweet spot' whereby birth is considered a normal (nonpathological) event that women can systematically prepare for emotionally, mentally, and physiologically, while also recognising that pain medications and other interventions are sometimes necessary to prevent trauma, injury, and death of a mother and/or infant? How does culture shape what people think that 'sweet spot' is? While I began with physician perspectives of sophrology, the next steps of my research will buttress those and also aim to apprehend patient experiences and expectations of sophrology specifically and prenatal/birth care in rural Japan in general. Why do patients choose sophrology clinics? Why *this* clinic? How do factors other than sophrology use such as staff reputations, proximity, and food/accommodations intersect to influence patient choices about where they give birth? How do these fit larger narratives about what it means to be healthy in Japan?

Conclusions: Critical-Reflexive Bricolage and Frames of Legitimacy

Anthropologists study humans over geographic space and across time with particular attention to culture. Several decades ago, medical anthropologists applied Appadurai's concept of the 'social life of things' to materia medica (Whyte et al 2003). Because humans are innovators and bricoleurs, medicines and items used in medical settings are used in ways that reflect local settings. The rationale for their creation does not always travel with them (Whyte et al 2003). This chapter is an example of the social lives of ideas. Knowledge production, including knowledge production about health and wellness, is a sociocultural process. Sophrology-influenced birth practices in a Japanese clinic provide a window into the making of medical knowledge as a product of culture – something in constant flux and completely dependent on who engages with ideas and how. At a time when people, in general, are being encouraged to reflect on their privileges and what is missing from the narratives they consume, this case helps highlight the challenges in tracing intellectual lineages, protecting intellectual property, and trying to make claims about appreciation, appropriation, and essentialism. It highlights how neologisms, rather than necessarily always being an entirely new entity, can be recontextualisations, recombinations, and reimaginations of previously held ideas.

This chapter also shows that understanding how knowledge is produced means going beyond dichotomous labels like orientalism and occidentalism, lay and specialist, appreciation or appropriation – and not falling into traps that engender overly simplistic representations. In many cases, this requires a balance between acknowledging inspirations for ideas with a focus on the process and why a particular idea is attractive to a stakeholder in the first place. The use of sophrology demonstrates how that is clearly easier said than done, particularly when ideas cross disciplines, cultures, geography, and time: explaining the inspirations of sophrology such that it appears legitimate to various audiences has been challenging and often resulted in references that exoticised or erased them rather than do them justice.

This chapter also illuminates tensions between health science disciplines and other epistemologies, and between lay and formal education. It also raises more questions. What happens when people from other disciplines know something using epistemological tools that are perceived to be incompatible or foreign from those in one's own discipline? How does one use, question, and authenticate that information? Does information that cannot be authenticated get coded as unscientific and thus dropped, adopted uncritically, or ignored? Does information that might be useful in scientific inquiries but hasn't been proven get coded as belief or as something else? Years ago, medical anthropologist Dan Moerman examined clinical trial results in which people given placebos improved more than people given no treatments; in theory, this should be impossible because placebos are by definition inert. Moerman (2002) argued that clinical trials inadvertently measure 'meaning response' – the power of belief – when they compare reactions to placebos to reactions to no treatment. But these findings went unnoticed in medicine until he reported it, and it's still common to report responses are 'no better than placebo' – most likely because belief is much less predictable than lab-tested pharmaceuticals and therefore less able to be 'scientised'. After all, belief in general requires faith, and science requires evidence. Similarly, Caycedo and other practitioners like him wanted to refocus psychotherapy, but rather than changing one aspect, they wanted to change the whole perspective. To do that required finding ways to frame what he learned outside his training, what he believed worked, into a theory and method that he could prove through evidence. What better way to do that than to convince other people to work with him to try to test it? To describe it as exotic and proven useful elsewhere? In science, there is always an element of belief.

In closing, I suggest that moving forward, readers and writers – scholars and nonscholars alike – adopt a practice of reflection that encourages them to consider what information they are using, where it comes from, in what context it was created, and why they want to use it themselves should they choose to include it in their own writing. In the same way that we consider implicit bias related to positionality (as a function of race, gender, class, religious background, sexual orientation, relationship status, ability status, and a number of other aspects of personhood) when we do research, we should apply a similar critical reflexivity to information consumption. Students in particular should be asking themselves when they read what the intended audience seems to be (pharmaceutical sceptics?), what occasion prompted its publication (trends in public interest in mind-body health?), what type of writing it is (a trade publication?) and what the purpose is (marketing a product?) before including it as a resource in something they write. As stated earlier, humans are innovators and bricoleurs, and knowledge is a sociocultural process not a set of static facts. Learning to practice a critical-reflexive bricolage when reading and writing can, perhaps, help alleviate some of the issues I have outlined here.

I myself found it challenging to parse the sources and present Caycedo's influences in a balanced way – particularly when defining sophrology. It is important to consider that this critical lens is being applied to Caycedo's work retroactively, and Western scholars were not thinking about the problematic dichotomisation of East vs. West when he conceptualised and popularised sophrology. Caycedo's work was a product of its time. It is the uptake and consistent circulation – that continues to this day in both popular and academic genres – that merits critique, and I have attempted to highlight that. I took care to use Caycedo's own words and the words of his primary students and collaborators to define what he meant and taught in a sociocultural context (as being social facts), rather than fall into the trap of repeating their words as objective facts in the ways that current writings do. And as much as Sofrocay may want to be the owner-experts of sophrology, these ideas have taken on new meanings in new contexts (particularly medical ones) – I have tried to acknowledge that as well. I hope this chapter then provides an example of how to utilise a critical-reflexive bricolage perspective, an explanation of the many facets of sophrology itself, and some sense of what questions about its use remain in maternity clinics in Japan in particular.

Bibliography

Allison, Anne. 1991. 'Japanese Mothers and Obentōs: The Lunch-Box as Ideological State Apparatus'. *Anthropological Quarterly* 64: 4, 195–208. https://doi.org/10.2307/3317212.

Antiglio, Dominique. 2021. 'Alfonso Caycedo, Founder of Sophrology'. BeSophro. Accessed on 26 November 2021. https://be-sophro.com/alfonso-caycedo-founder-of-sophrology/

Bancroft, W. Jane. 1982. 'Suggestopedia, Sophrology, and the Traditional Foreign Language Class'. *Foreign Language Annals* 15, no. 5: 373–79. https://doi.org/10.1111/j.1944-9720.1982.tb00965.x.

Bertrand, Anne-Sophie, Antoine Iannessi, Sandrine Buteau, Xiong-Ying Jiang, Hubert Beaumont, Benoit Grondin, and Guillaume Baudin. 2018. 'Effects of Relaxing Therapies on Patient's Pain During Percutaneous Interventional Radiology Procedures'. *Annals of Palliative Medicine* 7, no. 4: 455–62. https://doi.org/10.21037/apm.2018.07.02.

Bonapace, Julie, Guy-Paul Gagne, Nils Chaillet, Raymonde Gagnon, Emmanuelle Herbert, and Sarah Buckley. 2018. 'Physiologic Basis of Pain in Labour and Delivery: An Evidence-Based Approach to its Management'. *Journal of Obstetrics and Gynaecology Canada* 40, no. 2: 227–45. https://doi.org/10.1016/j.jogc.2017.08.003.

Botes, Michelle. N.d. 'How Sophrology Can Help: Coping with stress the Natural WAY'. Age-well.org. Accessed on 20 January 2023. http://www.age-well.org/sophrology.html.

Caycedo Institute (Sophrocay). N.d. 'What is Sophrology?'. Accessed on 20 January 2023. https://caycedoinstitute.com/what-is-sophrology/.

Crandon-Malamud, Libbet. 1991. *From the Fat of Our Souls: Social Change, Political Purpose and Medical Pluralism in Bolivia*. University of California Press: Berkeley.

Good, Byron, and Mary-Jo DelVecchio Good. 1992. 'The Comparative Study of Greco-Islamic Medicine: The Integration of Medical Knowledge into Local Symbolic Contexts'. In *Paths to Asian Medical Knowledge*, edited by Charles Leslie and Allan Young, 257–71. Berkeley: University of California Press. https://doi.org/10.1525/california/9780520073173.003.0012.

Moerman, Daniel E., and Wayne B. Jonas. 2002. 'Deconstructing the Placebo Effect and Finding the Meaning Response'. *Annals of Internal Medicine* 136, no. 6: 471–76. https://doi.org/10.7326/0003-4819-136-6-200203190-00011.

Horden, Peregrine, and Elisabeth Hsu. 2013. *The Body in Balance: Humoral Medicines in Practice.* New York: Berghann Books.

Ivry, Tsipy. 2010. *Embodying Culture: Pregnancy in Japan and Israel.* New Jersey: Rutgers University Press. https://doi.org/10.36019/9780813548302.

Japan Sophrology Association. Accessed on 15 January 2023. https://www.sophrology.jp/step.html.

Kasai, Noelle. N.d. New Horizon Institut. Accessed on 20 January 2023. https://new-horizon-institut.com/en/.

Kim, Hyun Hee, Alejandro A Nava-Ocampo, Sun Kyung Kim, Seo Hui Kim, Yun Ju Kim, Jung Yeol Han, Hyun Kyong Ahn, Hyun Mee Ryu, Jae Hyug Yang, and Moon Young Kim. 2008. 'Is Prenatal Childbirth Preparation Effective in Decreasing Adverse Maternal and Neonatal Response to Labor? A Nested Case-Control Study'. *ACTA Biomedica* 79: 18–22.

Lyons, Niamh. N.d. American Sophrology. Accessed on 20 January 2023. https://www.americansophrology.com/.

Kuriyama, Shigehisa. 1992. 'Between Mind and Eye: Japanese Anatomy in the Eighteenth Century'. In *Paths to Asian Medical Knowledge*, edited by Charles Leslie and Allan Young, 21–43. Berkeley: University of California Press. https://doi.org/10.1525/california/9780520073173.003.0002.

Ledger, Emma. 2017. '"Learning to Live": Why Sophrology is the New Mindfulness'. *The Guardian,* 12 November.

Liu, Dan, and Wan-Liang Hu. 2019. 'SLK Triple Therapy Improves Maternal and Fetal Status and Promotes Postpartum Pelvic Floor Function in Chinese Primiparous Women'. *Medical Science Monitor* 25: 8913–19. https://doi.org/10.12659/msm.917330.

Lock, Margaret. 1984. *East Asian Medicine in Urban Japan: Varieties of Medical Experience.* Berkeley: University of California Press.

Maharaj, Dushyant. 2009. 'Eating and Drinking in Labor: Should It Be Allowed?' *European Journal Obstetrics, Gynecology and Reproductive Biology* 146, no. 1: 3–7. https://doi.org/10.1016/j.ejogrb.2009.04.019.

Malina, Debbie. 2011. 'Dynamic Relaxation'. *Dancing Times,* November: 34–37.

Mamba, Augustin Mubiayi. 2018. 'Complicated Childbirth Aid Protocol Inspired by Luba-Kasai Therapeutic Practice'. *Perinatology & Pediatrics* 2, no. 1: 6.

Moreau, Johan, Kathleen Lavastre, Huguette Romieu, Francoise Charbonnier, Sophie Guillaumont, Charlene Bredy, Hamouda Abassi, Oscar Werner, Gregoire De La Villeon, Anne Requirand, Annie Auer, Stefan Matecki, Clement Karsenty, Aitor Guitarte, Khaled Hadeed, Yves Dulac, Nathalie Souletie, Philippe Acar, Fanny

Bajolle, Damien Bonnet, Laurence Negre-Pages, Thibault Mura, Maria Mournier, Pierre-Emmanuel Seguela, Julie Thomas, Xavier Iriart, Jean-Benoit-Thambo, and Pascal Amedro. 2020. 'Impact of Sophrology on Cardiopulmonary Fitness in Teenagers and Young Adults with a Congenital Heart Disease: The SOPHROCARE Study Rationale, Design, and Methods'. *IJC Heart and Vasculature* 27: 100489. https://doi.org/10.1016/j.ijcha.2020.100489.

Nichter, Mark, and Margaret Lock, eds. 2002. *New Horizons in Medical Anthropology: Essays in Honor of Charles Leslie.* London: Routledge. https://doi.org/10.4324/9780203398517.

Pandey, Rakesh. 2009. 'Editorial: Four Decades of Sophrology and Its Scientific Status'. *Indian Journal of Social Science Researches* 6, no. 1: 1–3.

Paxon, Heather. 2016. 'Rethinking Food and Its Eaters: Opening the Black Boxes of Safety and Nutrition'. In *The Handbook of Food and Anthropology*, edited by Jackob A. Klein and James L. Watson, 268–88. New York: Bloomsbury Academic. https://doi.org/10.5040/9781474298407.0021.

Romieu, Huguette, Francoise Charbonnier, Dora Janka, Aymeric Douillard, Valerie Macioce, Kathleen Lavastre, Hamouda Abassi, Marie-Catherine Renoux, Thibault Mura, and Pascal Amedro. 2018. 'Efficiency of Physiotherapy with Caycedian Sophrology on Children with Asthma: A Randomized Controlled Trial'. *Pediatric Pulmonology* 53: 559–66. https://doi.org/10.1002/ppul.23982.

Runestad, Pamela. 2016. 'The Medical Anthropologist as the Patient: Developing Research Questions on Hospital Food in Japan through Auto-Ethnography'. *Asia Network Exchange* 23, no. 1: 66–82. https://doi.org/10.16995/ane.161.

Runestad, Pamela. 2023. 'Feeding Mothers, Making Citizens: Japanese Maternity Clinic Meals as Treatment, Care and Identity'. *Verge: Studies in Global Asias* 9, no. 2: 157–85. https://doi.org/10.1353/vrg.2023.a903026.

Sandberg, Shana Freuhan. 2019. 'Resisting Intervention, (En)trusting My Partner: Unmarried Women's Narratives About Contraceptive Use in Tokyo'. In *Intimate Japan: Ethnographies of Closeness and Conflict*, edited by Allison Alexy and Emma E. Cook, 54–72. Honolulu: University of Hawaii Press.

Silva, Hugo Jario de Almeida, Jose Cortez Assuncao Junior, Franciele Santos de Olivera, Jaine Maria de Pontes Oliveira, Glauko Andre Figueiredo Dantas, Caio Alano de Almeida Lins, and Marcelo Cardoso de Souza. 2019. 'Sophrology Versus Resistance Training for Treatment of Women with Fibromyalgia: A Randomized Controlled Trial'. *Journal of Bodywork and Movement Therapies* 23: 382–89. https://doi.org/10.1016/j.jbmt.2018.02.005.

The Sophrology Institute. N.d. Accessed on 26 November 2021. https://sophrology.institute/.

Suzuki, Michiko, Seiji Isonishi, Osamu Morimoto, Masahisa Ogawa, and Kazuhiko Ochiai. 2012. 'Effect of Sophrology on Perinatal Stress Monitored by Biopyrrin'.

Open Journal of Obstetrics and Gynecology 2, no. 2: 176–81. https://doi.org/10.4236/ojog.2012.22036.

Tournaire, Michel, and Anne Theau-Yonneau. 2007. 'Complementary and Alternative Approaches to Pain Relief During Labor and Delivery'. *Evidence-Based Complementary and Alternative Medicine* 4, no. 4: 409–17. https://doi.org/10.1093/ecam/nem012.

Van Rangelrooij, Koen, Rafael Solans-Buxeda, Maria J. Fernandez-Garcia, Natalia Caycedo-Desprez, Rejina M. Selvam, and Antoni Bulbena. 2020. 'Effectiveness of a 4-Week Sophrology Program for Primary Care Patients with Moderate to High Anxiety Levels: A Randomised Controlled Trial'. *Actas Espanolas de Psiquiatria* 48, no. 5: 200–208.

Whyte, Susan Reynolds, Anita Hardon, and Sjaak van der Geest. 2002. *The Social Lives of Medicines.* New York: Cambridge University Press.

Zhen, Willa. 2019. *Food Studies: A Hands-on Guide.* New York: Bloomsbury.

Biography

Pamela Runestad is an assistant professor in the Department of Sociology and Anthropology at Elon University. Pamela is a medical anthropologist and Japanologist with interests in infectious disease, nutrition, gendered health narratives, and critical pedagogies.

8 The Influence of Traditional Chinese Medicine on Brazilian Naturology

Fábio L. Stern

Abstract: This chapter delves into the influence of Traditional Chinese Medicine (TCM) on the field of Brazilian naturology over the past 15 years. It examines the incorporation of TCM principles and practices into naturology courses in Brazil, shedding light on the historical and cultural factors that have shaped this healthcare movement. The chapter contends that the integration of TCM has left a significant mark on the trajectory of naturology in the country, providing valuable insights into its ongoing development. Nevertheless, it highlights a crucial point – that the TCM training in Brazilian naturology falls short of the recommendations set forth by the World Health Organization. Additionally, it explores how TCM knowledge has been appropriated through Orientalism, often relegating China-born instructors to the role of mere attractions for students rather than empowering them to devise effective teaching strategies for the subject.

Keywords: Traditional Medicine, Brazil, China, religion and health, Platonic Orientalism

This chapter will analyse the impact of Traditional Chinese Medicine (TCM) on courses of naturology in Brazil over the past 15 years. Naturology is a health movement similar to but distinct from naturopathy,[1] with a romantic and esoteric outlook that emerged in Southern Europe during the 19th century in response to the increasing industrialisation of medicine, which was seen as harsh and rationalistic. Naturologists are therapists who use folk and alternative medicines – which they classify as 'natural' – rather than so-called 'allopathic remedies' (i.e., pharmaceuticals, biomedical drugs),

1 This difference will be elaborated upon later in the text.

Gaitanidis, Ioannis, Luis Fernando Bernardi Junqueira, Avery Morrow, and Sangyun Han (eds), *Therapy, Spirituality, and East Asian Imaginaries*. Taylor & Francis Group 2025
DOI: 10.5117/9789048559015_CH08

vaccines and surgery, which they perceive as aggressive, artificial, and unnatural. To understand the origins of naturology, one must comprehend the formation of medical science, its genealogy of power from the 18th century onwards and its crisis after World War II, which made it possible to give space to therapeutic practices organised around ideals, discourses, and precepts different from those of modern biomedical science.

The flourishing of mercantilism in the Renaissance made Western European countries devote more attention to their citizens' health. The gold and silver crisis of the 17th century in the colonies precipitated a shift in Europe's economic production approach. The continent was overwhelmed by an influx of precious metals from the Americas, leading to widespread inflation. This situation rendered Spain and Portugal, the leading colonial powers of that era, increasingly reliant on importing these metals. As the century progressed, the depletion of mines exacerbated their economic woes, given that their militaries were largely financed through the wealth derived from these colonies. Consequently, European nations were compelled to overhaul their production strategies, aiming to engage the majority of their populations in generating goods to fund their military expenditures. Pressured by this demand, public administration gave birth to social medicine, a movement concomitant with urbanisation, growth, and unification of power in the cities (De Barros 2008, 50). The Renaissance also triggered a scientific revolution. From Leonardo da Vinci to Andreas Vesalius, Europe systematised the human body by dividing it into parts to better understand it (Neves 2011, 27). This way of thinking, later popularised by Cartesians, began influencing medicine in the 17th century.

In the 18th century, the proximity between medicine and the university dictated more and more the tone of medical advances, creating a gap between academic and folk views of healthcare (De Almeida 2009, 45). The new class of educated doctors predominantly came from the aristocracy, who also served as their chief clientele, as the fees for instruction and treatment made early medical science unavailable to the poor. As such, folk practitioners had to meet the medical demands of the less affluent (Porter 1988). When erudite physicians developed the first pretensions of a monopoly of medical practice, their proximity to the dominant classes was a determinant of the discrimination and persecution of folk practitioners. To ensure the supremacy of university medicine and guarantee market reserves, Europe legally established the standardisation of medical practice at the end of the 18th century (Pickstone 2006). This process was marked by the exclusion or subordinate assimilation of certain rival groups, such as Jewish doctors and women (De Almeida 2009, 45). Thus, these other healers came to be classified as charlatans and superstitious. This schism generated the notion of 'official medicine' – hence 'true medicine' – that would relegate the symbolic dimension of illness to the sideline (Laplantine 2010).

The 19th century saw the emergence of counter-Enlightenment movements such as Romanticism, which valued emotion, subjectivity, imagination, and individuality, rescuing folk practices that the Enlightenment had once relegated to the background. This interest had a significant impact on medical science. In the 19th century, medicine had already standardised its practice by the Enlightenment's scientific approach, but some Romantic physicians began documenting and studying folk healing practices, including herbs and home remedies. This movement fostered many new forms of therapies, such as Ignaz von Péczely's (1826–1911) iridology in Hungary, Thomas Allinson's (1858–1918) hygienic medicine in Scotland, Daniel David Palmer's (1845–1913) chiropractic in the U.S., and Benedict Lust's (1872–1945) naturopathy in Germany.

At the beginning of the 20th century, North America and Europe became increasingly demanding concerning health, developing expectations that academic medicine could not keep up with. The discovery of penicillin in 1928 promoted one of the greatest revolutions. Previously deadly pathologies, such as syphilis and tuberculosis, began to be cured, consolidating a profound transformation in how society approached pain, disease, ageing, and suffering. The body's well-being, once rarely addressed, became more prevalent, and citizens began to demand it as a fundamental right (Serres 2003, 25). Parallel to this, at the end of World War II, the idea of welfare to be provided by the state as a public benefit gained prominence (Neves 2011, 29). Health insurance demands intensified as this became popular among the newly created United Nations, leading to the founding of the World Health Organization (WHO) in 1948 to promote a positive and distinctive approach to health, which included welfare and mental health.

The conjunction of these three factors – Romanticism, the demand for well-being due to the pharmaceutical revolution, and the promotion of social welfare by the WHO – were essential to the revival of other forms of healing that attempted to encompass dimensions that academic medicine had neglected for at least two centuries in Europe and North America. Not coincidentally, numerous alternative therapies with a romantic allure did not gain widespread acceptance in broader society until after the 1960s.

Naturology is one of these cases. Although it resembles naturopathy – originated in Germany around the same time during the 19th century – naturology was initially a distinct movement typical of Italy and the Iberian Peninsula (Correia 1950; Ventura 1999). As both had similar goals, it was almost inevitable that naturology and naturopathy would eventually converge as they do today. However, the origins and initial proponents of naturology in Southern Europe were distinct from those of naturopathy in Northern Europe. For instance, Correia (1950) explains that because naturology developed among strongly Catholic countries, it was amalgamated with the values and conducts of Catholic morality until at least the 1940s. Unlike naturopaths, naturologists aimed to find harmony between their practices and Christian principles, deemed essential for promoting 'civilised' coexistence. In other words, naturology, at its inception, looked significantly more colonialist and Christocentric compared to naturopathy.

From their emergence to the mid-20th century, naturologists based their practices on vitalism and parapsychology, mixing esoteric Christianity with folk healing practices. Their 'natural' techniques – such as diets, baths, massages, and medicinal herbs – had already been traditional in Southern Europe for centuries before the term 'naturology' was coined (De Castro 1986). For instance, naturologists promoted a diet rich in fruits, vegetables, olive oil, fish, and wine to maintain good health. Likewise, the advocacy for therapeutic bathing stems from the deep-rooted Iberian and Roman tradition of soaking oneself in thermal waters. This practice expanded significantly after the Moors arrived in the eighth century CE, introducing the use of medicinal herbs, oils and other natural ingredients with healing properties into the bathing rituals.

After the New Age movement, however, European naturology turned away from parapsychology and Christianity toward New Age esotericism, which led Pessoa Jr. (2011, 293) to consider 'quantum mysticism' as the current foundation of naturology. As Teixeira (2013, 107) explains, nowadays, 'naturologists deny an esoteric, mystical or religious character to naturology. [...] Naturology does not want to be esoteric or mystical. It wants to be scientific, but a new science'. That is, although other healthcare professionals tend to classify naturology as esoteric, naturologists themselves do not wish to be perceived in that manner. This has led some naturologists to resist the inevitable identification of naturology with the New Age and other esoteric trends. Although they adopt esoteric healing practices such as Bach flower remedies, Kirlian photography (cf. Chapter 1), and Anthroposophy, naturologists regard those therapies as science, in the spirit of 'mythologies of science' as described by Hanegraaff (1996) to explain how New Agers creatively appropriate scientific symbols. In other words, while these partial appropriations of symbols and nomenclature are invoked as 'scientific', they do not operate by established scientific methods.

In the context of Asia, the perceptions within naturology can be grasped through the lens of 'Platonic orientalism', a concept first proposed by

Walbridge in 2001. This framework helps explain how Plato represented 'the East', notably Persia and Egypt, in his writings. Unlike typical Orientalist perspectives, which often cast 'the East' in a uniformly negative light, Plato acknowledged the wisdom and significance of these cultures whilst simultaneously perpetuating stereotypes about them. For instance, in *The Republic*, Plato (2016) portrays the Persians as a martial people whom the superior Greeks could easily subdue. Historically, such stereotypes have been leveraged to justify Western domination, from Ancient Greece to the present day. Although contemporary humanities now critique such viewpoints, Platonic orientalism remains commonplace among Western esotericists, who often pair it with the idea of the 'noble savage', romanticising 'the East'. In Saif's words, '"the Orient" represented an adherence to allegorical and symbolic interpretations of revelatory and experiential modes of obtaining knowledge of Being, in addition to commitments to "theurgy" and "white magic"' (Saif 2020, 72).

Despite Western esotericists acknowledging the value of Asia's wisdom, their method of appropriation still constitutes a form of Orientalism. According to Said (1990), Orientalism involves a simplistic portrayal of other cultures, often lumping them together as a singular 'East'. In the selective syncretism practised by Western esotericists, complex spiritual traditions are distilled to merely isolated elements devoid of their historical and philosophical grounding. This approach fails to appreciate the depth and wholeness of these traditions. Moreover, Orientalism suggests a power dynamic where 'the West' asserts dominance over 'the East'. By haphazardly picking and mixing elements from various Asian traditions, Western esotericists exert control, moulding Asia to fit their own agendas while frequently overlooking these sources' authenticity and original authority. For instance, it was not Hindus who gained recognition and financial benefit from Theosophy but Helena Blavatsky (1831–1891), who at most had a peripheral association with India's religious figures (Fuller 1988; Meade 2012).

As a secularised form of Western esotericism, the New Age also adopted Platonic orientalism. Whereas not every form of orientalism is New Age, as D'Andrea (2000) reminds us, naturology embraces it when dealing with Asian therapeutic practices. That means naturology associations are much more influenced today by Platonic orientalism than by Christian esotericism – as we will see in the following pages. Indeed, the initial pro-nature Christian stance characteristic of 19th-century naturology has largely faded. Even in Portugal, a predominantly Catholic country where naturology societies in the 1910s were firmly esoteric Christian, the majority of naturology organisations have shifted away from their original Christian discourse.

Although Western health practices such as thermalism, radionics, Bach flower remedies, and chiropractic are still considered part of naturology, present-day naturologists primarily use therapies from China such as acupuncture and *tuina*, a form of massage, as well as Ayurveda and yoga from India. Naturology clinics may also cite Arabic techniques like Unami medicine and Japanese techniques like *ryodoraku*, *shiatsu*, and *reiki* (cf. Chapters 1 and 2). Some Western-originated therapies with an Orientalist allure may also be noted, like *chua k'a*, a form of South American massage purportedly derived from exercises developed by Mongolian warriors to dispel fear in battle. However, there is no evidence backing this narrative, as no sources corroborate it before the famous Bolivian esotericist Oscar Ichazo (1931–2020), the initial promoter of *chua k'a*. It is highly probable that Ichazo crafted these historical origins as part of an invented tradition to legitimise his therapy.

In this chapter, I explore Brazilian naturology, focusing specifically on how Brazilian university education in naturology has integrated Chinese medicine in dialogue with the New Age movement. I will also examine the resulting tensions of this attempted integration within the Brazilian academic community. Although more naturology courses are currently authorised by Brazil's Ministry of Education (as of 2023), it is worth noting that the data collection for this study ended in August 2018. Back in 2018, only two universities had recognised naturology courses in Brazil: Universidade do Sul de Santa Catarina (UNISUL) in southern Brazil, and Universidade Anhembi-Morumbi (UAM) in São Paulo. Since the end of my data collection, several other naturology courses have been established in the country. For instance, the Universidade da Região de Joinville (UNIVILLE) established its naturology course in August 2018 and the Centro Universitário de Belo Horizonte (UNI-BH) established its own in February 2020. Today, Brazil's Ministry of Education lists 13 higher education institutions authorised to offer naturology courses. The recent growth of Brazilian naturology is linked to the creation of a private higher education monopoly. A major economic conglomerate, which acquired the two universities discussed below, subsequently launched naturology courses across other institutions within its network.

Early Naturology in Brazil

Studying naturology in Brazil has some peculiarities not found elsewhere. Spain, Portugal, and Italy have always had reservations about regulating naturology since it is not a health practice guided by evidence-based medicine. In the case of Portugal, in 1993, the Escola Superior de Biologia e Saúde in Lisbon initiated a naturology course, which the Ministry of Science, Technology and Higher Education of Portugal had never before recognised as a valid higher education degree. In 2003, Portugal chose not to regulate alternative health practices, and in 2009 the Portuguese State decreed the immediate closure of the Escola Superior (Carvalho 2009). In Brazil, however, naturology has been a university course recognised by the Ministry of Education since 2002 (Santa Catarina 2002). Hence, despite facing setbacks from government regulations and being unable to establish state-recognised college programmes in Europe, Brazil officially approves and recognises bachelor's degrees in naturology. This makes the flow of naturology in Brazil rather unique, bringing it closer to similar academic legitimacy-seeking movements such as osteopathy and naturopathy in the United States.

There are no precise records of how exactly naturology was introduced in Brazil. Nevertheless, there is empirical evidence of its widespread presence across Brazilian society since at least the 1980s (e.g., De Castro 1986), coinciding with the legitimisation and institutionalisation of alternative healthcare approaches, particularly after the establishment of the Brazilian Unified Health Service (Serviço Único de Saúde, or SUS) (Brasil 2006; cf. Chapter 5). Moraes (2007) asserts that the establishment of an alternative healing market in Brazil predates the aforementioned period and aligns with the country's growing inclination towards new religious movements. This inclination became more evident after 1946, when the Brazilian Constitution was updated to include that 'the freedom of conscience and belief is inviolable, and the free exercise of religious services is assured' (Brasil 1946, Art. 141).

Initially, the consumers of these therapies were white people from privileged social classes in the most populous Brazilian urban cities, such as state capitals. A survey in São Paulo, Brazil's largest city, revealed that most establishments offering those services were mainly in upper-middle-class neighbourhoods (Magnani 2000, 28). Another study indicated that about 80% of the alternative therapies' clientele in Recife (Northern Brazil) were white women, and more than 72% had a college education (Martins 1999) – at a time when only 14.4% of the Recife population had a college education (IBGE 2010a) and only 45.7% was white (IBGE 2010b).

In 1985, the State University of Rio de Janeiro (UERJ) and the Brazilian government reached an agreement to incorporate homoeopathy into the public health system (Brasil 2006). The aim was for all alternative therapies to remain under the control of 'official physicians' (i.e., medical graduates), safeguarding their market reserve – a policy that limits open competition in specific economic areas, thereby benefiting a select group – through state corporatism. Legal restrictions or regulations may enforce market reservation by limiting or prohibiting certain entities from operating freely within a particular market. In the healthcare sector, this policy is applied through government regulation, which specifies who is qualified to undertake medical roles. Professional practice of medicine is reserved for licensed physicians, with unlicensed individuals facing prosecution and potential imprisonment for unauthorised medical practices. In Brazil, the state outsources regulatory responsibilities to regional and federal councils. These bodies are tasked with recognising the qualifications of healthcare professionals and actively engage in political lobbying to ensure that specific medical procedures remain exclusive to their members.

Consequently, when the Inter-Ministry Commission for Planning and Coordination of Health Actions issued Resolution No. 9 on March 8, 1988, outlining the guidelines for introducing acupuncture and medicinal herbs into public health services, it explicitly stated that these practices were to be permitted only when performed by medical graduates (Brasil 1988). The end of the Brazilian military dictatorship in 1985 led to a new constitution that guaranteed universal health service access through a range of social and economic policies. In 1990, the Brazilian Ministry of Health implemented the Unified Health System (SUS) to promote this service nationwide. With health becoming a citizen's right, patients could demand healthcare, sometimes under the threat of a lawsuit (Serres 2003, 25). This has considerably increased the country's maintenance cost, requiring administrative alternatives. Thus, a series of actions by the Brazilian Ministry of Health encouraged the promotion of alternative medicines.

In 2000, the 11th Brazilian Health Conference recommended incorporating nonconventional health practices in the Community Health Agents and Family Health programmes. In 2003, the Brazilian Pharmaceutical Assistance Conference report emphasised the importance of expanding access to medicinal herbs and homoeopathy in the Unified Health System. It led to the formation of the Working Group on Natural Medicine and Complementary Practices to elaborate a national policy for these therapies. In 2004, the working group was included as a strategic niche within the Brazilian Agenda for Research Priorities. In 2005 a pilot project of social thermalism[2] was set up in Natural Medicine and Complementary Practices.

2 Social thermalism refers to public access to thermal mineral water establishments for preventive, therapeutic, and health maintenance purposes. In Brazil, all aquatic environments,

A presidential decree also created a working group on medicinal plants to elaborate a national policy (Brasil 2006). In 2006 the Working Group on Natural Medicine and Complementary Practices assumed the current nomenclature of 'Integrative and Complementary Practices'. Then, on 3 May 2006, Ordinance No. 971 approved the National Policy for Integrative and Complementary Practices (PNPIC, in its Portuguese acronym). A survey by the Department of Primary Healthcare of the Healthcare Attention Secretary confirmed five practices to be implemented in the Brazilian Unified Health System: (1) Chinese medicine (including acupuncture), (2) homoeopathy, (3) herbal medicine, (4) thermalism/crenotherapy, and (5) Anthroposophic medicine. The study showed that at least one of these practices was offered in 232 municipalities across all 26 Brazilian states (Brasil 2006).

Brazilian Naturologists only became aware of the National Policy for Integrative and Complementary Practices one year after its official release in 2006. It means that they were not involved in developing or discussing the policy. They only realised it when the first Brazilian naturologists pursued a master's degree in Collective Health. The creation of the first naturology undergraduate courses happened parallel to this. As previously noted, Brazilian public policies continued to safeguard market reserves for medical graduates, hence national policies omit any reference to bachelor's degrees in naturology, despite their existence.

The proper insertion of naturology into Brazilian higher education occurred in 1994 and was directly linked to the rise of Traditional Chinese Medicine and the New Age movement (cf. Chapter 5). Their first college programme was instituted at Faculdades Integradas Espírita, a Spiritist private college in Curitiba, an important capital city in Southern Brazil (Da Silva 2012; Teixeira 2013). Originating in France, Spiritism has fully developed into a religion in Brazil over the course of the 20th century. It is Brazil's third-largest religious group, ranking only behind Catholicism and Protestantism, with the country housing the world's largest Spiritist community. Furthermore, Brazilian Spiritism has significantly contributed to spreading various alternative therapies throughout Brazilian society. Many Spiritist centres offer healing and counselling services; some incorporate alternative therapies such as crystal healing, colour therapy, and *reiki*, the latter of which strongly appeal to Spiritists because it resembles the practice

including beaches, rivers, aquifers, and lakes, are the property of the Brazilian Navy and cannot be privatised. Consequently, no one is entitled to purchase and restrict access to a hot spring, for example.

of laying on of hands traditionally performed in Spiritist rituals (Aureliano & Cardoso 2015; Hess 1991).

According to Varela and Corrêa (2005, 151–53), the founding director of Faculdades Integradas Espírita, Octávio Melchíades Ulysséa (1931–2009), personally invited a medical professor and acupuncturist named Jorge de Morais Barbosa to design a course in traditional Chinese medicine for the college. The goal was for the course to cover Chinese massage (*tuina* 推拿, *guasha* 刮痧), bone setting (*dieda* 跌打), herbal medicine, physical exercises (*qigong* 氣功, *liangong* 練功), cupping (*baguan* 拔罐), moxibustion (*jiu* 灸), and acupuncture, with a greater focus on medicinal plants. Barbosa was an Umbanda practitioner, an acupuncturist, and a biomedical professor in Recife, northern Brazil. Despite no historical connection between acupuncture and Umbanda – a Brazilian religious synthesis of Spiritism and African diaspora spiritualities – Barbosa's religious affiliation was a key reason for the owner of a Spiritist private college to invite him. Thus, the history of this first Brazilian naturology course commenced with an acupuncturist working to create a Traditional Chinese Medicine undergraduate course in a Spiritist college. It is worth pointing out that although Brazil is a secular state, the educational system allows for institutions to be confessional because the Catholic Church founded most of the first Brazilian schools. Closing all those historical schools after adopting the secular state would, it was believed, be impractical. Instead, the state allowed other religions to open their own schools.

As in many other countries, the medical profession is highly regulated in Brazil. The Brazilian Federal Council of Medicine is among the most powerful professional-class councils, perhaps second to the National Bar Association. As such, medical graduates are lobbying to maintain state market reserve and power hegemony over health practices. For instance, pressure from the Brazilian Federal Council of Medicine was decisive for Jair Bolsonaro – 38th president of Brazil, from 2019 until 2022 – to expel Cuban physicians in the first year of his mandate, under the pretence that this would ensure a market reserve for Brazilian doctors (Pinheiro 2019). When the course designed by Barbosa was submitted to the Brazilian Ministry of Education for official accreditation, it was unable to retain the title 'Traditional Chinese Medicine'. This was because the Brazilian Federal Council of Medicine deemed the term 'medicine' contentious, given existing legislation in Brazil stipulating that only courses directly regulated by the Council of Medicine are permitted to use this title. At that moment, the Academic Council of the Faculdades Integradas Espírita looked for alternatives and discovered the existence of Portuguese naturology. Since naturology in Portugal had already incorporated therapies from Traditional Chinese Medicine, changing Barbosa's course name to 'naturology' was not a significant issue.

At first, students and teachers looked to New Age authors such as Fritjof Capra (1939–), Deepak Chopra (1946–), Ken Wilber (1949–), and Amit Goswami (1936–) to explain the rationality behind the therapies they were using. According to Teixeira (2013, 24), initially, 'the training in naturology was thought from the triad "art", "education" and "health", where these elements would articulate a new, more integral and expanded vision of healing'. The first teachers in the programme sincerely believed in transforming society through differentiated teaching based on the quality of life, integration, interdisciplinarity, holism, environmental education, philosophy, quantum physics, and affection. Also, as my doctoral research has revealed, three former teachers attested that the course's first teachers were admittedly New Agers – that is, self-claimed to be adherents of the New Age movement (Stern 2019).

In this first programme, there was significant resistance to the standard scientific method, which naturologists denounced as an outdated scientific model that needed reconsideration. Varela and Corrêa (2005) documented that even faculty members used to proclaim that naturology should have never entered the university since academia does not allow students to, in their own words, 'experience the process' (cf. Chapters 3 and 4). In other words, they intended to highlight their students' personal development, exploration, and self-discovery against the typical irrelevance of subjective experience in science. To do so, they encouraged their students to resort to nonacademic or even unorthodox methods for a university curriculum, such as tarot, astrology, circular dance, shamanism, crystals, entheogens, numerology, laying on of hands, hiking, pendulums, transpersonal psychology, philosophical readings of quantum physics, enemas, tree-hugging, rebirthing, and various religious rituals; all these in syncretism with the teachings of TCM. Teachers also used to offer weekend workshops to further explore topics that they could not teach at the university.

Despite Barbosa's formal education in biomedicine, several faculty members of the naturology course did not possess formal academic qualifications in healthcare. Instead, they acquired their knowledge of the therapies they taught through informal means, such as public courses or personal investigation. Brazilian legislation mandates that individuals must have at least an undergraduate degree to teach in higher education. While this rule does not specify the need for a degree in a related field, a professor's qualifications must be directly relevant to their teaching subject. For example, a professor of statistics is expected to have at least a degree in mathematics, and a professor of politics to hold at least a degree in social sciences. In earlier naturology courses, however, it was common for people with degrees in academic areas as diverse as law, philosophy, or literature to be responsible for health classes on *qigong*, *liangong*, *yin-yang* 陰陽, *wuxing* 五行 (five agents), *zangfu* 臟腑 (Chinese theory on inner organs), *jingluo* 經絡 (meridian network), *liuyin* 六淫 (six pathogenic factors), colour therapy, or chakras.

Even so, the Curitiba course was a commercial success. In 1996, it was already exported to a private university in Santa Catarina, UNISUL, where it became a bachelor's degree in 1998, but with no institutional clarity of what kind of environments students should be in when they arrived at their internships. During my doctoral research (Stern 2019), one of the former professors disclosed that the first bachelor's in naturology had many gaps regarding what naturology is, what it does, where naturologists work and their role in society. On this point, Brazilian legislation gives freedom to universities to create new bachelor's courses, authorising them automatically. After the graduation of the first class, the course must then be submitted to the State Secretary of Education, where it is evaluated whether it will be recognised or not. For instance, Barbosa's programme in Curitiba, the first one, was denied recognition by the Secretary of Education on every application and was finally discontinued in 2013.

In Santa Catarina, on the other hand, naturology became one of the most sought-after courses, with more than 800 students enrolled. After the graduation of the first class in 2002, the secretary of education visited the institution. Its audit clarified the lack of structure of the naturology pedagogical project and demanded major adjustments. First, the university changed the programme's coordination, replacing a New Age sympathiser with a sceptical biologist. Secondly, they organised an ad hoc team to align the programme with the other health programmes. Though a complete adaptation has never occurred, naturology teachers became more concerned with trying to do, or appear to be doing, some kind of science. Consequently, those faculty members who continued to advocate for a closer relationship with New Age esotericism were rapidly silenced or dismissed. As explained by Teixeira (2013, 28), the university no longer regarded discussions about New Age spirituality valid, under the allegation that this could open margins for questioning the scientificity of their training, hindering any future recognition by the Ministry of Education. The curriculum and the syllabi had to be reformulated, under protest from many students. Not everything was lost, though. Naturologists managed to persuade the university that naturology must keep 'energy healing' (cf. Chapters 1 and 5), convincing the programme coordinator that all alternative medicines are in some way grounded in traditional vitalistic principles. As of 2004, following the endorsement of the second pedagogical project, Brazilian naturology started to identify itself as being based on a threefold foundation of traditional medicines: TCM, Ayurveda, and shamanism (Hellmann and Wedekin, 2008).

In contrast to the aggressive repression of New Age esotericism, Chinese medicine itself was never considered academically invalid or scientifically irrelevant. Even though TCM has been popularised in Brazil, thanks primarily to the New Age movement (Moraes 2007), the Secretary of Education and the UNISUL never contested it as an appropriate subject for the naturology course. Teaching Chinese medicine has always been a central pillar of Brazilian naturology, even under biologistic programmes.

Training of Traditional Chinese Medicine in Naturology

TCM has been taught in Brazil throughout all naturology courses. Chinese massage, meditation, and body practices such as *liangong*, *qigong*, and *taiji* (also spelt *tai chi*) have been an integral part of its history. For instance, Passos (2015) attested that 61% of Brazilian naturologists stated that they always work with TCM. Moreira (2016) also pointed out that Chinese medicine is Brazil's most common subject of naturology papers. In 2016, 85% of the academic supervisors of Brazilian naturology courses had some technical training in TCM.

The importance of TCM in Brazilian naturology is such that practitioners even mingle non-Chinese practices with it. Some prominent examples are colour therapy, crystal healing, dowsing, clay therapy, art therapy, and shamanic healing. None of those is part of the traditional corpus of Chinese healing listed by the World Health Organization (WHO 2022). The WHO lists 3,415 standard terms for TCM whose therapeutic practices they summarise in the following categories: exercises, meditation, massage, acupuncture, moxibustion, cupping, and diet therapy. However, in a highly creative manner, Brazilian naturologists blend alien techniques into the Chinese system, resulting in very distinctive and innovative forms of Orientalist therapies. To a large extent, this is because naturologists use the terms 'complementary medicine', 'alternative medicine', and 'unconventional medicine' interchangeably with 'traditional medicine'. The theoretical origins of naturology are rooted in New Age authors such as Capra (1982), who distinguishes conventional (allopathic) medicine from all other forms of medicine, thus creating two categories: alternative medicine and allopathic medicine. As Hanegraaff (1996) observes, traditional medicine and alternative medicine are virtually synonymous in the New Age milieu.

Naturology offers a unique perspective on health and wellness, which enables practitioners to engage in constructive dialogue with diverse healing systems and therapeutic practices, integrating them seamlessly to promote a form of holistic healing. Naturology's cosmology aims to restore the inherent link between spirituality and healing, which practitioners perceive as being rooted in 'tradition' (cf. Chapter 5). It matters little to them if new alternative techniques and technologies are being developed. If a therapy is not 'allopathic', it is immediately conceived of as traditional and interchangeable with other alternative methods. To do so, Brazilian naturologists operate in the typical New Age way: they superficially combine different knowledge pieces into one big synthesis. In some cases, after they make this creative bricolage, naturologists themselves may deny the influences from which they drew such practices in the first place. The most prominent example is Peter Mandel's (1941–) chromopuncture, the application of coloured light pens to specific points on the body for therapeutic purposes. Acupuncture heavily reoriented Mandel's chromopuncture to the extent that the points to which the coloured light pen is applied are the same as the acupuncture meridians. The creator himself, nonetheless, denies the connection between Chinese acupuncture and the therapy he supposedly invented.

Brazilian naturologists strongly identify themselves with TCM, embodying a typical form of Platonic orientalism. They hold a deep appreciation for elements from Asia but through a lens that aligns with the West's positive perception of it as mystical, wise, ancient, legendary, and magical. Brazilian naturology often disregards the perspectives of East Asian scholars regarding their own culture. Despite the presence of teachers from China who delivered lectures in Portuguese at Brazilian naturology university courses, they were not regarded as authoritative sources on Chinese medicine by Brazilian naturologists themselves (for a similar phenomenon, cf. Chapter 4). Chinese professors tended to present a different view of Chinese medicine, which may seem incompatible with the orientalist imaginations of Brazilian naturologists. Differences in philosophical underpinnings, in what is considered culturally authentic or what are the 'correct' diagnostic and treatment methods and their 'proper' integration with Western medicine, have created a conflict between the practice of TCM in China and its interpretations by the New Age movement. New Age renditions may seem to oversimplify TCM methods, neglecting their rich philosophical and cultural background and occasionally merging them with spiritual and esoteric elements foreign to China. This results in what critics consider a diluted, exoticised version of TCM lacking the depth, effectiveness, and cultural authenticity of its 'traditional' counterpart. However, as New Age enthusiasts adapt TCM to their preferences, it aligns more closely with what Western audiences seek in an 'Eastern' practice. Despite the World Health Organization's endorsement of China's model, Brazilian naturology programmes have typically marginalised professors from China due to this ontological conflict.

For instance, professors Yu Tao and Li Qiyong relocated from China to Southern Brazil in the late 2000s to teach TCM to naturology students. However, they were only given minor roles in developing lesson plans, syllabi, and teaching methods, despite being allegedly hired for these purposes. Indeed, they were not actively involved in teaching classes or supervising clinical practices. My analysis suggests that Brazilian naturology universities primarily hired Chinese professors as tokens to attract students. But as the Chinese medicine practised by these professors does not align with the idealised vision of an 'enchanted East' advocated by Brazilian New Agers, they are disregarded or sidelined. Moreover, during mass layoffs in Brazilian naturology courses (as discussed later in this chapter), these professors were among the first to be dismissed.

Since the creation of the first bachelor's degrees in naturology, Brazilian universities have also offered professional training in acupuncture. Even so, there is some controversy regarding acupuncture's teaching for naturologists. As previously noted, medicine is a strongly regulated profession in Brazil with a powerful Federal Council. For over two decades, the Brazilian Council of Medicine has fought for acupuncture to be a physician's exclusive practice. The Workers' Party's (PT) past governments had barred attempts to reserve the market for medicine in Brazil (Larcher and Cronemberger 2013). It means that, at least for now, it is still possible for other professionals, such as nurses or physical therapists, to practice acupuncture in the country. This dispute has nonetheless split the Brazilian naturology collective. While some naturology universities teach basic needling techniques to undergraduate students, others adopt the more conservative stance that acupuncture is an invasive treatment that should only be introduced at the graduate level. Besides avoiding unnecessary conflicts with the Council of Medicine, the latter group maintains that acupuncture requires a much larger workload to form safe professionals.

As Brazilian naturology has become more pluralistic over time, today Chinese medicine no longer constitutes half of the training in naturology as it used to in its early phase. By focusing on training generalists, Brazilian naturology programmes launch into the market professionals who know a bit of everything but can only work deeply with something if they take extra courses. Chinese medicine shares space with several other practices in the Brazilian naturology programmes, such as iridology, aromatherapy, yoga, natural food, and floral medicines. Despite this, Brazilian naturology still dedicated an average of 600 hours to TCM in 2017 (Stern 2017, 422–41). Given that Brazilian law stipulates that a bachelor's degree must have at least 2,400 hours (Brasil 2007), and that undergraduate naturology courses have circa 3,600 hours (Stern 2017, 422–41), Chinese medicine represents one-sixth of a naturology undergraduate degree. By 2017, no other subject enjoyed that many hours in Brazilian naturology programmes.

Nevertheless, the number of hours of TCM training in Brazilian naturology is inferior to those in the WHO's benchmarks for training *tuina* and acupuncture (WHO 2020; 2021). The WHO recommends at least 400 hours of supervised clinical practice with a focus on TCM (WHO 2020, 11; WHO 2021, 11). In 2017, Brazilian naturology offered 450 hours of supervised clinical practice. Noteworthy, these hours were not limited solely to Chinese medicine but encompassed all naturology therapies (Stern 2017, 435, 441). In addition, the WHO recommends at least 416 hours of basic theory in TCM (WHO 2020, 11); Brazilian naturology courses do only 150 hours (Stern 2017, 441), one-third of the international recommendation.

This raises a critical issue in the training of naturologists in Brazil. Despite the significant attention given to TCM in these courses, naturology graduates are not recognised as 'traditional Chinese therapists' according to international standards. They only receive basic training, with a curriculum that falls short of the recommendations set by the WHO. While public discourse in Brazil regarding the regulation of naturology has stalled in the National Congress for several years, Brazil's membership in the WHO means that the Brazilian Ministry of Health generally adheres to its directives and recommendations. This poses a challenge for naturologists seeking to practice TCM solely with their undergraduate training. In Brazil, naturologists must pursue specialisation to meet international standards; their undergraduate degrees alone are insufficient.

Future of Brazilian Naturology

As I was completing my fieldwork in 2018, a monopolization of higher education was taking place in Brazil. Today, the country has the world's largest monopoly in private education, with one multinational group – which understands education as a commodity – owning more than one-third of all Brazilian universities (Beraldo 2016). Although there is strong resistance to this utilitarian usage of higher education in Brazilian public universities, there are no naturology programmes in public universities; private institutions offer all the courses authorised by the Brazilian Ministry of Education. In other words, public universities do not offer valid degrees in naturology; not even short courses are available. All naturology training in Brazil is in the hands of one company in the private sector.

In 2005 UAM was sold to the US-based Laureate Education. About 80% of the faculty members were fired in the process, with the company replacing doctors with lower-degree teachers to increase its profit margins. Later the Ânima group bought UAM, and in 2019 UNISUL was also acquired by them. Even other universities with more recent naturology courses are owned by Ânima, such as the UNIVILLE. In all of them, the process of mass layoffs to increase shareholder profits has been the rule. Today, naturology courses in Brazil are made up of a minority of professors trained in naturology, who are perceived largely as a locus to make money by selling their training. Material evidence of the lack of concern with these programmes' quality is that of the 13 naturology courses officially listed by the Ministry of Education, only four require in-person attendance. Brazilian universities are selling distance learning courses training to professionals dealing with other people's health, with complex practices such as massage, acupuncture, and potentially toxic herbs that can cause adverse effects. Imagine a physical therapist or a nurse trained only through the Internet. Although a federal bill (PL 5.414/2016) is being processed in the Brazilian House of Representatives to ban distance learning courses in health, the bill has not yet been approved in all instances. Hence, in the case of naturology, two-thirds of the programmes listed in the Brazilian Ministry of Education (as of 2023) are still distance learning courses.

Before 2020, there was momentum towards regulating naturology in Brazil, with naturology associations often enlisting the support of far-right congressmen for this endeavour. Naturologists desired that the state recognise the naturologist occupation as a health science profession. However, the COVID-19 pandemic exposed the far-right's stance against vaccines and their promotion of ineffective treatments and healing through prayer. These factors significantly contributed to Brazil recording one of the world's highest death tolls from the virus, with over 700,000 fatalities attributed to these policies. As a result, Brazilian public opinion has labelled the far-right as anti-science. Consequently, any further attempts to advocate for naturology regulation under their aegis have risked associating naturology itself with pseudoscience in the public eye. This initial regrettable choice to align with far-right representatives has compelled naturology associations to suspend their regulatory efforts temporarily. They have now recognised that this strategic alignment has made the political climate unsupportive and hostile towards advancing the naturology cause.

Establishing a monopoly over all courses has also made the future of naturology university courses challenging to ensure. Currently, most Brazilians who have training in naturology work with something else, and one of their very few professional fields finds itself in shambles. Naturology associations are weak; they could not even prevent mass layoffs during such a takeover. Furthermore, since all Brazilian legislations on integrative and complementary health practices prioritise medical graduates, it is more economically advantageous to sell Chinese medicine to biomedical doctors. There is, therefore, no guarantee that there will still be naturology university courses a few years from now. Perhaps Brazilian naturology will follow in the footsteps of European naturology, where courses moved away from university settings to the informal learning sector. Prospective training groups may no longer be connected to formal education but to open courses in alternative spaces within the New Age milieu, such as holistic clinics and natural product stores.

Bibliography

Abrana, Apanat, and Sbnat. 2014. *Anais do Congresso Brasileiro de Naturologia*. Palhoça: University of Southern Santa Catarina.

Almeida, Cybele C. de. 2009. 'Do mosteiro à universidade: considerações sobre uma história social da Medicina na Idade Média'. *AEDOS* 2, no. 2: 36–55.

Aureliano, Waleska A., and Vânia Zikán Cardoso. 2015. 'Spiritism in Brazil: From Religious to Therapeutic Practice'. In *Handbook of Spiritualism and Channeling*, edited by Cathy Guttierez, 275–93. Leiden: Brill. https://doi.org/10.1163/9789004264083_014.

Barros, Nelson F. de. 2008. *A construção da medicina integrativa: um desafio para o campo da saúde*. São Paulo: Hucitec.

Beraldo, Beatriz. 2016. 'Fusão cria o maior monopólio de educação privada do mundo'. *Esquerda Diário*, 16 August.

Brasil. 1946. *Constituição da República dos Estados Unidos do Brasil de 18 de setembro de 1946*. Brasília: Congresso Nacional.

Brasil. 1988. 'Resolução CIPLAN nº 9, de 8 de março de 1988'. *Diário Oficial da União*, 11 March.

Brasil. 2006. *Política Nacional de Práticas Integrativas e Complementares no SUS: PNPIC*. Brasília: Ministério da Saúde.

Brasil. 2007. 'Parecer CNE/CES N. 8/2007'. *Diário Oficial da União*, 13 August.

Capra, Fritjof. 1982. *The Turning Point: Science, Society, and the Rising Culture*. New York: Bantam.

Carvalho, Rita. 2009. 'Ministro ordena fecho de escola "superior"'. *Diário de Notícias*, 30 June.

Castro, José L. de. 1986. *Naturologia: a saúde integral do indivíduo e da sociedade.* Sintra: Europa-América.

Correia, António Mendes et al., ed. 1950. *Grande enciclopédia portuguesa e brasileira.* vol. 18. Lisboa: Editorial Enciclopédia.

D'Andrea, Anthony A.F. 2000. *O self perfeito e a Nova Era: individualismo e reflexividade em religiosidades pós-tradicionais.* São Paulo: Loyola.

Fuller, Jean Overton. 1988. *Blavatsky and Her Teachers: An Investigative Biography.* Washington: East-West.

Hanegraaff, Wouter J. 1996. *New Age Religion and Western Culture: Esotericism in the Mirror of Secular Thought.* Leiden: Brill. https://doi.org/10.1163/9789004378933.

Hellmann, Fernando, and Luana M. Wedekin, eds. 2008. *O livro das interagências: estudos de casos em naturologia.* Tubarão: Editora UNISUL.

Hess, David J. 1991. *Spirits and Scientists: Ideology, Spiritism, and Brazilian Culture.* University Park: Penn State University Press.

IBGE. 2010a. 'Amostra Educação: Recife'. Accessed on 27 February 2023. https://cidades.ibge.gov.br/brasil/pe/recife/pesquisa/23/22469.

IBGE. 2010b. 'Amostra Educação: Recife'. Accessed on 6 February 2024. https://cidades.ibge.gov.br/brasil/pe/recife/pesquisa/23/25888.

Laplantine, François. 2010. *Antropologia da doença.* 4th ed. São Paulo: WMF Martins Fontes.

Larcher, Marcello, and Daniella Cronemberger. 2013. 'Governo veta diagnóstico exclusivo em Ato Médico'. *Agência Câmara de Notícias*, 11 July.

Magnani, José G.C. 2000. *O Brasil da Nova Era.* Rio de Janeiro: Jorge Zahar.

Martins, Paulo H. 1999. 'As terapias alternativas e a libertação dos corpos'. In *A Nova Era no MERCOSUL*, edited by María Julia Carozzi, 80–105. Petrópolis: Vozes.

Meade, Marion. 2012. *Madame Blavatsky: The Woman Behind the Myth.* New York: Open Road.

Moraes, Maria R.C. 2007. 'A reinvenção da acupuntura: estudo sobre a transplantação da acupuntura para contextos ocidentais e adoção na sociedade brasileira'. Master's thesis, Pontífice Universidade Católica de São Paulo.

Moreira, Andrei M. 2016. 'As características metodológicas dos trabalhos de conclusão de curso da naturologia da UNISUL'. Bachelor's thesis, UNISUL.

Neves, Afonso C. 2011. 'Conceito ampliado de saúde'. In *Saúde integral: a medicina do corpo, da mente e o papel da espiritualidade*, edited by Paulo Bloise, 23–35. São Paulo: SENAC.

Passos, Mayara A. 2015. 'Perfil socioeconômico profissional dos naturólogos no Brasil'. Bachelor's thesis, Universidade Anhembi-Morumbi.

Pessoa Jr., Osvaldo. 2011. 'O fenômeno cultural do misticismo quântico'. In *Teoria quântica: estudos históricos e implicações culturais*, edited by Olival Freire Jr., Osvaldo Pessoa Jr. and Joan Lisa Bromberg, 281–302. Campina Grande: EDUEPB. https://doi.org/10.7476/9788578791261.0013.

Pickstone, John. 2006. 'Medicine, Society and the State"'. In *The Cambridge History of Medicine*, edited by Roy Porter, 260–97. Cambridge: Cambridge University Press.

Pinheiro, Beatriz J. 2019. 'Mais médicos: o lobby da classe médica que influenciou a decisão de encerrar o programa'. *El País Brasil*, 7 February 2019.

Plato. 2016. *The Republic*. Cambridge: Cambridge University Press.

Porter, Roy. 1988. 'Before the Fringe: "Quackery" and the Eighteenth-Century Medical Market'. In *Studies in the History of Alternative Medicine*, edited by Roger Cooter, 1–27. London: MacMillan. https://doi.org/10.1007/978-1-349-19606-7_1.

Said, Edward. 2003. *Orientalism: Western Conceptions of the Orient*. New York: Penguin Classics.

Saif, Liana. 2020. 'That I Did Love the Moor to Live with Him: Islam in/and the Study of Western Esotericism'. In *New Approaches to the Study of Esotericism*, edited by Egil Asprem and Julien Strube, 67–87. Leiden: Brill. https://doi.org/10.1163/9789004446458_005.

Santa Catarina. 2002. 'Decreto nº. 5.572, de 27 de agosto de 2002: reconhece curso de educação superior'. In *PUB DOSC*, 3. Florianópolis: ALESC.

Serres, Michel. 2003. *Hominescências: o começo de outra humanidade?* Rio de Janeiro: Bertrand Brasil.

Silva, Adriana E.M. da. 2012. 'Naturologia: um diálogo de saberes'. PhD thesis, Pontífice Universidade Católica de São Paulo.

Stern, Fábio L. 2017. *A naturologia no Brasil*. São Paulo: Entrelugares.

Stern, Fábio L. 2019. 'Cosmologia xamânica: a ressignificação do xamanismo na naturologia brasileira'. PhD thesis, Pontífice Universidade Católica de São Paulo.

Teixeira, Diogo V. 2013. 'Integridade, interagência e educação em saúde: uma etnografia da naturologia'. Master's thesis, Universidade Federal de Santa Catarina.

Varela, Daniele M., and Mariana A. Corrêa. 2005. 'Estudo sobre a Naturologia no Brasil e no mundo'. Bachelor's thesis, Universidade Anhembi-Morumbi.

Ventura, Carlos C. 1999. 'Naturologia: pontos nos Is'. *Jornal Espaço Público*, 3 February.

Walbridge, John. 2011. *The wisdom of the mystic East: Suhrawardī and Platonic Orientalism*. Albany: SUNY Press.

WHO. 2020. *WHO Benchmarks for the Training of Tuina*. Geneva: WHO.

WHO. 2021. *WHO Benchmarks for the Training of Acupuncture*. Geneva: WHO.

WHO. 2022. *WHO International Standard Terminologies on Traditional Chinese Medicine*. Geneva: WHO.

Biography

Fábio L. Stern is associate professor in the Programme for the Study of Religions at the Pontifical Catholic University of São Paulo, Brazil. His academic pursuits revolve around New Age spiritualities, the intersection of religion and health, and the applied study of religions. He has been elected as one of the national coordinators for the editors' forum of Brazilian Journals on Religious Studies and Theology for the 2023–2026 term. His doctoral research, which centred on the development of naturology in Brazil, was a pioneering effort, being only the second study of its kind in the country.

9 Constructing a Modern Esoteric Buddhist Breath Therapy

Nathan Jishin Michon

Abstract: Combining esoteric Buddhist breathing techniques and visualisations, contemporary psychology and chaplaincy, and various world meditations, the meditative therapies used with clients of Japan's Ōshita Daien 大下大圜 (1954–) and Takayama Seiei 高山誓英 (1948–) are case studies in entangled influences and modern adaptation. Ōshita Daien is a profoundly influential figure in the field of 'spiritual care' in Japan. Takayama was his student and further developed these methods for his own contexts. After briefly introducing their Shingon 真言 tradition and contextualising the term esoteric Buddhism, the chapter delves into the stories of these two priests with a focus on their individual paths and how their therapies came about. Finally, the chapter will reflect on their complex webs of influence and impact in terms of this volume's larger themes.

Keywords: Esoteric Buddhism, Contemporary Shingon, Spiritual Care, Meditation Therapy

The 'World Harmony Meditation Centre' (*Sekai heiwa meisō sentā* 世界平和瞑想センター)[1] sits in a location of limited access, in what might appear to be near the top of the world. Completed in 2019, it lies on the grounds of Senkōji 千光寺, a Shingon Buddhist temple near the top of a mountain range at the edge of the Japanese Alps, overlooking the town of Hida 飛

1 The official name in Japanese more literally translates to 'World Peace Meditation Centre' rather than using the word 'harmony', but Ōshita preferred to use the word 'harmony' in English after considering the multiple connotations of the word and thought it showed his connections to music. Although Japanese has a similar term with multiple connotations, at that point it was too late to change the officially registered Japanese name, so it was kept as 'peace'.

Gaitanidis, Ioannis, Luis Fernando Bernardi Junqueira, Avery Morrow, and Sangyun Han (eds), *Therapy, Spirituality, and East Asian Imaginaries*. Taylor & Francis Group 2025
DOI: 10.5117/9789048559015_CH09

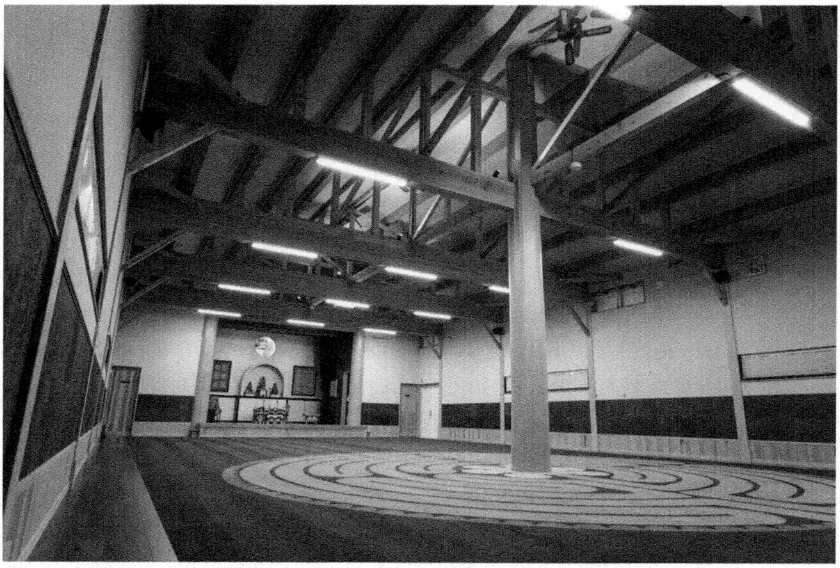

Figure 9.1. Inside the World Harmony Meditation Centre. Photo by Ōshita Daien.

騨 in Gifu Prefecture, central Japan. One must drive about a half hour up a winding mountain road to reach it. The centre is a single building with the capacity to seat around 300 people. It is a new structure on the grounds of a 1,250-year-old temple; yet being constructed from local wood of the mountain it was built upon helps it to blend in relatively well in its surroundings. There is also a curious eclecticism on the path to the building. Despite the old traditional Japanese style of most buildings, there are prayer wheels from Bhutan and a stupa from Sri Lanka that one passes on the way there. Inside the World Harmony Meditation Centre, after an entryway resembling a log cabin surrounded by locally sourced wood on six sides, the main hall is covered by a large, cushy, green carpet. The centre of the floor is dominated by the trunk of a 150-year-old pine tree which stands in the middle of a European Christian-style meditation walking labyrinth.

At the far end of the hall is a stage area which rises a couple of feet above the rest of the floor and can be used for either religious or secular purposes. On the stage are Shingon-style mandalas and sets of Taiwanese Buddhas on either side and three sizable Buddhas in the middle of a semi-altar-like space. Yet there is also a large screen which can come down, covering the buddhas for videos, PowerPoints, and other forms of presentation. This curious and intriguingly diverse building somehow all fits well together within its mountain environment.

Besides housing retreats, one of the centre's primary purposes is to host its founder's trainings in his unique 'clinical' meditation (*rinshō meisō* 臨床瞑想) for doctors, nurses, social workers, chaplains, and other care providers. Although the centre is still relatively new, Ōshita Daien began writing and training people over a decade before it opened; he began early discussions and development of his clinical meditation process even a decade prior to that, during the 1990s.

In many ways, this structure serves as a microcosm to encapsulate the primary theme of this chapter, exemplified by the case studies that follow: there are vastly interwoven webs of influences which transcend any narrow vision of 'East' and 'West' as monolithic forces that impact each other. As the following story of Ōshita Daien will come to show, the ways in which he formulates his systems of breathing, chanting, and meditative therapy involve myriad layers of complex transcultural interactions. This chapter then introduces one of Ōshita's students, Takayama Seiei 高山誓英, showing his own influences and ingenuity in further developing a meditative therapy in an effort to meet the needs of his local community. Both figures are Shingon Buddhist priests in contemporary Japan, yet this chapter will show that their place and role within the global dynamics are far more complex than a basic 'Easternisation' or 'Westernisation' phrase might suggest. Prior to examining these case studies, however, this chapter will first provide a brief introduction to Shingon and esoteric Buddhism as the pillars upon which these figures initially stand.

Shingon as 'Esoteric Buddhism'

Shingon Buddhism dates to the early ninth century in Japan, when Kūkai 空海 (774–835) brought a set of teachings and practices back to Japan from his journey to China. The word Shingon literally means mantra and reflects the emphasis on sacred or even apotropaic words and chanting which are common within the tradition. Although Kūkai himself did not establish a separate sect of Buddhism in Japan, his writings clearly show that he understood it as a distinct form of practice compared to the Buddhism that already existed in Japan at the time. One could say Kūkai was incredibly influential on two levels, both as a historical individual and as a hagiographic archetype. Ryuichi Abe asserts Kūkai 'was indisputably the single most popular Buddhist saint in medieval society. No other Buddhist figure has been more intensely legendized' (Abe 1999, 3). Countless myths of him healing the sick, banishing demons, and myriad other achievements are found so often throughout Japan that he would have had to live many lives to complete all these activities. Takamura Hiroki 高村弘毅 and Kōno Tadashi 河野忠, for example, found and diagrammed more than 300 wells and sources of water throughout Japan which all proclaim to have provided healing waters from Kūkai (Takamura and Kōno 2006, 40). The hagiography did not, however, bloom and grow from nothing.

Kūkai's historical influence was also immense. He transformed Japanese Buddhism so thoroughly during his life that many such imprints remain influential today. He transformed Japanese linguistics. He was called on by the courts for advice on topics ranging from architecture to medicine. He was recognised as one of the three most famous calligraphers of mediaeval Japanese society. He was able to systematise ritual and practice in ways that were both so novel and thorough that such shifts in many ways allowed for and formed the basis of subsequent popular forms of Japanese Buddhism to develop. Ritual connections he established with the aristocracy and the emperor continue between Shingon priests and the Japanese imperial household to this day.[2]

Whereas the previous Buddhist establishment placed its emphasis on textual study and philosophy, Kūkai shifted the emphasis to ritual and practice. The esoteric dimension involved mastery of the 'three mysteries' (*sanmitsu* 三密) of body, speech, and mind. Such mastery was completed, respectively, through practices of mudra, mantra, and visualisation. Another critical idea was *sokushin jōbutsu* 即身成仏, or enlightenment in this very body. Along with the notion that awakening was possible in one's present lifetime, Kūkai spread an idea which gradually gained dominance throughout Japanese Buddhism: that the Dharmakaya (*hosshin* 法身, 'true body' [of the Buddha]) is preaching constantly through all aspects of nature. In this case, the Dharmakaya was personified as Mahāvairocana Buddha, who rather than being a historical Buddha, was a representation of purity and light of the entire cosmos.

Kūkai primarily identified those teachings as *mikkyō* 密教, which is often translated as 'Esoteric Buddhism'. As Abe deftly illustrated, Kūkai was able to present such teachings as a new understanding and classification for other Buddhists of his time rather than a separate school per se. This allowed him to gain support and work with the Nara Buddhist establishment that held power, gaining the foothold he needed within early Heian Japanese Buddhism (794–1185).

2 Studies pertaining to Kūkai's historical influence on Japanese religion and society are vast. This paragraph provides only a short summary. See, for example, Abe 1999; Stone 2003, 11, 20–22; Fukuda 2014; Kōyasan daigaku sensho kankōkai 2006; Payne 2006; Tinsley 2011.

The translation of *mikkyō* using 'esoteric', however, deserves further treatment. *Mikkyō* consists of the characters *mi* 密, for 'secret', and *kyō* 教, meaning 'teaching', 'view', or 'belief'. The word is alternatively also translated as 'tantric Buddhism', though each translation is imperfect and comes with issues. Orzech, Payne, and Sørensen point out four different trends in scholars' views between the choices. Some see their choices as interchangeable, with little difference between them. Others view tantras as distinct texts and argue that esoteric refers to a stream of Buddhism prior to the appearance of those texts. Still, others view the terms as largely synonymous but beginning no earlier than the sixth century, referring to when a system of practices coalesced, accessed through *abhiṣeka* (empowerment) ceremonies which were guarded by a degree of secrecy. Finally, other scholars completely reject the use of tantra to describe premodern esoteric Buddhism in Asia. Despite such diverse positions and lack of agreement over better terms, 'esoteric' is still commonly accepted to identify *mikkyō* in English (Orzech, Payne, and Sørensen 2011, 5).

In this sense, esoteric Buddhism can refer to a range of traditions beyond Japan, let alone the Shingon tradition – and there is disagreement on precisely where the boundaries of the term lie. Some scholars believe it is a form of Buddhism that arose gradually as a distinct stream within Mahāyāna. Henrik Sørensen, for example, asserts that this form of Buddhism has its roots in India and 'is a movement centering on attaining its spiritual and worldly goals through ritual practices' (Orzech, Payne, and Sørensen 2011, 6; Sørensen 2011). Other scholars such as Ronald Davidson, however, conclude that esoteric Buddhism is a movement that began rapidly around the sixth century as a synthesis of other Mahāyāna developments which bore a longer history of development. Robert Sharf and Richard McBride provide further texture to these debates by challenging the notion that esoteric Buddhism existed as a separate 'school' within China. Even if it gradually became a more distinct school in Japan, such understandings were often read back into history through the lens of these later social structures[3]; nevertheless, the evidence in China suggests esoteric Buddhism was a more widespread movement which saturated much of the Buddhist

3 Esoteric Buddhism remained dominant in Japan throughout the Kamakura Period (1185–1333), but other schools began a slow formation and rise to prominence. During the Kamakura Period, many monks still held lineages with multiple teachers from what would become different schools or sects. On a popular level, people also drew few distinctions. Thus, although new teachings and lineages emerged around this time, they were far less clearly separate than later writings might suggest. But the divisions that began forming in this period coalesced into more distinct schools as the period ended. See especially the essays in Payne 1998.

community regardless of affiliation with any particular school (Orzech, Payne, and Sørensen 2011, 6–7). Due to the ties Kūkai developed with the court, Japanese esoteric Buddhism was intertwined with the social elite, and ritual ties to the emperor remain to this day. Thus, it is distinct from European-based forms of esotericism that can refer more to 'discarded' or 'forbidden' forms of knowledge. Despite some of the variance in perspective, there is at least general agreement around the fact that the esoteric Buddhist movement was centred around ritual practices such as *dhāraṇi*, mantra, *abhiṣeka*, and mandala.[4]

As Shingon was already a system of esoteric Buddhism that made its way from India via China, there were considerable layers of cultural synthesis within its practices. The discourse around mandalas within the tradition from Kūkai through contemporary Shingon priests often emphasised a syncretic notion of inclusivity – all beings and teachings are said to be included within the Shingon mandalas – even if they also presented a clear hierarchy of such views. Kūkai himself convinced the emperor to let him found a public school which taught burgeoning Shingon priests and others free of charge not only Buddhist but Confucian and Daoist teachings as well. Contemporary priests regularly refer to the mandalas and to this school of Kūkai's when rationalising the adaptation or inclusion of new and different traditions and practices within their Shingon framework. One contemporary priest reaching out and mixing myriad elements with his own Shingon lineage more than most is Ōshita Daien.

Ōshita Daien's Clinical Meditation and Breath Therapies[5]

Ōshita Daien was born not far from Senkōji temple in 1954 and became inspired to become a Buddhist priest after experiencing multiple family deaths by the age of 12. The abbot of the temple at the time told Ōshita that he might find some of the answers to his questions about life by going through priestly training. Ōshita became his student and a priest within the Shingon tradition. He went on to study at the tradition's primary school,

4 For further background and discussion on the range of meanings for esoteric Buddhism, see R. Sharf 2003; Orzech 1996; McBride 2004; Sharf and Sharf 2002; Sharf 2002; Chou 1945; Payne 1991; Orzech 1989; Orzech, Sørensen, and Payne 2011.

5 Unless otherwise noted, information on Ōshita Daien's life and activities within this profile is woven together primarily from interviews. However, some interview questions were based on biographical details provided by two texts he authored (Ōshita 2019b; 2019c; 2012, 17–21; 2005, 1–2).

Koyasan University, and also to spend time as a monk in Sri Lanka, gaining more experience in Buddhist cultures and meditation traditions beyond Japan. A Sri Lankan friend whom he originally met in Japan also introduced Ōshita to Sri Lankan Buddhists who were providing humanitarian relief and care. Upon returning to Japan, he also experienced his teacher's terminal illness and hospitalisation. Ōshita was disappointed at the impersonal aspects of care in the medical system and, after conversations with a few others who shared his concerns, he decided to get more directly involved. He trained to become certified as a music therapist and began volunteering at a local hospital. Music therapy is an evidence-based form of therapeutic interventions accepted by medical establishments within contemporary clinical environments but can include a diverse range of such interventions based on the psychotherapeutic approaches and the range of activities its practitioners employ; activities can include listening, writing, and making music, as well as singing and dancing, but is generally geared to needs, interests, and capabilities of the patient. While it began as a formal psychotherapeutic intervention in the United States, it is also now firmly established in Japan with training and certification.

Because of Shingon's own emphasis on mantras and the role played by vibration from sounds of the mantras, the use of music therapy may have been a natural fit for Ōshita. He stated that he believes chanting and music can have 'healing power' (*iyashi no pāwā* 癒しのパーワー) and that the music needs to be tuned to the patient in order to reach them in a special way.

The official certification in music therapy helped allow him to gain positions caring for people in local hospitals and clinics. Yet no matter your other qualifications, contemporary Japan is not an easy place for a Buddhist priest to help in hospitals, especially if they dress in customary priestly attire.[6] Historically, Buddhist temples often served as local clinics and even hospices or infirmaries; priests served not only in their ritual capacity but as local doctors, counsellors, and healers; typically the only individuals who could read in a village, they provided medical advice, mixed medicinal herbs, and distributed such medications (Miyagi 2018, 103–7; Yoshida and Hasegawa 2001; Japanese Association for Buddhist Social Welfare Studies 2006, 100). Since the Meiji Restoration (1868–1889), Buddhism lost most of its roles within Japanese society outside of funerary ritual functions. Thus,

6 Mark Rowe covers the development of the association of modern Japanese Buddhist priests with death and funerals in detail within his volume *Bonds of the Dead: Temples, Burial, and the Transformation of Contemporary Japanese Buddhism* (2011). For more specific looks at issues for Buddhists working in hospices and clinical environments, see Benedict 2022.

Buddhist priests became largely associated with death for the average contemporary Japanese. Surveys in Japan report that a religious professional is one of the least desirable people to meet on their deathbed.[7] Those who are sick often report that the presence of a Buddhist priest might mean they are about to die. Likewise, when Ōshita Daien first went into a hospital to volunteer with the sick during the 1990s, a security guard stopped him and said, 'I'm sorry, but the morgue is in the other direction' (Ōshita 2005, 3).

In time, Ōshita became a familiar face both in his own city of Hida, Gifu Prefecture and in numerous other facilities throughout Japan. He helped to establish several discussion and working groups locally and became a regular caring for terminally ill cancer patients at hospitals and clinics in the region. At first, there were no training programmes available like the various ones he would come to create, so he spent considerable time reading on his own in a variety of fields. Ōshita says that during this period, he was particularly influenced by Margaret Newman's (1933–2018) theories, which helped expand notions of health within nursing and hospice care to reimagine health as a more holistic notion, centred in the state of consciousness rather than only on physical measures. He also draws from Freud, Jung, and numerous other European and American psychotherapists. Gradually, he developed a keen interest in transpersonal psychology. He spent two years as a researcher at Kyoto University under the direction of Carl Becker, a renowned scholar of death, dying, and medical ethics in Japan. There, he examined different contemplative practices around the world and studied the scientific impacts of their practice. His readings involved in-depth examinations of numerous Buddhist traditions as well as mystics from Abrahamic traditions and their practices, Emanuel Swedenborg, and even contemporary figures like Ken Wilber.

In 2002, he began teaching courses on spiritual care at Koyasan University, the first such courses offered at a university in Japan. The idea proved to be a little too far ahead of its time and the programme folded soon after. However, he shifted efforts to creating his own organisation around the theme. By 2006, he founded the Japan Spiritual Care Workers Association

7 A 2006 survey, for example, conducted by the Japan Hospice Palliative Care Foundation only underscored this impression. Even when facing death, clergy of any kind are not thought of as a bedside comfort. One of the questions on the survey asked, 'If you had a terminal illness and were facing death, who do you think you would want supporting your heart?'. The survey allowed for multiple responses. Partners and children were the two most common at 69.2% and 61.7%, respectively. Friends, doctors, people who shared the same illness and nurses followed. Religious clergy (*shūkyōsha* 宗教者) were nearly last, tied with social workers at 4.2%. This was only ahead of 'nobody' at 4.1% and workplace colleague at 2.5% (Takamatsu 2006, 99–100).

(JSCWA, *Nihon supirichuarukea wākā kyōkai* 日本スピリチュアルケアワーカー協会) as an early chaplaincy education and certification organisation, which would later become a part of larger Japanese chaplaincy certification organisation that was formed a decade later. Along the way, he developed a system of 'Clinical Meditation' (*rinshō meisō* 臨床瞑想), or 'meditation therapy' (*meisō ryōhō* 瞑想療法), and then a training programme to certify doctors, nurses, and other clinicians in using the process. Over that time, Ōshita authored or coauthored more than a dozen books which outline his thoughts and practices. They include popular volumes about meditation and living more stress-free lives, nonfiction books that detail his theory and application of meditation therapy in different settings, and specialised training volumes directed at nurses and other clinical workers.

In building his Clinical Meditation system, Ōshita Daien attempted to organise a broad range of contemplative practices sourced from traditions around the world into four categories: relaxation, observation, energising, and releasing. As it sounds, *relaxation* exercises are for general relaxation of the body and mind. There is little need to exert particular concentration, but just bring oneself to greater ease. *Observation* exercises require a little more concentration and keen mindful attention to physical, emotional, and thought-based constructs. They can involve careful examinations of one's personal history and memories or close observation of the effects of breathing in a particular way. *Energising* meditations are typically visualisations; they bring about a sense of energy in the body and lead to heightened alertness. These can include focusing on mandalas or light, like meditating in front of a candle and imagining its light merging with one's own body or doing a similar activity outside while visualising the energy (*enerugī* エネルギー) of a nearby tree or mountain. Ōshita compares these meditations to the Shingon practices of *nyūga-ga'nyū* 入我我入 or *jiririta* 自利利他 in which one merges with Buddhas or other images of a mandala as part of a visualising and attaining of that deity's power or a broader perception of blending in with one's surroundings. *Releasing*, like relaxation exercises, refers to meditations that bring about a greater sense of ease, but these refer to meditations that work on a deeper level – closer to the cognitive sources of stress and suffering – and allow a longer-term effect after such 'release'. There are, of course, overlapping activities that might fit into more than one category. But this four-fold categorisation helped Ōshita organise a broad swath of meditations from different contemplative traditions into a system that could be more readily conveyed to not only patients but also clinicians who could learn to guide the practices. Through this systematisation, Ōshita attempted to combine a sort of flexibility which could adapt to different clinicians and patients' needs, while also providing enough structure to help them develop and, ideally, experience greater results over continued practice.[8]

Rather than limit the therapeutic practices to a single tradition of meditation practices, Ōshita is content to borrow from a variety of systems, theories, and practices depending on the needs of clients. However, one can see the overall dominance of his background in Shingon Buddhism and Sri Lankan Theravada Buddhism within his writings and offerings. There is also a subtle hierarchical structure which suggests a greater depth to the Shingon-based practices. The first two categories contain numerous meditations he encountered and practised in Sri Lanka as well as basic breathing and relaxing meditations from other world religions. His descriptions of energising meditations become increasingly full of Shingon-influenced practices, while releasing meditations are almost exclusively Shingon or Shingon-based descriptions. It is also suggested that these latter practices can be more advanced. Thus, although Ōshita reaches out broadly into other traditions, there is still an underlying value favouring his Shingon tradition and somewhat reminiscent of the ranking systems that Kūkai and other famous teachers of East Asian Buddhism commonly put forward while trying to gain favour from the respective rulers of their times and places. Kūkai's own *Ten Abiding Stages of Mind According to the Secret Mandala* (*Himitsu mandara jūjūshinron* 秘密曼荼羅十住心論) was, in a sense, very inclusive, incorporating the teachings of numerous other Buddhist schools and non-Buddhist teachings and giving them valid places along his path of practice. Yet they were placed into ten categories of mind that represented ever higher stages of cultivation and development.[9] The *mikkyō* teachings were at the top. Ōshita's own system is likewise very inclusive of different practices, while also favouring the Shingon practices as its pinnacle.

The overall client process from his music therapy background also shows through his client engagement and teaching. Yet, this background also lends itself to the novelty of the system. He might, for example, combine counselling of music therapy with traditional Shingon chanting and taiko drumming, mixing in breathing practices and guided visualisations all in a single session. He typically begins with an 'intake' session, getting to know the patient, their issues, needs, and preferences. He is careful never to force

8 More detailed explorations of this system can be found in Ōshita 2016a, 39–67; 2012, 177–94; 2016b, 160–77; 2019a, 66–89; 2021, 30–59; 2014, 92–113. An earlier form of the system and descriptions of the multitudes of practices he includes can be found in Ōshita 2010, 3–53.

9 More analysis of sectarian interpretations of the Ten Abiding Stages of Mind According to the Secret Mandala can be found in Abe (1999, 326–27).

anything overtly Buddhist or religious on any patient, only offering such options if the patient is open to it and if the setting allows (legal restrictions within some clinical settings can prevent providing certain religious-based therapies even if a patient requests it). As a licensed music therapist, he may offer secular music or traditional Buddhist chanting. He tries to find the volume, pace, rhythm, and style suitable to each patient employing a variety of breathing techniques and visualisations to help his patients relax further.

Ōshita asserts that combining chanting with music therapy was his own creation and that he had not seen any previous literature on the topic when he began to carry out such modes of therapy. However, he does say he was at least partly inspired by the use of *goeika* (御詠歌) chanting in traditional Japanese healing approaches prior to the use of modern therapies. *Goeika* is a form of Japanese Buddhist chanting performed along with rhythmic chimes of handbells and mallets striking small metal plates, often done in groups. Although little research has been done on *goeika*, discourse around Koyasan typically associates its background with healing, and introductory books for practitioners mention the link between such music and its capacity to relieve stress and heal (Kōyasan Kongōkō Sōhonbu 2015, 1–3). Ōshita emphasises that as opposed to many religious ceremonies, the application of chanting to contemporary therapy is typically performed on a one-on-one basis, being thus highly individualised. Qualities of the sound within the chanting are customised to meet the individual needs and preferences of each patient. 'Should it be louder or softer? Faster or slower? What about the rhythm? I must tune the music to the patient in many subtle ways. Without that sort of music therapy technique, it is not therapy'. He then laughed while I spoke with him, admitting such chanting was certainly not for everyone. Again, many of the patients are not religious and although some may prefer the traditional Japanese sound that such chanting provides, others may be averse. Ōshita again emphasised that this was why listening carefully during the initial assessment was so important.

If the patient is interested in learning some of the more contemplative tools, he will often start by simply saying, 'Shall we practice breathing together?'. He usually helps count breaths for the patient and breaths with them at their pace for the first eight to ten breaths. He then guides a relaxation practice for another five to ten minutes. As with the music, Ōshita's choices of meditation vary heavily depending upon the assessment of his patient. If the initial discussion showed that the patient particularly enjoys mountains, beaches, or some other place, he may ask them to imagine relaxing in such a scene, in combination with the music and breathing exercises. But he also states that there is a feel to the timing of when to incorporate different practices which require keen and continuous observation of the patient's physical and verbal responses and reactions. He adds that there is also an element of experience and that continual assessment and reflection after each session are critical to growth as a therapist.

If it is a Buddhist patient who shows interest in chanting, Ōshita may also teach them a mantra. He provided the following sample conversation during an interview:

> Do you know Avalokitesvara's mantra?
> No, I'm not familiar with that
> *On arorikya sowaka*
> Oh that's a different way than I'd think
> Right!? Let's practice chanting that: *On arorikya sowaka*

Ōshita adds that his patients may not have great technique at first, but that they practice chanting the mantra a few times together until getting the pattern down. 'Ok, shall we try chanting that repeatedly for a minute?'

Ōshita is also careful to point out that there are significant differences in the range of care that takes place within a hospital or public facility compared to the minority of patients who are able to directly visit his temple.[10] The patients who visit his temple tend to be more religious or more desperate – with an illness or condition that no clinical facilities can heal. He is relatively freer in the range of religious practices he may include within the temple, and sometimes he merges his more typical forms of patient care with *kajikitō* 加持祈祷 ritual healing ceremonies or *taiko* drumming while chanting. *Kaji* itself is a Japanese term commonly referenced in Shingon Buddhism and derives from the Sanskrit term *adhisthāna*, or 'empowerment'. *Kajikitō* are more specifically prayer-like rituals to help with a wide variety of both general and specific ailments and afflictions. The Shingon tradition has many compendiums of such rituals that developed over the centuries, each ritual generally designed to treat a particular ailment.[11] Most elements of such rituals are structured around the 'three mysteries' mentioned above, including a series of mudras, mantras, and visualisations.

No matter the setting, as he sees the same patient more often, Ōshita will work on gradually more complex breathing techniques and visualisations.

10 While working with Kyoto University, Ōshita also ran several studies of meditation applied to caring for people's needs in an elementary school, athletic training programme, doctors, and nurses from a palliative care ward. These studies are all included in Ōshita 2010, 117–36.

11 For overarching theory and categorisation of such rituals see, for example, Mitsui 2016.

Although not always a straight progression, he typically advances people through the four categories of his clinical meditation system with the options he provides. Every meditation begins with some relaxation, but as the patient becomes more experienced, they may shift to an observation or energising meditation after a few minutes.

In training others within his system, Ōshita Daien created a three-part certification process. It involves reading literature he's written and participating in three multiday retreat trainings. The first two trainings each cover two meditation categories within the system. They consist of lectures about meditation styles, guided meditations, and discussion sessions around the experiences of meditation, difficulties within the practice, and nuances of how to apply it in different participants' own lives and workplaces. Prior to participating in the third workshop, students must prepare sample meditations to guide patients during role-playing activities. The final training session involves splitting into pairs to not only actualise such role-play activities but also to go through levels of feedback and processing of the experience of guiding a meditation so that each participant can refine their guidance styles. The students who role-play as patients may provide feedback like, 'Your speech was a little too fast', 'Maybe be a little more gentle with the sound of your voice' or 'Don't hit the meditation bell quite so hard'. Ōshita adds that these are gradual processes and students are obviously not expected to begin as experts. 'Everybody fails in the process numerous times, but through plenty of practice and feedback, everyone slowly refines their technique'.

Takayama Seiei's Clinical Meditation and Breath Therapies[12]

One of the students Ōshita trained in his clinical meditation courses was a fellow Shingon priest named Takayama Seiei. Takayama lived most of his life in Hokkaido, the northernmost of Japan's islands, and became the abbot of Naritasan Shinnyoin 成田山真如院, a temple in Sapporo, Hokkaido's largest city. Whereas many Japanese temples are run through membership systems that connect families to the temple for funerals and memorial services, not all temples have such memberships or sources of financial sustenance.[13]

12 The details about Takayama's life and work come from two interviews with him (Takayama 2019a; 2019b).

13 For a detailed look at the business and monetary side of temple funerary practices in contemporary Japan, see Rowe 2011.

Since its founding in the year 1900, Naritasan had never had traditional members and was always run as a *kitō* temple, providing specialised rituals and services for people with particular needs at different times in their lives. Many of these dealt with healing-based services for those with physical or mental illness, but people also came to ask for blessings for good business, study success, love, and a variety of other needs. Hokkaido is already a very rural island and by being on the outskirts of Sapporo in the 1900s, Naritasan was barely connected to the main city. Many soldiers came for protective blessings before heading into war in one of the many fronts that existed during the first half of the 20th century. Those who were injured or traumatised by the war in various ways also came to the temple for aid. Naritasan especially took care of prostitutes and military partners who no longer had a place to go after their male counterparts left for war. It was, thus, a small temple that took care of many of Sapporo's socially disadvantaged during Japan's imperialist period and its aftermath.

After taking over as abbot, Takayama tried as much as possible to continue this tradition through his focus on the physically and mentally ill. However, at one point he found himself counselling a woman who had come for support after a troubled marriage and divorce. Although the woman was gracious and kind, after a while he stopped hearing from her. Takayama discovered she had committed suicide. The shock of the incident overwhelmed him. His feelings of inadequacy to provide for the people who asked for his counselling also grew to a tipping point. His training as a Shingon priest was primarily about contemplative rituals and chanting. Even though he served many people with mental illnesses or troubling life issues, much of his approach was based on instinct rather than specialised training. He says that the woman's suicide shined a light on his weaknesses, yet it inspired him to seek out numerous forms of training. He attended different chaplaincy programmes in Japan and, over a period of six years, was ultimately certified through three different organisations: Spiritual Care Workers Association, Japan Society for Spiritual Care 日本スピリチュアルケア学会, and Japan Society for Interfaith Chaplains 日本臨床宗教師会.[14] Through these trainings, he studied the psychotherapeutic theories and counselling styles of Jung, Freud, and Rogers; he learned spiritual care from the viewpoints

14 Although Takayama completed the study and service required to earn certificates from each of these organisations, he did not follow through in maintaining any of those certifications. He appreciated the training he received from them, but his situation was different from chaplains serving in public settings. He did not feel his clientele sought such certificates, and his own practice within a temple providing religious and healing rituals alongside the spiritual care of chaplaincy crossed ethical boundaries with some of the organisations (Takayama 2019a).

of Simonton Method, thanatology, and nursing (Takayama 2018, 12–13). Takayama also examined both Buddhist and Christian perspectives on spiritual care. He felt Ōshita Daien's clinical meditation programme would be a perfect complement to his work from the perspective of a Shingon priest who already was using his tradition's rituals and contemplative practices and completed that programme as well. His Buddhist spiritual care courses were taught by Ōshita Daien, but Ōshita Daien had included a course taught by Kubotera Toshiyuki 窪寺俊之within the Spiritual Care Workers Association curriculum. Kubotera is a Protestant minister and professor Seigakuin University in Osaka who previously trained in chaplaincy in the United States. Kubotera was thus able to impart both the Christian origins of chaplaincy and different theological perspectives on spiritual care. In both the United States and Japan, professional chaplaincy training often involves learning about other religions and theologies different from one's own tradition. This is not only meant to help broaden one's capacity to care for people from more religious traditions but also to help provide comparative perspectives that help one look at their own tradition in new ways and with new questions.

After completing all this training, back in his home temple, he established the Heart Recuperation Centre (Kokoro no ryōyōin 心の療養院). He began seeing a wider variety of cases. He said many people came to him to speak about mental depression, but he also had visitors with various physical disabilities, struggles with autism, and families grieving from a suicide. He added that most people come to his temple after already having visited hospitals or other clinics for care but feeling like they need something in addition, as if there was something missing. Some are patients who have been told they will not recover from their illness and are either looking for a miraculous alternative or a way to cope and live with the illness. In comparison to clinical facilities that say they cannot do anything more for a patient's condition, he says that 'because this [i.e., his temple] is not a hospital, I can't turn anyone away. I must accept everyone. I listen deeply, offer some advice and try to help people calm their minds'.

He says that often conversations will start out lightly. But because Naritasan is a Buddhist temple, he asks if his patients would like to try breathing exercises or meditative visualisations without much hesitation soon after the sessions begin. There are exceptions. If an individual has had trouble sleeping, meditation will typically just put them to sleep, so he may avoid it in such cases. Takayama is careful to say that meditations are not a panacea and are not right for all people. 'For example, with depression, as much as possible, I don't do meditation with them. Maybe just basic breathing meditation for 10 minutes. But if you do a deep meditation, it can potentially be dangerous'. With certain other mental illnesses, he asserts, meditation can also be dangerous. He draws a line between the type of help he tries to provide and stresses that he does not want people to confuse his temple as an actual clinic – which could even put him in legal trouble.

In most cases, though, Takayama begins with a style that he developed after adapting some of the techniques he learned from Ōshita Daien. After some brief introduction, he helps lead the individual in a meditation, typically for about 10 minutes. He asks beginners to try counting their breaths for the entire time. If they total around 50 breaths, he often asks them to try only about 20 breaths during the next 10-minute session, and to see if it helps them to relax further. Between meditation sessions, he asks questions about how they are doing or how they feel. They might go back and forth with the guest answering his questions for a few minutes. When there seems to be an impasse developing, he will transition back to a meditation session. He says that after meditation, people are often far more ready to open up and express themselves, moving deeper into their own experiences.

Because these activities were still a function of his temple, rather than basing most of his work at a hospital like Ōshita Daien, he could generally operate with more freedom from legal rules and facility policies. His work therefore included far more mixture of the therapeutic breathing and counselling with esoteric Buddhist rituals, mantras, and other more overtly religious subject matter. If an individual is interested in *kajikitō*, for example, he will perform a variety of types depending on their issues and requests, including exorcisms (*yakubarai* 厄払い) and *goma* 護摩 fire rituals – ritual categories in the Shingon tradition that have many forms depending on the type of illness and other factors. Thus, the Shingon aspects in Takayama's own care tend to be far more overtly Buddhist and Shingon than the services provided by Ōshita Daien.

Dependant Originations and Entangled Syntheses

Neither Ōshita Daien nor Takayama Seiei speak more than some basic words outside of their native Japanese, and almost the entirety of both their work is based within Japan. They are ordained within a Japanese Buddhist tradition and access it as a primary source of inspiration for their care and therapeutic practice. Yet, as these case studies demonstrate, there is a deeply complex entanglement of influence and conscious contribution to the worlds around them.

Ōshita Daien's life included abundant, interconnecting streams of inspiration and influence. Despite being a Shingon Buddhist priest, he experienced life as a Theravada monk in Sri Lanka. The journeys in Sri Lanka provided inspiration for Ōshita in the way he saw Buddhist practices being applied to help everyday people. He began to do this in his own way back in Japan, albeit through therapeutic formats and processes that came to Japan from the US (hospice care, transpersonal psychology, music therapy, etc.). Even these therapies brought to Japan from the US themselves were developed with various threads of influence from around the world over time. Ōshita also interacted with and researched many other forms of Buddhism, as well as figures and teachings from other world contemplative traditions while at Kyoto University. Along the way, he was constantly synthesising knowledge from these various streams and presenting them in newly combined forms. His numerous writings, organisations, public talks, and trainings showed a continuous evolution of this interplay and his role within it.

Takayama Seiei may not have the public persona and overall societal impact of a figure like Ōshita Daien, but his story equally exemplifies these intertwining influences and impacts at a more local level. To a degree, he is impacted by all the various networks and influences of Ōshita as his student. But Takayama takes those lessons alongside the other programmes he trained in and his Shingon background, creating new systems to try and meet the needs of those in his local sphere.

Further social and historical layers of complexity only compound these. Contemporary Shingon Buddhism itself, for instance, is not found in a bubble or in a simple slow attainment of historical accoutrements from India to China and then Japan. There were intricate exchanges with a variety of practitioners throughout Japanese history. Even in modern history, the sophisticated interplay across the Atlantic was impacting US and European culture just as such cultures have been changing and transforming the Shingon tradition. As indicated in the Introduction of this edited volume, the mind-cure movements and the flow of Asian teachers into North America and Europe during the late 19th and early 20th centuries led to the categories of 'mind' and 'mental health' for understanding health and sickness in new ways. These critical exchanges had an immense historical impact on the fields that Ōshita and Takayama would come to enter. Occult movements in the US and Europe also have a complex history of intercultural exchange with esoteric Buddhism and other Asian traditions (Tweed 2005; Jaffe 2004). The innumerable complexities added by historical layers would be impossible to fully track in a book-length volume, let alone a section within a chapter. Yet even these brief examples help express the point.

Ōshita and Takayama have both taken in countless streams of influence, but both have played active roles in how they sought such information, accessed it, and adapted and transformed it on their own terms. The extreme complexities in such webs of influence are far more than any simple tidal flow from East to West could ever manage to indicate. As the examples above show, there are no linear streams of influence that flow into their esoteric Buddhism from 'the West'. Both these men primarily identify as Shingon Buddhist priests and follow ritual practices purportedly passed down for over a thousand years as part of the healings they offer (Takayama more so). The esoteric Buddhism they present, though, is itself a web of many influences. Around and within that, they pull from readings and trainings that have been cross-culturally developed. They apply that to their own therapies which develop over time. Ōshita, in particular, borrows from other schools of Buddhism and different contemplative practices around the world. Takayama serves as an example of how Ōshita is impacting those around him in Japan as well. Takayama has learned from Ōshita and incorporated aspects of that experience into his own breathing therapies with patients on the northernmost main island of Japan. Yet Takayama also learned from and incorporated the spiritual care training of a Christian minister and various other psychological and therapeutic approaches. If anything, a more apt image might be a deeply entangled net of neurons in the brain constantly firing signals in an explosive communicative dance.

Bibliography

Abe, Ryuichi. 1999. *The Weaving of Mantra: Kūkai and the Construction of Esoteric Buddhist Discourse*. New York: Columbia University Press.

Benedict, Timothy O. 2022. *Spiritual Ends: Religion and the Heart of Dying in Japan*. Berkeley: University of California Press. https://doi.org/10.1525/luminos.136.

Chou, Yi-liang. 1945. 'Tantrism in China'. *Harvard Journal of Asiatic Studies* 8, no. 3/4: 241–332. https://doi.org/10.2307/2717819.

Fukuda, Ryōsei 福田亮成. 2014. *Kūkai shisō to sono tenkai* 空海思想とその展開 [Kūkai's Thought and its Development]. Tokyo.

Jaffe, Richard M. 2004. 'Seeking Śākyamuni: Travel and the Reconstruction of Japanese Buddhism'. *Journal of Japanese Studies* 30, no. 1: 65–96. http://doi.org/10.1353/jjs.2004.0019.

Kōyasan daigaku sensho kankōkai 高野山大学選書刊行会 ed. 2006. *Gendai ni ikiru Kūkai* 現代に生きる空海 [Kukai in Our Time]. Kōyasan Daigaku Sensho vol. 5. Kōyachō: Kōyasan daigaku.

Kōyasan Kongōkō Sōhonbu 高野山金剛講総本部. 2015. *Kōyasan Kongōryū Goeika Q&A* 高野山金剛流ごえいかQ&A [Koyasan Kongo School of Goeika Q&A]. Kōyachō: Kōyasan Shingonshū Kyōgakubu.

McBride, Richard D. 2004. 'Is There Really "Esoteric" Buddhism?'. *Journal of the International Association of Buddhist Studies* 27, no. 2: 329–56. https://poj.peeters-leuven.be/content.php?url=issue&journal_code=JIABS&issue=2&vol=27.

Mitsui, Eikō 三井英光. 2016. *Kajikitō no genri to jisshū* 加持祈祷の原理と実修 [Principles and Practice of Blessing Prayer]. Koyacho: Kōyasanshuppansha.

Miyagi, Yōichiro 宮城洋一郎. 2018. *Nihon kodai bukkyō no fukushi shisō to jissen* 日本古代仏教の福祉思想と実践 [Welfare Thought and Practice in Ancient Japanese Buddhism]. Tokyo: Iwatashohin.

Nihon Bukkyō Shakai Fukushi Gakkai 日本仏教社会福祉学会 ed. 2006. *Bukkyō shakai fukushi jiten* 仏教社会福祉辞典 [Buddhist Social Welfare Dictionary]. Tokyo: Hōzōkan.

Orzech, Charles D. 1989. 'Seeing Chen-Yen Buddhism: Traditional Scholarship and the Vajrayāna in China'. *History of Religions* 29, no. 2: 87–114.
https://doi.org/10.1086/463182.

Orzech, Charles D. 1996. 'Maṇḍalas on the Move: Reflections from Chinese Esoteric Buddhism Circa 800 C.E'. *Journal of the International Association of Buddhist Studies* 19, no. 2: 209–44. https://poj.peeters-leuven.be/content.php?url=issue&journal_code=JIABS&issue=2&vol=19.

Orzech, Charles D., Richard K. Payne, and Henrik Sørensen. 2011. 'Introduction: Esoteric Buddhism and the Tantras in East Asia: Some Methodological Considerations'. In *Esoteric Buddhism and the Tantras in East Asia*, edited by Charles D. Orzech, Henrik Sørensen, and Richard K. Payne, 1–18. Boston: Brill.
https://doi.org/10.1163/ej.9789004184916.i-1200.6.

Orzech, Charles, Henrik Sørensen, and Richard Payne, eds. 2011. *Esoteric Buddhism and the Tantras in East Asia*. Boston: Brill. https://doi.org/10.1163/ej.9789004184916.i-1200.

Ōshita, Daien 大下大圓. 2005. *Iyashi iyasareru supirichuaru kea: Iryō, fukushi, kyōiku ni ikasu bukkyō no kokoro* 癒し癒されるスピリチュアルケア：医療・福祉・教育に活かす仏教の心 [Healing and More Healing Through Spiritual Care: The Buddhist Mind in Medicine, Welfare, and Education]. Tokyo: Igakushoin.

Ōshita, Daien 大下大圓. 2010. *Kea to taijin enjo ni ikasu meisō ryōhō* ケアと対人援助に活かす瞑想療法 [Meditation Therapy for Care and Interpersonal Assistance]. Tokyo: Igakushoin.

Ōshita, Daien 大下大圓. 2012. *Isagiyoku ikiru: Bukkyōteki shinpuru raifu* いさぎよく生きる：仏教的シンプルライフ [Living with Rigor: A Simple Buddhist Life]. Tokyo: Nippon hyōronsha.

Ōshita, Daien 大下大圓. 2014. *Jissenteki supirichuaru kea: Nāsu no ikikata o kaeru 'jiririta' no kokoro* 実践的スピリチュアルケア：ナースの生き方を変える'自利利他'のこころ [Practical Spiritual Care: 'Self-Reliance and Altruism' to Change Nurses' Way of Life]. Tokyo: Nihon kango kyōkai shuppansha.

Ōshita, Daien 大下大圓. 2016a. *Rinshō meisōhō: Kokoro to shintai ga yomigaeru yottsu no mesoddo* 臨床瞑想法：心と身体がよみがえる4つのメソッド [Clinical Meditation: Four Methods to Revive Mind and Body]. Tokyo: Nihon kango kyōkai shuppansha.

Ōshita, Daien 大下大圓. 2016b. *Mikkyō tairaku ni ikiru waza: sōgō meisō ga anata wo kaeru* 密教大楽に生きるワザ：総合瞑想があなたを変える [Esoteric Dhyana Living with Ease: Comprehensive Meditation Transforms You]. Tokyo: Nippon Hyōronsha.

Ōshita, Daien 大下大圓. 2016c. *'Inochi' no omomi: Shōnikai to rinshōshūkyōshi ga kataru 'kokoro no shohōsen'* 「いのち」の重み：小児科医と臨床宗教師が語る「心の処方箋」 [The Weight of Life: A Pediatrician and a Clinical Religious Practitioner Discuss 'Prescription for the Heart']. Tokyo: Kosei Shuppan.

Ōshita, Daien 大下大圓. 2017. *Kūkai no meisō de mayoi ga kieru! Chōkenkō ni naru!* 空海の瞑想で迷いが消える！超健康になる！ [Kukai's Meditation Will Make Your Doubts Disappear! You Will Become Super Healthy!]. Tokyo: Makino shuppan.

Ōshita, Daien 大下大圓. 2019a. *Meisōryoku: Ikikata ga kawaru yottsu mo mesoddo* 瞑想力：生き方が変わる四つのメソッド [The Power of Meditation: Four Methods to Change the Way You Live]. Tokyo: Nippon hyōronsha.

Ōshita, Daien 大下大圓. 2019b Interview by author, 6 June. Senkōji Temple, Hida, Japan.

Ōshita, Daien 大下大圓. 2019c Interview by author, 7 June. Senkōji Temple, Hida, Japan.

Ōshita, Daien 大下大圓. 2021. *Sokushin jōbutsu kanhō* 即身成仏観法. Osaka: Seizansha.

Payne, Richard K., ed. 1998. *Re-Visioning 'Kamakura' Buddhism*. Honolulu: University of Hawai'i Press.

Payne, Richard K. 1991. *Tantric Ritual of Japan: Feeding the Gods: The Shingon Fire Ritual*. Delhi: Aditya Prakashan. https://doi.org/10.1515/9780824843939.

Payne, Richard K. 2006. 'Awakening and Language: Indic Theories of Language in the Background of Japanese Buddhism'. In *Discourse and Ideology in Medieval Japanese Buddhism*, edited by Richard K. Payne and Taigen Dan Leighton, 79–96. New York: Routledge.

Rowe, Mark M. 2011. *Bonds of the Dead: Temples, Burial, and the Transformation of Contemporary Japanese Buddhism*. Chicago: University of Chicago Press. https://doi.org/10.7208/chicago/9780226730165.001.0001.

Sharf, Robert H. 2002. 'Visualization and Mandala in Shingon Buddhism'. In *Living Images: Japanese Buddhist Icons in Context*, 151–97. Stanford, CA: Stanford University Press.

Sharf, Robert, and Elizabeth Sharf, eds. 2002. *Living Images: Japanese Buddhist Icons in Context.* Stanford, CA: Stanford University Press.

Sharf, Robert. 2003. 'Thinking through Shingon Ritual'. *Journal of the International Association of Buddhist Studies* 26, no. 1: 51–96. https://poj.peeters-leuven.be/content.php?url=issue&journal_code=JIABS&issue=1&vol=26.

Sørensen, Henrik. 2011. 'On Esoteric Buddhism in China: A Working Definition'. In *Esoteric Buddhism and the Tantras in East Asia*, edited by Charles D. Orzech, Richard K. Payne, and Henrik Sørensen, 153–75. Boston: Brill. https://doi.org/10.1163/ej.9789004184916.i-1200.51.

Stone, Jacqueline I. 2003. *Original Enlightenment and the Transformation of Medieval Japanese Buddhism*. Honolulu: University of Hawaii Press. https://doi.org/10.1515/9780824840501.

Takamatsu, Tetsuyū 高松哲雄. 2006. 'Shūkyō to iryō: Kanwa iryō to shūkyōsha no hatasu yakuwari 宗教と医療：緩和医療と宗教者の果たす役割' [Religion and Medicine: Palliative Medicine and the Role of the Religious]. In *Gendai ni mikkyō o tō* 現代に密教を問う [Questioning Esoteric Buddhism in Our Time] 3: 98–109. Koyasan University Anthology. Kōyachō: Kōyasan daigaku.

Takamura, Hiroki 高村弘毅 and Kōno Tadashi 河野忠. 2006. 'Kōbō Daishi to Mizu 弘法大師と水' [Water and Kōbō Daishi]. In *Gendai ni ikiru Kūkai* 現代に生きる空海, edited by Kōyasan daigaku sensho kankokai 高野山大学選書刊行会, 40–41. Kōyachō, Japan: Kōyasan daigaku.

Takayama, Seiei 高山誓英. 2018. *Kokuzō bosatsu gumojigyō kasō oyobi shakai de jissenshita rinsho jitsurei kiroku* 虚空蔵菩薩求聞持行回想及び社会で実践した臨床実例記録 [Recollections of the Ākāśagarbha Bodhisattva Mantra Recitation

Practice and Applications in Clinical Case Studies]. Sapporo: Naritasanshinnyōin Sapporobunin.

Takayama, Seiei 高山誓英. 2019a Interview by author. Sapporo, Japan.

Takayama, Seiei 高山誓英. 2019b Interview by author. Sapporo, Japan.

Tinsley, Elizabeth. 2011. 'Kukai and the Development of Shingon Buddhism'. In *Esoteric Buddhism and the Tantras in East Asia*, edited by Charles D. Orzech, Henrik Sørensen, and Richard K. Payne, 691–708. Boston: Brill. https://doi.org/10.1163/ej.9789004184916.i-1200.282.

Tweed, Thomas. 2005. 'American Occultism and Japanese Buddhism: Albert K. Edmunds, D.T. Suzuki, and Translocative History'. *Japanese Journal of Religious Studies* 33, no. 2: 249–81. https://doi.org/10.18874/jjrs.32.2.2005.249-281.

Yoshida, Kyūichi 吉田久一 and Hasegawa Masatoshi 長谷川匡俊. 2001. *Nihon bukkyō fukushi shisōshi* 日本仏教福祉思想史 [Japanese History of Buddhist Welfare Thought]. Tokyo: Hōzōkan.

Biography

Nathan Jishin Michon is a Japan Society for the Promotion of Science Visiting Scholar at Ryukoku University. His research particularly focuses on Buddhist chaplaincy and contemporary Japanese Buddhism. Among other works, they are the editor of *Refuge in the Storm: Buddhist Voices in Crisis Care* and coauthor of 'Buddhist Chaplaincy' in the *Oxford Research Encyclopedia*.

Part 4

Alternative Therapies and National Identities

Over the course of the 20th century, medicine emerged as a key avenue for modernisation and state-building in East Asia. The century was marked by a series of state-led campaigns aimed at curbing the activities of folk and ritual healers, deemed at odds with newly established scientific and biomedical paradigms. Concurrently, the period saw the invention of 'national medicines' – like Traditional Chinese Medicine and Korean Traditional Medicine – often celebrated as 'national treasures' that promised to reconcile Western science and Eastern knowledge. This dynamic between medical practices and state policies also resonated at the individual level. For example, following its economic reforms in 1978, China witnessed a surge in 'nurturing life' (*xiuyang* 修養) or 'self-cultivation' (*xiuxing* 修行) therapies focused on personal health, moral integrity, and individual autonomy.

As Anna Iskra, Fabian Winiger and David A. Palmer have observed (2020), the growing public interest in self-health, Traditional Chinese Medicine, and motivational literature has fostered a new type of subjectivity – one that views health and personal development as core elements of self- and, by extension, societal governance. Iskra, Winiger and Palmer contend that the rise of self-cultivation movements since the 1970s has been closely aligned with discourses on an escalating 'moral crisis' within the People's Republic of China, characterised as a deterioration of mutual respect and trust, rampant corruption, unethical business conduct, increased selfishness, radical materialism, and a decline in civic virtues, including patriotism. As the chapters in this final section illustrate, Mainland China is but one example of how East Asian therapies and spiritualities have become intertwined with cultural nostalgia, narratives of nationhood, and the quest for a redefined identity in the face of both galloping scientific progress and high levels of real or imagined globalisation.

Iskra, Anna, Fabian Winiger, and David A. Palmer. 2020. 'Remaking the Self: Spirituality, Civilization and the Chinese Quest for the Good Life in the Reform Era'. In *Handbook on Religion in China*, edited by Stephan Feuchtwang, 66–86. Cheltenham: Edward Elgar Publishing.

10 *Ki Suryŏn* in South Korea

Reclaiming the Term *Pigwahakchŏk* (Unscientific) to Challenge Scientific Supremacy

Victoria Ten and Michael Wharton

Abstract: Industrial growth and the development of a new middle class in South Korea around the 1980s went together with increased consumption and leisure culture, causing growing concerns with health and personal self-cultivation. *Ki suryŏn* 氣修練 are contemporary reinventions of South Korean self-cultivation practices similar to Indian yoga and Chinese *qigong*. This chapter focuses on an interview with Ch'oe Hyŏngsu, a trainee of GiCheon 氣天, one particular type of *ki suryŏn* practice. In the narrative of Ch'oe, the term *pigwahakchŏk* (unscientific), which he uses in a positive sense, embodies the conflict between the Korea of old and new: a way of life gone forever, yet reconstructed, idealised, and counterposed against modernity, understood as a combination of processes of Westernisation, globalisation, and the supremacy of scientific thinking.

Keywords: *ki suryŏn*, GiCheon, invented tradition, self-cultivation, New Age, body-mind

In this chapter, we will analyse an interview that Victoria Ten conducted with Mr Ch'oe Hyŏngsu, a trainee of GiCheon 氣天.[1] GiCheon is one of

1 Interview of 10.11.2010, Puch'ŏn, South Korea. Ch'oe Hyŏngsu gave Victoria Ten explicit permission to use his real name. This chapter contains elements from Chapters 1, 2, and 7 of the book by Victoria Ten published in 2020 (Ten 2020a). In 1998, Kich'ŏn Chungang Hyŏphoe 기천중앙협회 (Kich'ŏn Central Association) transcribed the term 기천 (氣天 McCune-Reischauer romanisation *Kich'ŏn*) into English as *Kichun*. The website http://www.kichun.co.kr was established by Pak P'yŏngsu on behalf of Kich'ŏn Chungang Hyŏphoe. In 2001, Lee Kit'ae (Yi Kit'ae), a disciple of Lee Sangwŏn, modified the transcription to *GiCheon* in order to distinguish Lee Sangwŏn's lineage from other branches of the practice. Consequently, in 2001, Kich'ŏn Chungang Hyŏphoe launched the website http://www.gicheon.com, which Lee Kit'ae managed on behalf of the association.

Gaitanidis, Ioannis, Luis Fernando Bernardi Junqueira, Avery Morrow, and Sangyun Han (eds), *Therapy, Spirituality, and East Asian Imaginaries*. Taylor & Francis Group 2025
DOI: 10.5117/9789048559015_CH10

many South Korean practices of mind-body cultivation. It represents one of the first *ki suryŏn* 氣修練 (training related to *ki*-life energy) groups established in South Korea in the early 1970s. We will examine *ki suryŏn* as a contemporary urban practice, which, much like Chinese *qigong* 氣功 (Palmer 2007; cf. Chapter 3) and Indian yoga (Van der Veer 2007), has been a modern reinvention that draws upon older Asian traditions. The notion of 'invented tradition' was first introduced by E.J. Hobsbawm and T.O. Ranger (1992 [1983]). However, Adam Chau highlights that all traditions are essentially constructed and invented. Consequently, he argues for embracing a dynamic, process-oriented, and context-specific comprehension of tradition within its actual social milieu (Chau 2011, 3). This aligns closely with the ethnographic approach we aim to employ in this chapter.

The sociologist Woo Hairan defines *ki suryŏn* as techniques directed towards moral and physical development. *Ki suryŏn* is supposed to lead to the harmonisation of the mind-body and the actualisation of an individual's hidden potential in the context of a union with the universe. *Ki suryŏn* groups focus on bodily practice, while selectively appropriating elements from various Korean religious traditions. Woo Hairan (2006b, 71–73) observes that techniques associated with *ki suryŏn* have spread beyond particular *ki suryŏn* groups, becoming a cultural product approachable by the majority of the Korean population. As part of popular culture, the cosmology and values of *ki suryŏn* have been interiorised by contemporary South Korean society through various means, including computer games, animation, and films. As a result, the terms *ki* 氣 and *ki suryŏn* have evolved into central keywords within contemporary Korean culture.

When examining *ki suryŏn* and similar East Asian (Chinese, Korean, and Japanese) practices in academia, we encounter a methodological problem: How should we tackle and classify them? What are they and how do we study them? In her work, Woo Hairan (2018) identifies *ki suryŏn* as part of an emerging New Age culture in South Korea. She defines New Age as a nonmainstream and noninstitutionalised religious/spiritual culture or, more precisely, as a set of practices that have gained global popularity since the second half of the 20th century. These techniques are particularly prevalent in industrial and urban societies and are centred around improving individuals' spiritual, mental, and physical capabilities. In her comparison

Since 2004, Lee Kit'ae has been teaching *GiCheon* outside of Korea, leading to the term *GiCheon* gaining recognition within the international *ki*-training community and accruing some social capital. Consequently, followers of other leaders, not limited to Lee Sangwŏn's disciples, now commonly use *GiCheon* as the transcription for 氣天.

of New Age cultures in Korea and Europe, Woo Hairan calls on researchers to devote greater attention to New Age phenomena in East Asia.

The belief in personal transformation that leads to the transformation of society and humanity as a whole has been identified as central to the New Age movement (Melton 1990, xiii; Chen 2006, 28–29, 35–38; cf. Chapter 5). While noting that *ki suryŏn* can be categorised as a part of New Age culture, we will primarily approach it as a culture of self-cultivation or, more precisely, as a Korean variant of East Asian *ki* practices (known as *qi* in Chinese; cf. Chapter 1). East Asian techniques related to *ki* are grounded in various physiological, psychological, and behavioural principles and often include healthcare, diet, massage, gymnastics, breathing exercises, meditation, and visualisation, as well as rules of daily behaviour (Despeux 2008). The Russian sinologist N.V. Abayev (1983, 1) approaches *ki* methods as a part of 'psycho-physical culture'. Abayev understands the goal of traditional East Asian culture as an orderly organisation of chaos into cosmos. This includes the complex organisation, governance, and cultivation of the physical and psychological lives of individuals, which can be achieved by the interiorisation of certain cultural values. Psycho-physical training aims to cultivate, or 'form', a person towards a culturally defined 'ideal'; this process of formation involves different methods of conscious, goal-oriented, and systematic regulation of psychic processes and corporeal practices. The level of psycho-physical development measures the progress the individual has made from an entry point, where the cultural development of that individual began. According to Abayev, psycho-physical culture constitutes a quintessential element of East Asian civilisations (Abaev and Shirokov 1991).

Michel Foucault (2001, 46) pointed out that similar techniques of self-transformation were shared by a number, if not by all, of civilisations around the world. He defined them as 'technologies of the self' that 'allow individuals to effect, by their own means or with the help of others, a certain number of operations on their own bodies and souls, thoughts, conduct, and way of being, so as to transform themselves in order to attain a certain state of happiness, purity, wisdom, perfection, or immortality' (Foucault 1988, 18). The practices in ancient Greece, based on which Foucault developed this concept, included rites of purification, concentration of the spirit/breath, techniques of retreat, and practices of enduring pain and hardship (Foucault 2001, 12, 46–47). East Asian techniques related to *ki* fit neatly into Foucault's definition of technologies of self. As discussed above, their goal is the transformation of the self. Likewise, they tend to focus on the purification of mind and body and include retreating from society – for example, into the mountains, as numerous Daoist hermits or Buddhist monks and nuns have done throughout history. Contemporary *ki suryŏn* is centred around breathing techniques. GiCheon positions, in particular, are painful to sustain. As has been argued elsewhere, pain as a transformative factor is an important element of many East Asian techniques of self-cultivation (Lobetti 2014), and GiCheon is one example of that (on suffering and transformation, cf. Chapter 6).

Pronounced as *xian* in Chinese, the character *sŏn* 仙 (immortality, immortals) has been traditionally associated with East Asian Daoism. It consists of two characters: *in* 人 (Ch: *ren*; human being) and *san* 山 (Ch: *shan*; mountain). The concepts of *sŏndo* 仙道 (Ch: *xiandao*; the way of immortals) and *sŏnpŏp* 仙法 (Ch: *xianfa*; techniques of immortality) are important parts of this East Asian culture of immortality. Korean *ki suryŏn* practitioners, including GiCheon students, widely use the terminology of Daoist internal alchemy, which is founded on practices of abdominal breathing. They also employ the term *tanhak* 丹學 (Ch: *danxue*; study of *tan*/*dan*), also referred to as *naedan* 內丹 (Ch: *neidan*). The character *tan* 丹 (Ch: *dan*), which means red colour or cinnabar, has also become a generic term for elixir of immortality achieved through external or internal alchemy (Kim Daeyeol 2000, 150). The term *tan* is a part of the word *tanjŏn* 丹田 (Ch: *dantian*; cinnabar field), subdivided into lower, middle, and upper according to the Daoist view of the body. In GiCheon and other similar East Asian practices, *tan'gong* 丹功 (*tan* power) is the process of strengthening the lower cinnabar field – located in the lower abdomen – and thereby increasing one's internal power, known as *kong* 功 or *naegong* 內功 (inner power).

The principles of alchemy in East Asia and Europe are alike in many ways. European alchemy evolved from ancient Greek and Arabic alchemy, and it appears that both were, in turn, influenced by East Asian alchemy (Smith 2014, 126). The objective of external alchemy is to produce an elixir that can transform any metal into gold and grant immortality. Similarly, internal alchemy also aims for immortality, but the elixir is created within the mind-body of the alchemist, typically through rituals and practices. Alchemy, therefore, would be another example of technologies of the self, as it seeks to transform the individual from mortal to immortal. In East Asian contexts, the term 'immortality' refers to processes of refining oneself and gaining a heightened understanding of reality through the advancement of one's physical, moral, spiritual, and cognitive faculties (Miura 2008a; Miura 2008b; Robinet 2008b; Kirkland 2008). As Don Baker (2007, 508) has noted, like other *ki suryŏn* groups, GiCheon can be easily classified as a school of internal alchemy.[2] The operational terms of the constructed tradition of

2 For more on GiCheon as a school of internal alchemy, see Ten 2020b.

GiCheon come from the ancient culture of internal alchemy, a classic form of self-cultivation in East Asia. Yet, these terms are utilised by contemporary practitioners in ways that reflect modern problems.

The character *ki*, a fundamental concept that underlies East Asian views of life, has been variously translated into English as energy, spirit, breath, or willpower (cf. Chapter 1). GiCheon instructors often talk about *ki* flow (*sunhwan* 순환) and *ki* blockage (*makhida* 막히다). These notions, common in the culture of *ki suryŏn*, are shared by *hanŭihak* 韓醫學 (Korean traditional medicine), which is part of the broader framework of East Asian medicine. *Hanŭihak* employs ideas from East Asian classics, such as the *Inner Canon of the Yellow Emperor* (*Huangdi Neijing* 黃帝內經), which are commonly used by Chinese medical doctors in China and Taiwan, as well as *kanpō* 漢方 medicine in Japan (Kim Taewoo 2010, 12, 30; Scheid 2002). During their training, many GiCheon practitioners identify *ki* with physical or mental-emotional abilities and describe *ki* as feelings of warmth, shaking or pain.

The term *suryŏn*, translated by Isabelle Robinet into English as 'cultivation and refinement', already forms part of the title of *Xiulian xuzhi* 修練須知 (Required Knowledge on Cultivation and Refinement), an anonymous Chinese work included in the Daoist Canon (Robinet 2008a, 557). Modern editions of the Daoist Canon trace their origins to an edition dating back to 1445 CE, which, in turn, was compiled based on the catalogues of Daoist writings prepared over a millennium earlier (Boltz 2008, 28). Therefore, East Asia has a longstanding, continuously evolving culture of self-cultivation, with Korean *ki suryŏn* re-invented in modern times as only one of its many avatars.

Before delving into the main subject of this chapter, it is essential to provide a brief overview of the methodology employed in this study. Victoria Ten (Jeon Yeon Hwa) has been practising and teaching GiCheon since 2001, and in 2006 she received the official title of *pŏmsa* (instructor) from the late GiCheon grandmaster Lee Sangwŏn (Yi Sangwŏn, usually referred to by his students as *Sabunim*) who passed away in 2007. Between 2010 and 2011, Victoria interviewed 61 GiCheon practitioners in South Korea, and based on these interviews, completed her doctoral thesis at Leiden University in 2017. While the study of *ki suryŏn* has gained increasing attention over the past two decades (Yang Ch'unho et al. 2000; Ch'oe Miyŏn 2008; Pak Misuk et al. 2003; Woo Hairan 2006a; 2006b), Victoria stands out as one of the few researchers who have extensively written about the subject in English (2015; 2020a; 2020b). Her research style fits the classic model of autoethnography as conceived by the anthropologist David Hayano in 1979. For Hayano, autoethnography meant a researcher writing an ethnography of her 'own people' while fully identifying herself with this group. This involvement entails enjoying full membership in the group, as acknowledged by both the researcher and the members of the group (Hayano 1979, 99–100). Victoria's research also falls under the categories of embodied knowledge and personal experience, reflexive ethnography, narrative ethnography, and self-ethnography (Ellis and Bochner 2000: 734, 740–42, 746; for a similar approach, cf. Chapters 2 and 3). For Victoria, the story of Mr Ch'oe is about how he experienced self-transformation in the cultural context of mountain immortality, a goal of GiCheon practice.

Michael Wharton became a GiCheon practitioner in 2019. As he is a novice, it might be difficult to classify him as a 'full member of the GiCheon community'. Nevertheless, Michael's own practice influences and forms his perception and understanding of GiCheon. When writing, Michael also writes about himself and his own experience. The ethnographic literature showcases a variety of writing styles used to express the self, with different approaches in how the ethnographer integrates himself into the text while providing feedback on others' statements (Brettell 1997, 225). This sheds light on the connections between the researcher and the individuals being interviewed (Gmelch 1991, 21, cited in Brettell 1997, 225). The personal background and societal position of researchers always influence the type of research agenda they create and pursue (Motzafi-Haller 1997, 204–16). Michael is also an active member of the UK Green Party. He conceives of GiCheon as providing a conceptual and ideological inspiration for experiencing the body as a microcosm and the community as a macrocosm; as GiCheon purifies the body, so we have to actively clean and heal the environment. GiCheon positions can be physically demanding, just like engaging in 'green activities' such as litter-picking on the beach and tree planting. Despite the physical challenges, both these endeavours are essential for reclaiming physical and environmental well-being. Michael understands that the contemporary scientific method tends to separate humanity from nature, positioning us as mere observers of natural phenomena. To restore a sense of connection with nature, humanity must learn to coexist harmoniously with the natural world. For Michael, Mr Ch'oe's story is about environmental concerns, pollution, and the protection of nature.

GiCheon as One of the First *Ki Suryŏn* Practices in South Korea

The first GiCheon teacher Pak Chŏngnyong (later called by his students Taeyang Chinin 大洋眞人, lit. Perfected Person Taeyang), first appeared in Pusan, South Korea, in the early 1970s, where he started teaching GiCheon positions and martial arts. He claimed that he was raised and taught in the mountains by Wŏnhye Sangin 元慧上人 (Superior Person Wŏnhye), a mountain immortal who possessed extraordinary powers (Pak and Ch'oe, n.d.). In 2010, Victoria received an unpublished manuscript from the late GiCheon teacher Kim Hŭisang. Kim learned that a writer, Ch'oe Hyŏn'gyu, had conducted interviews with Taeyang Chinin over several months, eventually composing a manuscript based on those interviews. Kim had obtained the manuscript from other GiCheon practitioners and believed that Ch'oe Hyŏn'gyu was the original author. Later, Victoria met Ch'oe Hyŏn'gyu, who confirmed that he was indeed the author and granted her permission to read and use the manuscript. Ch'oe Hyŏn'gyu had submitted the manuscript to Han'gyŏre Publishing Company, which rejected it. However, as some GiCheon practitioners who worked at the publishing house found the manuscript interesting, they circulated it within their community. The manuscript details Taeyang Chinin's childhood in the mountains and his later reintegration into South Korean society.

GiCheon was one of the first *ki suryŏn* groups that emerged in South Korea in the 1970s. GiCheon matured as a movement in the 1980s, coinciding with a broader trend of self-improvement becoming popular among the middle classes. This 'New Age culture' (Woo Hairan 2018) was largely a result of the middle classes' new-found leisure time and disposable income, made possible by the booming economy of the 1980s. The popularity of GiCheon and other *ki suryŏn* groups stemmed from a cultural movement, seeking life improvement as a response to the adverse impacts of industrial pollution and urbanisation. This quest involved re-establishing a connection with nature, particularly the mountains. As a result, while Koreans have long enjoyed mountain trips and hiking, this cultural trend has experienced a revitalisation since the 1980s, gaining a new lease of life (Dax 2015).

GiCheon training includes static and dynamic positions. The main static GiCheon position is called *naegasinjang*. It is considered the foundation of the practice and is performed as follows: the legs are spread with the feet shoulder-width, the ankles are turned outward at about 45 degrees, the knees are bent down and inward, a fist apart from each other, squatting, with the pelvis pointing down and the upper spine straight and perpendicular with the ground. The hands are held just in front of the face, elbows at shoulder level, palms facing forward and the wrists bent backwards to an uncomfortable degree (see Figure 10.1).

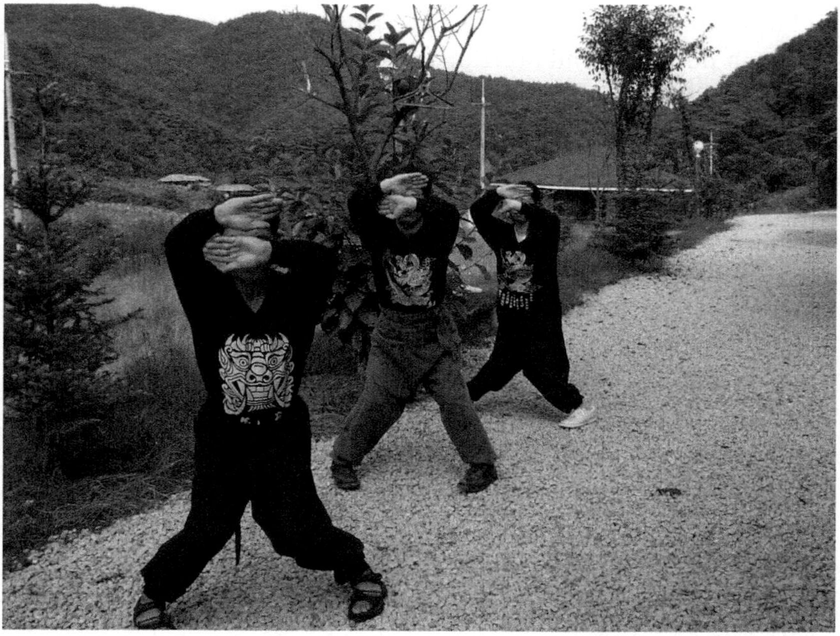

Figure 10.1. GiCheon students performing *naegasinjang* position at GiCheon Munmak mountain centre. Photo provided by SangMuWŏn organisation, used with permission.

The maximal bending of the joints in *naegasinjang* and other GiCheon positions is called *yŏkkŭn* 易筋.[3] Joints are considered *ki* gateways, and application of the *yŏkkŭn* principle is believed to facilitate the flow of *ki* throughout the body and mind, thus improving health. GiCheon instructors state that *naegasinjang* alone is sufficient for achieving perfect health, final enlightenment, and even complete immortality.

Life Choices of *Ki Suryŏn* Teachers in South Korea Today

Ch'oe Hyŏngsu, a small business owner in his early 50s at the time of the interview in 2010, was the first GiCheon student in the Puch'ŏn studio of the late GiCheon grandmaster Lee Sangwŏn back in 1995.[4] As revealed in his interview, Ch'oe displayed a remarkable talent for GiCheon, desiring to become a GiCheon teacher if the circumstances were different. Initially, he was concerned that taking on the role of a GiCheon teacher might result in

3 The character 易 (*yŏk*) is usually translated as 'change' and 筋 (*kŭn*) as 'muscle' or 'applying strength'.

4 Puch'ŏn is one of the satellite towns of Seoul.

a loss of income. Teaching GiCheon does not offer a steady salary, so Ch'oe could not afford to take this risk because he had a family of six to support. It was also a challenging period for Lee Sangwŏn; he had just opened his studio and had to reside there without a hot water boiler. At that time, Lee Sangwŏn's wife issued him an ultimatum: either he must stop practising GiCheon or he would have to leave their family home permanently. Lee Sangwŏn made the difficult decision to choose the latter option: carrying only a small bag of clothes, he left his wife and two children behind. Until that point in his life, he had been working in a successful dress-making business managed by his wife. Lee Sangwŏn's wife harboured a strong aversion to GiCheon, finding it obscure and unfamiliar. She struggled to accept how much it occupied his attention and diverted his focus from their business. This story, which Lee Sangwŏn himself described to Victoria as sad and tragic, is viewed by Ch'oe and other GiCheon practitioners as a representation of what happens to those who choose GiCheon over an apparently 'normal' lifestyle.

Victoria lived in South Korea from 2000 to 2004, and then again from 2007 to 2011. During her time there, she observed the highly competitive nature of Korean society (Lett 1998). Within this context, she noticed that GiCheon teachers, including figures like Lee Sangwŏn, Kim Mansŏng, Lee Kit'ae, and others, were both respected and pitied by their students. Most of the students, primarily from the middle classes, expressed sympathy for their teachers because of the relatively low income generated from instructing GiCheon. When talking about Kim Hyŏnt'ae, another GiCheon teacher and land-owner who generated rental income from his property, the students always made a remark along the lines 'but he has another source of income'. Indeed, the relatively low income of GiCheon teachers was initially seen by students – and Korean society more broadly (Lett 1998; Kendall 1996) – as a hindrance to social status, marriage prospects, and happiness. A few years later, however, this situation would begin to change.

As mentioned above, GiCheon and other *ki suryŏn* practices significantly developed in the 1980s. In 1997, the International Monetary Fund (IMF) crisis broke out in South Korea, bringing about the collapse of the economic system, massive short-term unemployment, and the bankruptcy of many small and medium enterprises, thus causing long-lasting social and psychological damage. Many couples divorced and/or abandoned their children. Woo Hairan argues that these factors contributed to the sharp rise of *ki suryŏn* popularity in the early 2000s. With individual anxiety and existential identity crises on the rise, people were compelled to seek self-transformation, often turning to *ki suryŏn* as a pathway (Woo Hairan 2018, 26). These practices promised to assist individuals in exploring their inner selves, reevaluating their beliefs and habits, and finding meaning in their lives.

By the early 2000s, *ki suryŏn,* as a mass social phenomenon, was attracting widespread attention from Korean academia. This is evidenced by the large number of articles published during that time (ex., Yang Ch'unho et al. 2000; Ch'oe Miyŏn 2008; Pak Misuk 2003; Woo Hairan 2006a; 2006b). Within this context, GiCheon and similar practices gained much more social prestige in Korean society, and Lee Sangwŏn became one of the most well-known GiCheon leaders. Despite a lack of financial stability, he garnered respect and admiration from the broader Korean community. In 2005 – ten years after their divorce – the health of Lee's former wife began to deteriorate and she reached out to her ex-husband, asking him to become one of his students. Despite the years spent apart, she aimed to mend their relationship and suggested reuniting for the sake of their now grown-up children. Ultimately, Lee Sangwŏn did not agree to remarry but graciously accepted her as a student, patiently offering his guidance and support.[5]

Imagining an Alternative World Where Mountain Immortals Live

Ch'oe believed that GiCheon seamlessly integrates various aspects of Korean tradition, religion, philosophy, and etiquette, expressing deep sorrow over the current state of GiCheon in contemporary Korea. In his interview, he lamented the increasing influence of Westernisation and the pervasive computerisation of Korean society, which, in his view, have impacted the essence of GiCheon. In the following excerpts from an interview conducted in Korean, Ch'oe recalls his beginnings as a GiCheon practitioner:[6]

> Victoria: How did you know about GiCheon training, and when did you start practising?
> Ch'oe: [...] since I was small [...] as we, Koreans, grow up [...] obscure (*magyŏnhan*) ideas of traditional martial arts, *sanjung suryŏn* 山中修練 (training in the mountains). [...] More than this vague idea of martial arts, how should I call it, *toga* 道家 (Daoism) [...] the stories we hear from elders, what we feel when we read books ... there is this kind of yearning.

5 Victoria Ten heard this story from Lee Sangwŏn many times before his death in 2007.

6 We have made an effort to keep Ch'oe'story as it was conveyed in the interview, in short, truncated sentences.

> [...] People of my age mostly have it [...]. However, working and leading a social life [...] Also, since there was no such thing in my immediate environment, there was no opportunity to come into contact with it. [...] By chance, when I was 39, I discovered GiCheon [...] it was 1995. There was this advertisement of GiCheon in the newspaper, the paper that was circulated to the postboxes of every shop, every house. [...] So, I went there and met Sabunim [grandmaster Lee Sangwŏn]. I was his first student at Yŏkgok training studio, Puch'ŏn, the very first. [...] While practising GiCheon, first my body got healthier. [...] And also my thoughts. [...] Shall I say that the thoughts that were scattered before that, have consolidated and settled, a little bit? [...] The most important thing: I had this disc problem in my back. [...] I fixed it through the training.

Here, he refers to his early life and how he initially became interested in Korean mountain mythology. Ch'oe goes on to then explain how he experienced positive changes in the state of his mind-body only one month after starting the practice:

> One month after starting the training, my body got very light; my back stopped hurting. [...] Also, my steps got very light when I walk. [...] Also, in everyday life, I usually don't fight with people, but [...] I got this self-confidence, like a young person's, that I can fight with two or three people and win. And also [...] I got a peace of mind and confidence that I can talk with anyone and keep my peace of mind; I got this kind of pride, [...] courage. [...] So GiCheon became part of my everyday life. [...] In my heart, I got peace of mind, composure, self-confidence, things like that. [...]

Ch'oe also mentions that, as his self-confidence grew, he felt ready to fight if needed. His ability to maintain his composure and emotional state also improved. He goes on to postulate that his youthful desire to be unique and have something that nobody else had was also satisfied by his GiCheon practice.

> Before that, I had a vague [...], what I wanted to do in the everyday life, a longing. [...] Like a dream. A dream about GiCheon; what I wanted to become. All men pass through this stage as they mature. In middle and high school, during my adolescence, that vague [...] in my body, I wanted to have an ability different from what other people have. [...] Despite the fact that I knew that it was impossible. But I had such a desire. What made this desire stronger, is that our Taeyang Chinin often came [to

> our training studio] and showed us unusual things. [...] Like cutting a newspaper with a toy knife, as if with the scissors. [...] That is the result of his practice. Now we call it *naegong* 内功 (inner power). I saw things like that with my own eyes. [...] This is like in a film, like in a story from a novel, but [I realised that they are] real. [...] I started GiCheon too late. Had I started as a young child, when the bones are still soft [...] then I could have become like that man [...] maybe, and achieve similar results?

Ch'oe laments that he did not begin his GiCheon practice earlier in his life when it would have had a more transformative effect on his body and its development. He also carries on his point by explaining that he would have preferred to study GiCheon at a point in an imagined history when the practice would have been appreciated more than in the contemporary world.

> If our contemporary lifestyle, our modern society was agricultural, like 100 years ago [...] GiCheon would have achieved great power and success. The person who studies it [...] there inside [GiCheon] tradition, knowledge, philosophy is contained. Talent and science are generated by my own body. But isn't the world of today a place that does not need it at all? Although I can achieve health through that [...] But can I make a handphone with it? Can I make dollars with it? No. So it is getting slightly weaker, getting less [...] it's a waste, I think [...]. If I become a *toin* 道人 (persons who follow the Way) now, and develop amazing power, in this society, simply speaking, like in manga [...]. Civilization has developed too much. [...] The efficacy of GiCheon has diminished in comparison with those times.

Ch'oe is critical of contemporary South Korean society and believes that it does not encourage pursuits such as GiCheon, but instead focuses entirely on material wealth gain under capitalism. The gains of GiCheon practice, in terms of social capital, would have been greater in the imagined past, than in this modern age. The 'efficacy' in terms of advancement in society is lessened due to modernity and its contempt for the 'unscientific':

> Contemporary society has become very diversified and complicated. In the past, after you were born and reached a certain age, you just studied a bit [...] and did what? The only thing you could do as a Korean person was agriculture. Some people could occupy an official position. [...] The society was, to that degree, simple. [...] In GiCheon, we have fields of study and philosophy. All the things that are melted in our [Korean] lifestyle and culture, they are in GiCheon. [...] It is not possible to study

> these things deeply in contemporary society. There are too many other things one has to do apart from GiCheon.

Here Mr Ch'oe talks about the elite members of society, the *yangban* 兩班, a class of Confucian scholars and their descendants who formed the aristocracy during the Chosŏn dynasty (1392–1910) and served as the primary source of recruitment for the state bureaucracy. Ch'oe conveyed a strong sense of nostalgia for an envisioned simpler time, which he connects to the Chosŏn dynasty, a time with less stress, where being physically fit was the primary requirement. He longed for a time when he could dedicate more of his energy solely to GiCheon. However, in the present, his attention has to be divided among numerous other responsibilities:

> During my childhood I heard many stories about stepping on clouds and flying. These stories are unscientific (*pigwahakchŏk*), but we always had this longing, our generation [...]. So, when I heard that there is such a thing, immediately [...] I thought that I have to study this. [...]

In South Korea, as in other regions, people often recall their own childhood as a touchstone of cultural legitimacy. The desire for a space of reminiscence generates a sensation of grief and bereavement and is occasionally viewed as an unavoidable outcome of modern circumstances. This wistfulness frequently centres around things considered 'folkloric' and 'traditional', playing an active role in creating histories and mythologies (Kendall 2009, xviii, xxiv). The same sentiment has permeated the lives of older generations who have witnessed Korea's significant transition from a predominantly agrarian society to an industrialised one. Many present-day Koreans can relate to this type of yearning, which provides context and reasoning for the resurgence, revival, and reinvention of practices such as *ki suryŏn* and GiCheon, conceived as containing the essence of 'authentic' Korean culture.

The term *pigwahakchŏk* (*pi:* un-, *kwahak:* science, *kwahakchŏk:* scientific) was widely used during the era of Pak Chŏnghŭi, the South Korean dictator in power from 1961 to 1979. This discourse followed the ideas of the Japanese colonisers, stating that Korea was backward and needed to 'catch up' with modernity and Western civilisation (see, for example, Yuh 2010). This perspective included viewing certain elements of traditional Korean culture, such as shamanism, as outdated and superstitious (Hwang 2007). For example, traditional Korean acupuncture was restricted under Japanese rule (Na Seonsam 2012, 47).

Ch'oe called the stories about people stepping on clouds and flying *pigwahakchŏk* (unscientific) while alluding to *sinsŏn* 神仙, divine immortals who dwell in the mountains. As explained above, GiCheon and other *ki suryŏn* groups share ideas of mountain immortality with traditional East Asian Daoism, and the belief in the existence of mountain gods and immortals remains widespread in contemporary Korea (Mason 1999; Kang Sŏngbok and Pak Chongik 2010; Kim Sŏnp'ung 2003; Kim Yŏngja 2005).

Ch'oe also associated GiCheon and traditional acupuncture methods with *pigwahakchŏk*. He expressed his disappointment with the current legal restrictions on acupuncture in South Korea, where its practice is limited to officially licensed Traditional Korean Medical Doctors. Indeed, it is difficult for ordinary Koreans to become a Traditional Korean Medical Doctor, as it requires a university degree in Traditional Korean Medicine, which is an expensive and time-consuming project. Therefore, for most people acupuncture became an illegal or forbidden occupation (Na Seonsam 2012, 48). Ch'oe contrasted this situation with contemporary Japan, where the laws on acupuncture are more lenient, allowing a broader range of professionals to practise it. Ch'oe further linked contemporary difficulties with achieving licensing to practise acupuncture to its historical restriction during Japanese rule. For him, it symbolises how a modern, Western lifestyle promoted by the Japanese colonial era has overshadowed and disregarded 'traditional' Korean values, which he associated with an idealistic vision of a simpler, agricultural world, where practitioners of GiCheon would attain social success. Ch'oe's imaginary vision is intricately linked to the ideals of mountain immortality. In his interview, he highlighted how one can touch upon that bygone world and become a part of it to some extent:

> Not only GiCheon, but in our country, there are different kinds of Korean [...] should I call it martial arts? There are different kinds of *sŏndo* 仙道 (the way of immortals), *sŏnpŏp* 仙法 (techniques of immortality) and the basis of all of them is breathing. That is *tanjŏn* 丹田 (cinnabar field) breathing. Through *tanjŏn* breathing, we purify our body, organise our thoughts, and increase and cultivate *ki*.

When Ch'oe points out that we 'purify our body, organise our thoughts, increase and cultivate our *ki*', he describes the process of internal alchemy, which is the way of active intentional self-purification. This process aims to bring us closer to the ideals of mountain immortals, who embody pure immortality. The way in which Ch'oe and others speak about GiCheon and Korea reflects the nation-building discourse from the Pak Chŏnghŭi era (1961–1979) and Japanese colonial times. Ch'oe, and older generations of practitioners weave GiCheon, an imagined 'traditional Korean culture', and the concept of the 'unscientific' together. Ch'oe includes beliefs and practices related to mountains, such as *sŏndo* (the art of immortality), *sŏnpŏp* (techniques of immortality), and *sanjung suryŏn* (training in the mountains) into this larger group, linking them with stories of walking on clouds, martial arts, Daoism, *tanjŏn* breathing, and the cultivation of *ki*.

Ch'oe defines GiCheon as 'unscientific' by looking back into an imagined Korean past. 'Unscientific' thus becomes, for Ch'oe, a tool of dissent, a way to disagree with the values and aspirations of contemporary life. He does not challenge the definition of 'science' itself, but his explanation of what is 'unscientific' and his positive evaluation thereof manifest a clear dissatisfaction with what is generally considered modern 'Western' science. He turns the concept of science upside-down, evaluating it negatively while praising the 'unscientific' as a saviour of Korean society.

Ki Suryŏn as a Core of Korean New Age Culture

Woo Hairan, one of the leading scholars of the Korean New Age, examines how contemporary societal issues in South Korea have contributed to the development of New Age culture and to the focus on self-cultivation (2018, 26). These social issues include the high level of competition in East Asian societies, previously discussed by Farquhar and Zhang (2012, 49) in the Chinese context and by Chen Shu-Chuan in Taiwan. Anthony Giddens (1991, 64, 119) describes modernity as a risk society which creates and sustains the threat of personal meaninglessness. Chen Shu-Chuan (2006, 82–84) sees New Age practices of self-transformation as a social reaction to such a threat, thereby defining them as both a reaction to and an expression of modernity.

Since the 1960s, significant progress has been made in the reconciliation of modern Western medicine with what was previously considered 'occult' and 'unscientific'. In mental health, meditation is now being promoted even by clinicians who would have recently written a prescription for a conventional pharmaceutical treatment (Basso et al. 2019; Harrington 2009; Hickey 2019; cf. Chapters 6 and 9). Exercise, a healthy diet, and trips to the countryside are becoming increasingly popular among psychotherapists in the West, thanks to advancements in psychotherapy, neurology, and psychiatry (Harrington 2009; Hickey 2019; Baker 2020). There has been a growing demand for alternative therapies instead of the more traditional talking therapy, which has evolved and developed since its initial pioneering by Freud and Breuer (Novotney 2017). Art therapy (Uttley et al. 2015), drama therapy (Chang et al. 2019), acupuncture (Samuels et al. 2008), therapeutic massage (Sherman et al. 2010), yoga (Maddux et al. 2017), and *tai chi* (Jiang et al. 2016) have all been clinically trialled and studied under the scrutiny of the Western scientific method as mechanisms to treat mental health conditions. These 'alternative therapies' are now becoming simply 'therapies' to treat patients.

As a means to challenge conventional Euro-American concepts of medicine, health, and illness, many New Age movements have drawn upon East Asia for inspiration (cf. Chapters 4, 5, and 8). Woo Hairan (2018) sees *ki suryŏn* as lying at the core of Korean New Age culture, which reached its golden age in the 1980s. She notes that Korean scholars often resist using the term 'New Age' because of its strong 'Western' connotations and prefer, instead, to adopt the Korean concept of *suryŏn munhwa* 修練文化 (training culture). Woo Hairan identifies the Korean New Age as a movement comprising five sectors, which she describes as five concentric circles, moving from the outermost to the innermost as follows:

(1) Well-being/healing culture: a substratum layer related to consumer culture which has accelerated the commercialisation of the New Age in Korea. The 'well-being boom' of the 2000s was related to economic stability placing a special emphasis on physical health.

(2) Yoga and *qigong* are considered important for well-being in Korea.

(3) Since the 1990s, transpersonal psychology/psychotherapy and Neuro-Linguistic Programming (NLP) have garnered increasing interest in South Korea. In 1993 the Avatar programme, a product of Star's Edge International, an American company offering self-development courses, was introduced to the country. What Woo defines as 'New Age Science' commenced with the Korean Society of Body-Mind-Spirit Science (*Hanguk chŏngsin kwahak hakhoe* 韓國精神科學學會), founded by natural scientists in 1994, and the Minaisa Club, an association promoting 'New Science', which came into being in 1997. They offered lectures on alternative medicine, consciousness development, and the new economic system.

(4) Self-development and meditation programmes, including traditional Buddhist meditation combined with psychotherapy.

(5) *Ki suryŏn* groups are at the heart of the Korean New Age movement. Many of them are well organised, operate under charismatic leaders, and their membership is usually based on the payment of a fee.

Woo Hairan (2018, 29) points out that *ki suryŏn* groups actively promote Korean national consciousness. The motif of fostering Korean national identity is a recurring and prominent theme in GiCheon literature (Kim

Hŭisang and Kich'ŏnmun Ponmun 2000; 1998) and is also evident in the narratives shared by GiCheon practitioners, as illustrated in the interview with Ch'oe. Although not explicitly stated, Ch'oe expresses a desire for Korean society to evolve positively, aligning more with what he perceives as traditional practices such as acupuncture and GiCheon. Contemporary practitioners of self-cultivation in China demonstrate a similar interest in societal issues (Palmer 2007; Farquhar and Zhang 2012), and ideas of national consciousness play a significant role in the New Age movement in Japan, a characteristic that distinguishes New Age in East Asia from its counterpart in Europe (Prohl 2007, 373; Shimazono 1999, 131). If, however, we consider GiCheon and *ki suryŏn* as techniques of the self, it is possible to identify commonalities in East Asia and Europe of how such techniques have been connected to an idealised past created by practitioners and intellectuals alike. In the following section, we argue, in fact, that in the same way that Michel Foucault imagined an idealised European past in which he found the roots of his techniques of the self, Mr Ch'oe also looked back into Korean history with a certain sense of nostalgia, comparing an idealised past with a decadent present that needs to bring back ancient Korean techniques of self-transformation to save itself.

Technologies of the Self: Ideas Banished from the Mainstream Western Thought

Foucault based his concept of technologies of the self on *epimeleia heautou*, 'care of the self', the theme appearing clearly in Greek philosophy, both Hellenistic and Roman, in the fifth century BCE and continuing until the fourth to fifth century CE. Socrates was a great adherent of *epimeleia heautou*. He said: 'You occupy yourself with various projects, your money, your reputation. You do not occupy yourself with yourself' (Foucault 2001, 7). Foucault explains that *epimeleia heautou*, care of the self, involves modification of one's attitude towards reality, towards others, and towards oneself (Foucault 2001, 12, 46–47). He suggests calling 'philosophy' the form of thought that examines what allows the subject to gain access to the truth. He also calls 'spirituality' the research, practice, and experience through which the subject carries out the transformations necessary for accessing the truth. In other words, only a transformed and purified self has the right to access the truth. Spirituality here is a view according to which the truth can be gained only by paying the price of modification or purification of the self. With a certain nostalgic sentiment, Foucault summarises the teachings of the Pythagoreans, Platonists,

Stoics, Cynics, Epicureans, and Neo-Platonists, stating that for them, the question of the truth was always connected to the problem of spirituality.

However, 17th-century Europe saw complications in the relationship between faith and reason. It was a turbulent period during which other subjects – like the nature of authority, the possibility of progress, the application of natural laws to the organisation of society, and the criticism of absolutism – were also brought to the fore and re-examined (Gaziyev 2016). Foucault, therefore, identifies the rise of a 'Cartesian moment' in the 17th century, which played a crucial role in shaping narratives of Western subjectivity. During this period, the older tradition of self-transformation was marginalised within mainstream Western intellectual thought but survived in the realm of the occult. According to Foucault, the concept of self-transformation lingered in the twilight of this realm, best exemplified by the figure of Faust and his rejection of scientific rationalism in favour of sorcery and magic (Foucault, 2001, 296–97). Indeed, according to Foucault, in modern Western thought, the notions of self-transformation were not entirely dismissed; instead, they made occasional appearances in various forms, such as psychotherapy and Marxism (Foucault 2001, 30).

The period from the 1960s to the 1980s was when Michel Foucault was most active as a scholar. Waves of the burgeoning movement later termed 'New Age' were sweeping across the globe. Many of these movements were centred around ideas of self-transformation (Melton 1990, xiii; Chen 2006, 28–29). It is, therefore, no coincidence that Foucault's conceptualisation of technologies of self seems to announce later concepts, such as 'self-spirituality' and 'reflexive self', widely discussed by New Age scholars (Heelas 1996; Chen 2006, 64–65). In fact, sociologists and religious studies scholars have considered 'self-cultivation' one of the defining elements of the New Age movement (Melton 1990, xiii; Chen 2006, 28–29, 35–38). For Foucault, self-cultivation becomes a concept he extracts from a reconstructed past to explain a present already infused with counter-cultural New Age ideas. His contemporaries in Korea did the same: reinventing and reconstructing modern traditions by invoking notions of self-cultivation allegedly stemming from ancient Asian cultures.

Conclusion: The Nostalgia of the 'Unscientific'

Foucault began producing his most renowned works in the 1960s (1961, 1963), a period of radical change when many fundamental concepts underpinning the structure of Western society were re-examined. As New Age movements matured in the 1970s, they gave rise to new, unorthodox approaches to science. Woo Hairan's research demonstrates how modern Koreans have adapted and expanded the idea of science through the introduction of New Age Science or New Science. In this cultural shift, *ki suryŏn* plays a central role. Contemporary individuals continue to shape this newly invented tradition, inspired by ancient practices of self-cultivation in East Asia, and utilise them as a source of legitimation.

This chapter has analysed an interview with Ch'oe, along with his vision of GiCheon, one of the first *ki suryŏn* practices of modern South Korea. Ch'oe describes this Korean discipline of self-transformation as *pigwahakchŏk* (unscientific), which he hails as a positive characteristic. Indeed, current research indicates that elsewhere in East Asia, the term 'superstition' was sometimes also used in a positive sense (Junqueira 2025; 2023). Ch'oe reclaims the term 'unscientific', infusing it with positive meaning, and directly associates it with GiCheon and the concept of immortals dwelling in the mountains. He links these mountain immortals with an imaginary Korean past, portraying a simple agrarian society with pure, unpolluted nature, untouched by the grime of modernity. Despite never having lived during that era himself, Ch'oe expresses deep nostalgia for this time when GiCheon would be a vital key to social success.

As discussed above, Foucault projects the idea of self-cultivation back into the past. Following the New Age movement, self-cultivation techniques are regaining legitimacy in both the East and West. Traditional East Asian self-cultivation practices, as well as contemporary reinvented traditions, align with Foucault's description of technologies of self. GiCheon is one such technique, a modern self-transformation practice centred around abdominal breathing and painful static positions. Ch'oe feels that GiCheon, similar to acupuncture, is not duly supported by modern 'Western' science, yet wishes for a world that acknowledges their cultural and social value. This sentiment closely connects Ch'oe and Foucault. Both delve into the past, whether real or imagined, to examine the culture of self-transformation, its legitimacy or lack thereof, and they both contemplate how such practices can challenge the supremacy of modern Western science. It is a sort of looping effect between scholars and New Age practitioners: 'self-cultivation' becomes a tool that practitioners like Ch'oe employ to talk about newly invented traditions, while scholars use the concept of 'self-cultivation' to explain how to understand the New Age (Melton 1990, xiii; Chen 2006, 28–29, 35–38), and philosophers like Foucault locate the origin of 'self-cultivation' in the ancient past. No one seems to be able to escape from the nostalgia of our 'unscientific' histories.

Bibliography

Abayev, N.V. 1983. *Chan-buddhism yi kultura psihicheskoi deyatelnosti v srednevekovom Kitae* Чань-буддизм и культура психической деятельности в средневековом Китае [Zen-Buddhism and Psychic Culture in Mediaeval China]. Novosibirsk: Nauka.

Abayev, N.V., and G.I. Shirokov. 1991. 'Chast 1: Shkola Wu-shu Sinsimak: nekotorie osobennosti sistemi psihofizicheskoi trenirovki Часть 1: Школа Ушу "Синсимак": некоторые особенности системы психофизической тренировки' [Part 1. Wu-shu School Sinsimak: Some Features of Psycho-Physical Training]. In *Metodicheskie posobia po sistemam psihofizicheskoi trenirovki zigun in ushu* Методические пособия по системам психофизической тренировки цигун и ушу [Manuals on the Systems of Psycho-Physical Training Qigong and Wushu], edited by N.V. Abayev and I.E. Garry, 3–7. Irkutsk: Vostochno-Sibirskaya Pravda.

Baker, Ian A. 2020. 'Cocaine in British Colonial Burma: Convergences of Commerce, Consumption, and Control'. PhD thesis, University of Strathclyde.

Baker, Don. 2007. 'Internal Alchemy in the Dahn World School'. In *Religions of Korea in Practice,* edited by Robert E. Buswell Jr., 508–13. Princeton: Princeton University Press. https://doi.org/10.2307/j.ctv346r61.41.

Basso, Julia C., Alexandra McHale, Victoria Ende, Douglas J. Oberlin, and Wendy A. Suzuki. 2019. 'Brief, Daily Meditation Enhances Attention, Memory, Mood, and Emotional Regulation in Non-Experienced Meditators'. *Behavioural Brain Research* 356, no. 1: 208–20. https://doi.org/10.1016/j.bbr.2018.08.023.

Brettell, Caroline B. 1997. 'Blurred Genres and Blended Voices: Life, History, Biography, Autobiography and the Auto/Ethnography of Women's Lives'. In *Auto/Ethnography: Rewriting the Self and the Social*, edited by Debora E. Reed-Danahay, 223–46. Oxford: Berg. https://doi.org/10.4324/9781003136118-13.

Boltz, Judith M. 2008. '*Daozang* and Subsidiary Compilations'. In *The Encyclopedia of Taoism,* edited by Fabrizio Pregadio, 28–33. New York: Routledge.

Chang, Wen-Lung, Yu-Shiuan Liu, and Cheng-Fu Yang. 2019. 'Drama Therapy Counseling as Mental Health Care of College Students'. *International Journal of Environmental Research and Public Health* 16, no. 19: 3560. https://doi.org/10.3390/ijerph16193560.

Chau, Adam Y. 2011. *Religion in Contemporary China.* New York: Routledge.

Chen, Shu-Chuan. 2006. 'Getting Healed from a Globalised Age: A Study of the New Age Movement in Taiwan'. PhD thesis, University of Warwick.

Ch'oe, Miyŏn 최미연. 2008. 'Kuksŏndo wa Han'guk ch'um ŭi sinmyŏng 국선도와 한국춤의 신명 (神明)' [Kuksŏndo and exhilaration in Korean dance]. Taehan muyong hakhoeji 大韓舞踊學會 54: 155-173.

Dax, Frank. 2015. 'Recreational Hiking in South Korea: Transforming the Body, Transforming the Land'. *Korea Journal* 55, no. 3: 80–102. https://doi.org/10.25024/kj.2015.55.3.80.

Despeux, Catherine. 2008. 'Yangshen 養生 Nourishing Life'. In *The Encyclopedia of Taoism*, edited by Fabrizio Pregadio, 1148–50. New York: Routledge.

Ellis, Carolyn, and Arthur Bochner. 2000. 'Autoethnography, Personal Narrative, Reflexivity'. In *Handbook of Qualitative Research*, 2nd ed., edited by N.K. Denzin and Y.S. Lincoln, 733–68. Thousand Oaks, CA: Sage Publications.

Farquhar, Judith, and Zhang Qicheng. 2012. *Ten Thousand Things: Nurturing Life in Contemporary Beijing*. New York: Zone. https://doi.org/10.2307/j.ctv14gphrg.

Foucault, Michel. 1961. *Folie et déraison: Histoire de la folie à l'âge classique*. Paris: Librairie Plon.

Foucault, Michel. 1963. *Naissance de la clinique: Une archéologie du regard médical*. Paris: Gallimard.

Foucault, Michel. 1988. 'Technologies of the Self'. In *Technologies of the Self: A Seminar with Michel Foucault*, edited by Luther H. Martin, Huck Gutman, and Patrick H. Hutton, 16–49. London: Tavistock Publications.

Foucault, Michel. 2001. *L'Hermeneutique du sujet: Cours au Collège de France (1981–1982)*. Paris: Gallimard.

Gaziyev, Masud. 2016. 'The Scientific Revolution and The Enlightenment: Conflict between Faith and Reason?'. Research Gate. Accessed on 11 February 2023. https://www.researchgate.net/publication/340933957_The_Scientific_Revolution_and_The_Enlightenment_Conflict_between_Faith_and_Reason.

Giddens, Anthony. 1991. *Modernity and Self-Identity: Self and Society in the Late Modern Age*. Cambridge: Polity Press.

Gmelch, Sharon. 1991. *Nan: The Life of an Irish Travelling Woman*. Prospects Heights: Waveland Press.

Harrington, Anne. 2009. *The Cure Within: A History of Mind-Body Medicine*. New York: W. W. Norton & Company.

Hayano, D. 1979. 'Auto-Ethnography: Paradigms, Problems and Prospects'. *Human Organization* 38, no. 1: 99–104. https://doi.org/10.17730/humo.38.1.u761n5601t4g318v.

Heelas, Paul. 1996. *The New Age Movement: The Celebration of the Self and the Sacralization of Modernity*. Oxford: Blackwell.

Hickey, Wakoh S. 2019. *Mind Cure: How Meditation Became Medicine*. Oxford: Oxford University Press. https://doi.org/10.1093/oso/9780190864248.001.0001.

Hobsbawm, Eric, and Terence Ranger, eds. 1992 [1983]. *The Invention of Tradition*. Cambridge: Cambridge University Press.

Hwang, Merose. 2007. 'The Mudang: The Colonial Legacies of Korean Shamanism'. In *Han Kut: Critical Art and Writing by Korean Canadian Women*, edited by

The Korean Canadian Women's Anthology Collective, 103–19. Toronto: Inanna Publications.

Junqueira, Luis F.B. 2025. 'Disembodied Spirits or Mental Suggestion? Psychical Research and the Redefinition of Superstition in Republican China'. In *Uncanny Beliefs: Superstition in Modern Chinese History*, edited by Emily Baum and Albert Wu. Cambridge, MA: Harvard University Asia Center.

Junqueira, Luis F.B. 2023. 'The Science of the Spirit: Psychical Research, Healthcare and the Revival of the Occult in a Modernising China, 1900–1949'. PhD thesis, University College London.

Jiang, Dongsheng, Weihong Kong, and Joanna J. Jiang. 2016. 'The Role of Tai Chi in Mental Health Management-Lessons Learned from Clinical Trials'. *Reviews on Recent Clinical Trials* 11, no. 4: 324–32. https://doi.org/10.2174/1574887111666160729100829.

Kang, Sŏngbok 강성복, and Pak Chongik 박종익. 2010. 'Kongju T'aehwasan sanhyangkye ŭi sŏnggyŏk kwa sansinje 공주 태화산 산향계 (山饗稧)의 성격과 산신제' [The Character of *sanhyangkye* at Kongju T'aehwa Mountain and Sansinje]. *Han'guk minsokhak* 韓國民俗學 51: 215–45.

Kendall, Laurel. 2009. *Shamans Nostalgias and the IMF: South Korean Popular Religion in Motion.* Honolulu: University of Hawaii Press.

Kendall, Laurel. 1996. *Getting Married in Korea: Of Gender, Morality, and Modernity.* Oakland, University of California Press.
https://doi.org/10.1525/california/9780520201989.001.0001.

Kim, Daeyeol. 2000. 'Le symbolisme de la force vitale en Chine ancienne : "modèles" et significations dans l'alchimie taoïste opératoire: études des pratiques alchimiques du Baopuzi neipian [The symbolism of the vital force in ancient China: 'models' and meanings in Taoist operative alchemy: studies of Baopuzi neipian alchemical practices]'. PhD thesis, Université de Paris-Sorbonne (Paris 4).

Kim, Hŭisang, and Kich'ŏnmun Ponmun 氣天門 本門, eds. 2000. *Kich'ŏn* 氣天. Seoul: Ch'orokpaemaejiksŭ.

Kim, Hŭisang 김희상, and Kich'ŏnmun Ponmun 기천문 본문. 1998. *Kich'ŏnmun immun* 기천문 입문 [Kich'ŏnmun Introduction]. Seoul: Yŏn'gusa.

Kim, Sŏnp'ung 김선풍. 2003. 'Tan'gun sinhwa wa T'aebaeksan, Mokmyŏksan, Samgaksan sinhwa ŭi taebi punsŏk 단군신화와 태백산・목멱산・삼각산신화의 대비분석' [A Comparative Study on Tan'gun Legend and the Legends of T'aebaek, Mokmyŏk and Samgak Mountains]. *Kangwŏn minsokhak* 강원민속학 17: 73–102.

Kim, Taewoo. 2010. 'Medicine Without the Medical Gaze: Theory, Practice, and Phenomenology in Korean Medicine'. PhD thesis, University at Buffalo.

Kim, Yŏngja 김영자. 2005. 'Sansindo e p'yohyŏntoen sansin ŭi yuhyŏng 산신도(山神圖)에 표현된 산신(山神)의 유형' [Various Types of Mountain Gods Depicted in Paintings]. *Han'guk minsokhak* 韓國民俗學 41: 187–223.
Kirkland, Russell. 2008. 'Transcendence and Immortality'. In *Encyclopedia of Taoism,* edited by Fabrizio Pregadio, 91–93. New York: Routledge.
Lett, Denise. 1998. *In Pursuit of Status: The Making of South Korea's 'New' Urban Middle Class*. Cambridge, MA: Harvard University Asia Center.
https://doi.org/10.1163/9781684173112.
Lobetti, Tullio F. 2014. *Ascetic Practices in Japanese Religion*. London: Routledge. https://doi.org/10.4324/9780203794852.
Maddux, Rachel E., Daiva Daukantaité, and Una Tellhed. 2017. 'The Effects of Yoga on Stress and Psychological Health Among Employees: An 8- And 16-Week Intervention Study'. *Anxiety Stress & Coping* 31, no. 2: 121–34.
https://doi.org/10.1080/10615806.2017.1405261.
Mason, David. 1999. *Spirit of the Mountains.* Seoul: Hollym International Cor.
Melton, J. Gordon. 1990. 'Introductory Essay: An Overview of the New Age Movement'. In *New Age Encyclopedia*, edited by J. Gordon Melton, Jerome Clark, and Aidan A. Kelly, xiii–xxxiii. Detroit: Gale Research Inc.
Miura, Kunio. 2008a. 'Shenren 神人 Divine Man; Spirit Man'. In *Encyclopedia of Taoism*, edited by Fabrizio Pregadio, 885–86. New York: Routledge.
Miura, Kunio. 2008b. 'Xianren 仙人 Immortal; Transcendent'. In *Encyclopedia of Taoism*, edited by Fabrizio Pregadio, 1092–94. New York: Routledge.
Motzafi-Haller, Pnina. 1997. 'Writing Birthright: On Native Anthropologists and the Politics of Representation'. In *Auto/Ethnography: Rewriting the Self and the Social*, edited by Debora E. Reed-Danahay, 195–222. Oxford: Berg.
https://doi.org/10.4324/9781003136118-12.
Na, Seonsam. 2012. 'East Asian Medicine in South Korea'. *Harvard Asia Quarterly* 14, no. 4: 44–56.
Novotney, Amy. 2017. 'Not Your Great-Grandfather's Psychoanalysis'. *Monitor on Psychology* 48, no. 11: 40.
Palmer, David A. 2007. *Qigong Fever: Body, Science, and Utopia in China*. New York: Columbia University Press. https://doi.org/10.13140/2.1.2859.9680.
Pak, Misuk 박미숙 and others. 2003. 'Ki suryŏn i sŭt'ŭresŭ panŭng e mich'i nŭn yŏnghyang 기(氣)수련이 스트레스 반응에 미치는 영향' [Effects of ki suryŏn on stress management]. Han'guk sŭp'och'ŭ simni hakhoeji 한국스포츠심리학회지 14, no. 3: 101-109.
Pak, Taeyang 박대양, and Ch'oe Hyŏn'gyu 최현규. *Sosŏl Kich'ŏnmun* 소설기천문 [*Kich'ŏnmun novel*]. Unpublished and undated manuscript.
Prohl, Inken. 2007. 'The Spiritual World: Aspects of New Age in Japan'. In *Handbook of New Age*, edited by Daren Kemp and James R. Lewis, 359–74. Leiden: Brill.

https://doi.org/10.1163/ej.9789004153554.i-484.128.
Robinet, Isabelle. 2008a. '*Jindan dayao* 金丹大要 Great Essentials of the Golden Elixir'. In *Encyclopedia of Taoism,* edited by Fabrizio Pregadio, 557–58. New York: Routledge.
Robinet, Isabelle. 2008b. '*Shengren* 聖人 Saint; Saintly Man; Sage'. In *Encyclopedia of Taoism,* edited by Fabrizio Pregadio, 879–81. New York: Routledge.
Samuels, Noah, Cornelius Gropp, Shepherd Roee Singer, and Menachem Oberbaum. 2008. 'Acupuncture for Psychiatric Illness: A Literature Review'. *Behavioral Medicine* 34, no. 2: 55–64. https://doi.org/10.3200/BMED.34.2.55-64.
Scheid, Volker. 2002. *Chinese Medicine in Contemporary China: Plurality and Synthesis.* Durham: Duke University Press. https://doi.org/10.2307/j.ctv125jgmn.
Shimazono Susumu. 1999. '"New Age Movement" or "New Spirituality Movements and Culture"?'. *Social Compass* 46, no. 2: 121–33.
https://doi.org/10.1177/003776899046002O.
Smith, Pamela. 2014. 'Knowledge in Motion'. In *Cultures in Motion,* edited by D. Rodgers, B. Raman, and H. Reimitz, 109–33. Princeton: Princeton University Press. https://doi.org/10.23943/princeton/9780691159096.003.0005.
Sherman, Karen J., Evette J. Ludman, Andrea J. Cook, Rene J. Hawkes, Peter P. Roy-Byrne, Susan Bentley, Marissa Z. Brooks, and Daniel C. Cherkin. 2010. 'Effectiveness of Therapeutic Massage for Generalized Anxiety Disorder: A Randomized Controlled Trial'. *Depression and Anxiety* 27, no. 5: 441–50.
https://doi.org/10.1002/da.20671.
Ten, Victoria. 2015. 'Encoding Visual Imagery of Ki Suryŏn Exported to the West'. *International Institute for Asian Studies (IIAS) Newsletter* 70 (Spring): 8–9.
Ten, Victoria. 2020a. *Body and Ki in GiCheon: Practices of Self-Cultivation in Contemporary Korea*. Würzburg: Ergon Verlag.
https://doi.org/10.5771/9783956507342
Ten, Victoria. 2020b. 'Transforming the Self in Contemporary Korean Ki Suryŏn 氣修練: Water, Wood, and Stone in Two GiCheon 氣天 DVDs'. In *Contemporary Practices of Citizenship in Asia and the West: Care of the Self,* edited by Gregory Bracken, 67–88. Amsterdam: Amsterdam University Press.
https://doi.org/10.2307/j.ctv11cwbd6.7.
Ten, Victoria, and Robert Winstanley-Chesters. 2020. *New Goddesses on Mt. Paektu: Transformation, Myth and Gender in Korean Landscape* [online].
http://www.gicheon.com/wp-content/uploads/2021/01/New-Goddesses-on-Mt.-Paektu-Transformation-Myth-and-Gender-in-Korean-Landscape.pdf.
Uttley, Lesley, Alison Scope, Matt Stevenson, Andrew Rawdin, Elizabeth Taylor Buck, Anthea Sutton, John Stevens, Eva Kaltenthaler, Kim Dent-Brown, and Chris Wood. 2015. 'Chapter 2, Clinical Effectiveness of Art Therapy: Quantitative Systematic Review. Systematic Review and Economic Modelling of the Clinical Effectiveness

and Cost-Effectiveness of Art Therapy Among People with Non-Psychotic Mental Health Disorders'. *Health Technology Assessment* 19, no. 18. Southampton: NIHR Journals Library. https://doi.org/10.3310/hta19180.
Van der Veer, Peter. 2007. 'Global Breathing: Religious Utopias in India and China'. *Anthropological Theory* 7, no. 3: 315–29.
http://doi.org/10.1177/1463499607080193.
Woo, Hairan (U Hyeran 우혜란). 2006a. 'Ki suryŏn tanch'e ŭi minjokjuŭi chŏk sŏnghyang kwa segyehwa kihoek: tanwŏldŭ rŭl chungsim ŭro 기수련 단체의 민족주의적 성향과 세계화 기획: 단월드를 중심으로' [Nationalistic Orientation and Globalisation Plan of ki suryŏn Groups: Focusing on Dahn World]. *Inmun kwahak yŏn'gu* 人文科學研究 11: 37–63.
Woo, Hairan (U Hyeran 우혜란). 2006b. 'Tong side Han'guk ŭi ki suryŏn munhwa wa musok 동시대 한국의 기수련 문화와 무속' [Contemporary Korean ki suryŏn Culture and Shamanism]. *Chongkyo yŏn'gu* 종교연구 9: 71–113.
Woo, Hairan (U Hyeran 우혜란). 2018. 'The New Age Movement in South Korea: Development and Scope'. *Alternative Spirituality and Religion Review* 9, no. 1: 20–30.
https://doi.org/10.5840/asrr201862644.
Yang, Ch'unho 양춘호 and others. 2000. 'Kuksŏndo *suryŏn* kwa salm ŭi chil e kwanhan yŏn'gu 국선도 수련과 삶의 질에 관한 연구' [The Study on Kuksŏndo Practice and Quality of Life]. *Han'guk sahoe ch'eyuk hakhoeji* 13: 27–38.
Yuh, Leighanne. 2010. 'Contradictions in Korean Colonial Education'. *International Journal of Korean History* 15, no. 1: 121–50.

Biography

Victoria Ten (Jeon Yeon Hwa) is a teacher of GiCheon, a Korean discipline for the health of mind and body, a scholar, and a lawyer. Victoria's PhD thesis, defended at Leiden University in 2017, is an anthropological research into GiCheon. She has published extensively on *ki suryŏn* and contemporary Korean society.

Michael Wharton is a philosopher, poet, writer, and professional proofreader/copyeditor, as well as an aspiring political candidate for the UK Green Party. He runs an online journal (*There is Always a Theory*), and he currently manages a charity shop for the UK housing charity Shelter.

11 Nationalism and the Legitimacy of Traditional Chinese Medicine in Macau: Colonial Legacy and Contemporary Imaginaries

Loretta I.T. Lou

Abstract: This chapter explores how colonial legacy and the transition of sovereignty influenced the legitimacy of Traditional Chinese Medicine (TCM) in Macau. Contrary to previous research suggesting that the legitimacy of TCM hinges on the creation of miracles, I posit that in Macau the credibility of TCM predominantly stems from empathetic healing and cultural nationalism, which repositions TCM as a source of national treasure and pride. Similar to the promotion of Confucianism, the internationalisation of TCM represents China's latest effort to use its traditional culture as a conduit of soft power. Through championing the dissemination of TCM across former Portuguese colonies, Macau not only contributes to China's intent to broaden its global influence, but it also accentuates the city's enduring role as a nexus between 'Chinese' and 'Western' medicinal practices, a legacy dating back to the 16th century.

Keywords: Traditional Chinese Medicine (TCM), Nationalism, Lusophone connections, Macau, Portugal, China

Scholars of Traditional Chinese Medicine[1] (TCM) have long noted that TCM is a project of nationalism – an imaginary and reinvented tradition of

1 In this chapter, I use the term Traditional Chinese Medicine (TCM) to refer to therapeutic practices endorsed by the People's Republic of China (PRC) during the mid-20th century. For therapeutic practices prior to this period, I refer to them generically as 'Chinese medicine' or 'Chinese therapies'.

Gaitanidis, Ioannis, Luis Fernando Bernardi Junqueira, Avery Morrow, and Sangyun Han (eds), *Therapy, Spirituality, and East Asian Imaginaries*. Taylor & Francis Group 2025
DOI: 10.5117/9789048559015_CH11

the People's Republic of China (PRC) (Croizier 1965; Farquhar 1996; Taylor 2004; Scheid 2007; Hsu 2008; Hsu 2021). Lauded as a remarkable national heritage, the Chinese government has supported and invested heavily in the institutionalisation and modernisation of Chinese medicine since the 1950s. Consequently, TCM is fully integrated into China's healthcare system and enjoys the same legal status as biomedicine (Farquhar 1996; Scheid 1999). Public support for Chinese medicine is also strong in the PRC (Scheid 1999). However, the same cannot be said for TCM outside of China. In places where biomedicine dominates the primary healthcare system, the legitimacy of TCM cannot be taken for granted. In recent years, researchers have explored how TCM practitioners established and grappled with the issue of legitimacy in Europe, North America (Zhan 2001; Zhan 2009; Lieber 2012; France and Rodriguez 2019), and Africa (Hsu 2002). Yet there is a lack of research on the legitimacy of TCM in peripheral Chinese regions, such as Hong Kong and Macau, former European colonies that became Special Administrative Regions (SARs) of the PRC in the late 1990s.

Drawing on my first-hand experience as a native Macanese and on my ethnographic research spanning over the past 17 years (2005, 2016, 2021, 2022), this chapter investigates how colonial legacy and the transfer of sovereignty have shaped the legitimacy of Traditional Chinese Medicine in Macau, where TCM has transitioned from being a local industry comprising small private practices to a national industry that receives support and promotion from the Chinese Central and Macau SAR governments. Firstly, I argue that while the laissez-faire governance of the Portuguese administration hindered TCM's official recognition prior to Macau's handover to China in 1999, its hands-off approach also prevented Chinese medicine from being eradicated from Macau's medical landscape. This allowed TCM practitioners to reinforce their legitimacy through empathic healing and mutual diagnosis with patients. Secondly, following Macau's 'return to the motherland', nationalism has played an increasingly pivotal role in legitimising TCM. My research highlights that while nationalism has undoubtedly elevated the profile of TCM in postcolonial Macau, TCM itself has also provided the Macau SAR government and local TCM practitioners with a platform to showcase their patriotism to China by spearheading the introduction of Traditional Chinese medicine to other former Portuguese colonies. Such efforts have not only contributed to China's aspiration to assert its soft power and global influence but have also reinforced Macau's self-imposed cultural identity as a bridge between 'Chinese' and 'Western' medicine since the 16th century.

Public Health in Macau: A History

After more than 400 years of colonial rule since 1557, Macau, a former colony of Portugal, was returned to the People's Republic of China under the constitutional principle of 'One Country, Two Systems' in 1999. Although folk and Chinese medicine had circulated and been practised long before the colonial era, the lack of historical research on Macau before the arrival of the Portuguese has led most historians to mark the start of Macau's medical history with the establishments of the Santa Casa da Misericórdia de Macau (Macau Holy House of Mercy), Hospital de São Rafael (St Raphael Hospital), and Igreja de São Lázaro (St Lazarus Church). These three historically significant institutions were all founded between 1568 and 1569 by a Portuguese Jesuit missionary named D. Belchior Carneiro, S.J., who sought to save not only the bodies but also the souls of the patients. St. Raphael Hospital, commonly known to the Chinese as the 'healing temple', was the first Western-style hospital in Asia and served as the site of the first smallpox vaccinations in China (Barnes 2007; Amaro 2008; Macau Memories 2019; Cultural Affairs Bureau 2023). Meanwhile, the Portuguese missionaries of St Lazarus Church established 'one of the first leper asylums on Chinese soil', providing care for both Chinese and European lepers from the 16th century to the 19th century (Leung 2009, 287).

Despite these medical developments, historians have shown that during the late 16th and 18th centuries, both Chinese and foreigners in Macau preferred Chinese folk medicine to 'Western' medicine, observing that there were few reliable and skilful Western doctors in the Far East (Barnes 2007; Amaro 2008; Macau Memories 2019). In fact, Matteo Ricci (1552–1610), an Italian Jesuit priest and the most important founding figure of the Jesuit China missions, wrote in his journal that Chinese medicine was just as effective as Western medicine (Tao 2010).

In the 19th century, biomedicine underwent rapid development, with significant advancements that have had a lasting impact on the field (Bloch 1988). During this period, the Portuguese in Macau constructed the Centro Hospitalar Conde de São Januário, commonly referred to as São Januário Hospital. Originally established as a military hospital in 1874, it was later converted into a public hospital, aiming to cater to the increasing healthcare needs of the local population. Concurrently, Chinese merchants in Macau established Kiang Wu Hospital (*Jinghu yiyuan* 鏡湖醫院) in 1871, marking the first ever hospital run by the Chinese in the city. While Kiang Wu Hospital primarily offered Chinese therapies, São Januário Hospital focused exclusively on biomedicine, reflecting the divergent medical approaches adopted by the Portuguese and the Chinese at that time.

The bubonic plague pandemic of the 1890s also compelled the typically hands-off Portuguese government to take action (Huang 2019; Huang 2021). Historians note that during this outbreak, the Macau-Portuguese government began regulating the city's hygiene and investing in preliminary healthcare services for the public (Huang 2019; Huang 2021; Afonso 2007). For example, at the height of the bubonic plague in 1895, the Portuguese established *Zhangkai yiguan* 長開醫館, literally 'long-hour clinic', which provided free medical care to the public. An official Portuguese doctor and a translator staffed the clinic. Some historians speculate that this clinic may have served as a precursor to the present-day Serviços de Saúde de Macau (Macau Health Bureau) (Wu, Tang, and Jin 2009, 2042).

By the early 20th century, the Macau-Portuguese government had already established a hospital and a limited number of medical stations, nurseries, and pharmacies (Wu, Tang, and Jin 2009). However, due to its laissez-faire approach, most Macau residents had to rely on private healthcare and local charities for medicine and treatments until the healthcare reform in the 1980s. It was not until 1979 that the Macau-Portuguese government finally established a health bureau, the Serviços de Saúde de Macau, to coordinate the activities of public and private institutions in the fields of health, medicine, and disease prevention (Decree-Law no. 4/79/M). This marked the beginning of Macau's medical modernisation. In 1984, an integrated healthcare system consisting of São Januário Hospital and a network of primary healthcare centres was established in response to a new wave of population growth. Until then, informal healthcare, both 'Western' and 'Chinese', had played a significant role in the lives of Macau residents.

The 1990s witnessed the continuous development of formalised biomedical care in Macau. Today, São Januário Hospital, which has been transformed into a modern facility offering a comprehensive range of medical services, is an illustration of this progress. Additionally, Macau now boasts several private hospitals alongside São Januário Hospital. While these private hospitals primarily focus on biomedicine, it is worth noting that they all incorporate a department for TCM (except for São Januário Hospital). In total, there are four hospitals in Macau, with São Januário serving as the only public hospital. These hospitals are accompanied by a network of 724 primary care premises, the majority of which are privately operated, as indicated by the health statistics of 2021 (DSEC 2021).

Given the prominence of biomedicine and the integration of TCM in private rather than public hospitals, it raises the question of where Chinese medicine – which once held a significant role in the city – fits within this evolving medical landscape.

The Legitimacy of Traditional Chinese Medicine in Macau

The status of TCM in Macau is intricately linked to the city's colonial legacy, its handover to China in 1999 and the rapid development of biomedicine in the 19th and 20th centuries. Unlike TCM doctors in Mainland China, who acquired a distinct professional identity as early as 1955 due to Mao's emphasis on self-reliance and scepticism toward Western medicine (Kirby 1989; Farquhar 1996; Kadetz and Stanley-Baker 2022), Chinese medicine was not integrated into Macau's public health service during the colonial era (Lou 2016). In fact, it was not until 1998, just a year before Macau's handover, that the Macau-Portuguese government faced pressure to mandate TCM doctors obtain a certificate from a recognised institution in Macau, Portugal, or Mainland China (Decree-Law no. 84/90/M; Meneses 2022, 66). During the same year, the government took a significant step to incorporate TCM services for the first time at one of the health centres. However, São Januário Hospital, the only public hospital in Macau, remains the sole facility to date without a dedicated department for TCM.

In his special report on Macau's TCM industry in January 2022, scholar-journalist João Paulo Meneses attributes this stagnation to the closed-mindedness of the Portuguese administration (Meneses 2022, 65). Nonetheless, a closer examination of publications and documents produced by the Association of Chinese Medicine in Macau suggests that the Portuguese administration may not have been as closed-minded as Meneses criticised. In fact, both the deputy secretary and the director of the Health Bureau attended the 25th-anniversary event of the Association of Chinese Medicine in Macau in 1991. Prior to that, the Health Bureau collaborated with the Association of Chinese Medicine in Macau in October 1989 to organise a series of public talks on Chinese and Western medicine. In her congratulatory remarks for the first issue of *The Journal of Chinese Medicine Doctors in Macau* (1991), Ana Maria Basto Perez, the Deputy Secretary for Health and Social Affairs of the Macau-Portuguese government (1991–1996), acknowledged TCM's significant contribution to alleviating human suffering. However, she also admitted the substantial challenges of integrating two fundamentally different medical systems into a unified health framework (cf. Chapter 8 on TCM in Brazil).

Although TCM is not officially integrated into Macau's healthcare system, it holds an important place in the history of Kiang Wu Hospital, the city's most renowned private hospital. In fact, the history of Kiang Wu Hospital serves as a micro-history of the rise, decline, and subsequent resurgence of Chinese medicine in Macau. Founded in 1871 by wealthy Chinese merchants, Kiang Wu Hospital initially operated as a traditional 'healing temple', exclusively providing Chinese therapies and medicical treatments to the public. However, in 1892, Dr Sun Yat-sen (1866–1925), the founding father of the Republic of China and a biomedical doctor, introduced 'Western' medicine to the hospital. Despite his efforts to promote biomedicine, it was met with resistance from the public (Buchillet 2010). The public's suspicion towards 'Western' medicine has a long history. It was most pronounced during the outbreak of the bubonic plague in Macau and nearby regions in 1895. At that time, the Macau-Portuguese government initially planned to isolate all infected patients at the barrack-hospital of Solidão. However, due to the strong resistance of Chinese patients to Western medical treatment, the barrack-hospital of Solidão was ultimately designated for the isolation and treatment of the Catholic population or whoever was willing to receive Western medical care (Buchillet 2010, 82). As Elizabeth Sinn pointed out, 'isolation as a precautionary measure against infectious diseases was strange enough to the Chinese, the idea of being taken to a ship was even more incomprehensible' (Sinn 2003, 162). There were numerous rumours about foreigners cutting up the Chinese bodies, and taking their liver, testicles, bones, and eyes out to make medicine (Platt et al. 1998, 37; Lou 2022). As a result, the majority of infected Chinese patients either succumbed to the disease at home or sought refuge in the quarantine wards established by Chinese doctors at Kiang Wu Hospital.

Despite these initial setbacks, 'Western' medicine gradually gained popularity among the Chinese population as the effectiveness of biomedical treatments improved in the 20th century. By the onset of World War II, the majority of patients at Kiang Wu Hospital opted for biomedicine for more immediate relief. Their decisions were also influenced by the shortage of Chinese herbal medicine caused by the Japanese army's blockade of Macau's land and waterways. Therefore, the hospital had to halt its Chinese Medicine service, marking the start of the eventual decline of this healthcare option at Kiang Wu Hospital. With dwindling business and a scarcity of herbal medicine, the Chinese Medicine department struggled to sustain its operations and ultimately ceased to operate altogether in 1945 following the resignation of two Chinese Medicine practitioners.

After more than 50 years of suspension, the board of directors of Kiang Wu Hospital announced their intention to reinstate the Chinese medicine outpatient service, including acupuncture and an herbal medicine pharmacy.

This move was undoubtedly motivated by the imminent return of Macau to Chinese sovereignty, where the concurrent use of Chinese and biomedicine is widely practised.

One of the primary challenges in the resumption of TCM services was the shortage of professional staff. To overcome this hurdle, on 17 February 1998, Kiang Wu Hospital signed a memorandum with the Chinese Medicine Hospital in Zhuhai. This partnership invited their TCM doctors to run a specialist clinic alongside Kiang Wu's own TCM doctors in Macau during the interim phase. Meanwhile, Kiang Wu Hospital continued its efforts to recruit new TCM doctors and provide further training opportunities for its staff. As the challenges surrounding the revival of TCM became more prominent, the Macau-Portuguese government could no longer ignore the issue. In 1998, just a year before Macau's handover to China, the local government finally took the necessary steps of implementing regulations on the licensing and qualifications of TCM providers.

On 23 March 1998, Kiang Wu Hospital officially reopened its TCM department after a prolonged hiatus. Despite the extended break, the demand for Chinese medicine in Macau remained strong. If you visit Kiang Wu Hospital's TCM department during the weekend, you will find a large crowd waiting patiently in the reception areas. In Macau, the demand for TCM has remained relatively stable since its handover to China (Meneses 2022, 62), and most locals incorporate both Chinese and Western medicine into their self-care routines. Before the reopening of Kiang Wu Hospital's TCM department in 1998, residents continued to seek TCM treatments from small private TCM clinics and rely on the service of Tung Sin Tong, a respected charitable society that has been providing uninterrupted TCM services to the people of Macau since 1892.

Thanks to the Portuguese government's laissez-faire approach, Chinese medicine has remained a part of the city's medical landscape, never facing eradication. Its ups and downs have been influenced by changes in political regimes and social conditions. Therefore, understanding the legitimacy of Chinese medicine in Macau requires considering multiple factors: not just the city's medico-legal system (or its absence) but also the trust and confidence patients place in Chinese Medicine.

When I embarked on this research in 2005, viewers in Macau, Hong Kong, and China were captivated by the television show *In Search of Reclusive Doctors* (*Xunzhao yinshi yishu* 尋找隱世醫術), a documentary about medical miracles performed by TCM doctors. In exalting the Chinese doctors' miraculous power to save people on their deathbeds, the documentary paradoxically placed great emphasis on the scientific validity of TCM (Lou 2016). In line with this, the anthropologist Mei Zhan's study of TCM doctors in Shanghai and San Francisco also found that the legitimacy of Chinese medicine is built upon its ability to treat difficult cases (Zhan 2001, 454). She argues that TCM doctors have used miracle-making to 'craft a niche' for TCM within a biomedicine-centric healthcare system: 'The everyday practice and discourse of traditional Chinese medicine has come to be "a site for the production of the extraordinary"' (Zhan 2001, 454).

In an environment where TCM faces fierce competition from biomedicine, it is understandable why some TCM practitioners feel they need to establish their legitimacy through miracle-making. However, my research in Macau suggests a different story. Although the Macau-Portuguese government had paid little attention to the legislation and development of Chinese medicine throughout the 20th century, miraculously, the majority of Chinese medical doctors in Macau have managed to carry on as private practitioners within the biomedicine-centric system, practising without the halo of miracles. How did they achieve this? While various factors contribute to the professional legitimacy of TCM in Macau, including accessibility and affordability, in this chapter, I want to focus on three key strategies. These strategies challenge the idea that the legitimacy of TCM in Macau relies on miracle-making. Instead, they are based on: 1) fostering empathy and establishing mutual medical references between TCM doctors and patients; 2) refashioning TCM with discourses of science and modernity; and 3) promoting TCM as a celebration of cultural nationalism.

Looking at Illnesses Together

If legitimacy is not produced through extraordinary events or miracles on deathbeds, how and where else is it produced? In my research, I found that the professional legitimacy of Chinese medicine was reinforced by the ordinary practice of 'looking at an illness' (*kanbing* 看病) with their patients (Farquhar 1996, 2). Particularly in smaller TCM clinics, both TCM practitioners and their patients actively contribute to establishing medical norms (Ferzacca 2000, 30). Patients are so knowledgeable about their conditions that they are able to use TCM jargons such as 'fire in the bones' (*guhuo* 骨火), 'depleted fire' (*xuhuo* 虛火), 'cold cough' (*hanhai* 寒咳), 'hot cough' (*rehai* 熱咳), 'dry' (gan 乾), 'wet' (*shi* 濕) to describe their states of health. They called this *jiubing chengyi* 久病成醫, suggesting that after coping with an illness for an extended period, one eventually becomes their own doctor. In fact, many TCM users claim they can interpret their own prescriptions, as illustrated in the following conversation:

> 'Licorice root (*gancao* 甘草) is *yaoyin* 藥引[2]'. Mrs Lam analysed her doctor's handwritten prescription for me while we were sitting in the waiting room.
> 'How do you know?' I asked.
> 'I've been eating Chinese medicine for many years now. *Jiubing chengyi* 久病成醫!'
> 'Do you think you would be able to read the Western medicine prescription?'
> 'How could I?' Mrs Lam laughed. 'I've only had five years of primary school education. I don't know English or Portuguese! How could I read it?'

TCM users are also proactive in self-diagnosis. When Mr Chan was diagnosed with sciatica by his doctor at the government hospital, he was certain that the doctor misdiagnosed him. 'I am pretty sure that it is rheumatism. I felt so much better after drinking the herbal tea you prescribed me last night.' Mr Chan told his TCM doctor. '*Xiyi* 西醫 (lit. doctors of Western medicine, that is, biomedicine) only know to give me pain killers!'

Similarly, when Mr Lee was diagnosed with a mental illness (*jingshenbing* 精神病) by a psychiatrist in the government hospital, he came to Dr Tam's clinic with a short article cut from a newspaper, titled 'The Ancient Way to Cure Epilepsy' (*zhidianzheng gufang* 治癲症古方). He urged Dr Tam to give him the treatments mentioned in the article because he appeared to suffer from the same symptoms.

> 'The psychiatrist said I have a mental disorder! I don't! I just have numb and tingling fingers!' Mr. Lee said angrily.
> 'I believe you! I believe you! The hospital is very wrong in prescribing you those drugs'. Dr. Tam tried to calm him down.

After Mr Lee left, Dr Tam sighed: 'Whenever a patient can't speak clearly, *xiyi* prescribe them psychotic drugs. Alas, even if he wasn't crazy, he certainly would be after taking those medications for such a long time!'

The practice of looking at an illness together (*kanbing*) (Farquhar 1996, 2) not only distinguishes Chinese medicine from Western (bio-)medicine

2 *Yaoyin* is also known as *yaoyinzi*. In Chinese Medicine, *yaoyin* serves as a conduit for certain medicines to reach their targeted organs, arteries, or veins.

in terms of doctor-patient relationship, but it also legitimises the need for a second opinion from Chinese medicine doctors. TCM doctors are more likely to embrace pluralism (Scheid 2002) and understand patients who often feel their personal experience of health and sickness is undervalued in the standardised processes of modern medicine (Lo and Stanley-Baker 2012). Shared cultural references in TCM enable both parties to engage and contribute to the understanding of health and illness. Chinese medicine knowledge is thus owned not only by the TCM doctors but also by Chinese patients who share the same cultural heritage. Unlike Western medicine doctors who sometimes feel the need to assume a different identity while on duty (Good 1993), TCM doctors strive to communicate in the language of their patients and openly express their personal side. It is this human touch that helps legitimise the cultural value of Chinese medicine in the absence of miraculous treatments (cf. Chapters 2, 3, and 4).

It's Not Miracles, It's Science

Given the delayed legislation surrounding the licensing of private healthcare services and the specific qualifications required to enter the field of TCM (Decree-Law no. 84/90/M), TCM practitioners in Macau feared being further marginalised as miraculous healers. Unlike their counterparts in San Francisco or Shanghai (Zhan 2001), Dr Tam was particularly annoyed when people said Chinese medicine can perform miracles: 'Do they really think Chinese medicine can cure everything? That's absurd! We are doctors, not deities! To expect us to fix everything is demeaning! A death case is a death case!'

Indeed, most TCM practitioners I interviewed shared the view that miracles are not easily made, if they can be made at all. While miracle-making may be seen as a sign of professional achievement by some TCM practitioners (Zhan 2001, 453), others take offence at the stereotype, as it implies that TCM is unscientific (Lou 2016).

However, the delayed regulation of TCM by the Macau government did cause anxiety among some TCM practitioners, particularly the *zhongyishi* 中醫師, who were recognised not through an accredited degree but by a committee chaired by a TCM professional body (Lou 2016). In Macau, the government distinguishes between a *zhongyisheng* 中醫生 (Chinese medicine doctor) – namely, a TCM practitioner with a university degree – and a *zhongyishi* (Chinese medicine master), a healer who is trained through the traditional apprentice system and practises without a university degree. The distinction originated during the colonial era but has gradually transitioned towards completely phasing out the licensing for Chinese medicine masters, thereby restricting the practice of Chinese medicine to those with accredited degrees. Not everyone welcomed this move. Veteran *zhongyishi* Dr Tam voiced his discontent during a 2005 interview:

> This policy goes against Chinese culture! Tell me, who do you think is more senior, *shi* 師 (teacher) or *sheng* 生 (student)? In Mainland China, they don't differentiate between Chinese doctors in this manner. The Portuguese divided us based on whether we had a degree or not. But let me ask you, what's more important, a diploma or experience? Chinese medicine is *jingyan yixue* 經驗醫學 (medicine based on experience). However, in Macau, the government views young doctors with a degree as more legitimate.

Having said that, Dr Tam's tone shifted noticeably when I asked him about his experience as his father's apprentice. Coming from a family of Chinese medicine doctors, Dr Tam's father was a renowned *zhongyishi* and received numerous honours for his contribution to Chinese medicine in Macau. One would expect Dr Tam to take pride in his background. However, he appeared uncomfortable discussing the apprenticeship system, as he considered it unprofessional and unsustainable for the long-term development of TCM.

> Look, we shouldn't dwell too much on the master-and-apprentice system of the past. Let's focus on the current state of TCM education. If you emphasise the old apprenticeship system, it might give the impression to Americans that our medicine is inferior to theirs.

With that, he went upstairs to retrieve a pamphlet from the Faculty of Chinese Medicine at Macau University of Science and Technology. 'Instead, I think you should highlight the 39 courses we currently offer to our TCM students', Dr Tam proposed. As one of the TCM programme advisors, Dr Tam urged me to share the TCM curriculum with my American colleagues. He was trying to convince me that TCM is not only as scientific as Western medicine but also superior in terms of breadth. 'We Chinese medicine doctors need to study Western medicine', Dr Tam said, 'but Western doctors only focus on Western medicine. Do you see what I'm getting at?'

Dr Tam's perspective resonated widely within the TCM community. Dr Wu, another TCM doctor who stressed the role of modern science in the legitimation of TCM, pointed me to this excerpt from *The Journal of Chinese Medicine Doctors in Macau* (1991):

> The scope of modern Chinese medicine is remarkably extensive, encompassing literature and history, animal physiology and plant ecology, meteorology and astronomy, geography and geology, chemistry and genetic engineering. Chinese medicine is a holistic discipline that incorporates advanced science and technology. It is imperative for us to leverage modern science and conduct research to discover new avenues for enhancing our field.

Within Macau's TCM circle, the term 'science' was used casually and synonymously with 'modern' – and being 'modern' was considered a good thing. The historian Sean Hsiang-lin Lei makes a similar point in his book *Neither Donkey nor Horse*, where he explores the transformation of Chinese medicine from being perceived as the opposite of modernity in the early 20th century to becoming a significant symbol and vehicle for China's own pursuit of modernity half a century later (Lei 2014). This attitude is closely related to Mao's successor Deng Xiaoping's determination to 'rejuvenate the nation through science education' (*kejiao xingguo* 科教興國), a development strategy to make science and technology (*keji* 科技) a national priority. Indeed, as Judith Farquhar remarks, 'medicine is the only indigenous Chinese science to continue into the twentieth century in a way that is institutionally and discursively prominent' (Farquhar 1996, 222).

So, what has Macau done to make Chinese medicine great again? In recent years, Macau has made significant strides in promoting TCM by positioning itself as a national and international hub in the field. Since 2011, Macau has been a member of the World Health Organization's Collaborating Centre for Traditional Medicine (CCTM), actively advocating for the integration of Chinese medicine into the primary healthcare system. Meanwhile, the Guangdong-Macau TCM Park (GMTCM Park) serves as a flagship industry park, facilitating collaboration between Macau and TCM enterprises from other regions of China. The park aims to not only standardise TCM within China but also internationalise it for overseas markets (Meneses 2022, 54). To bolster the impact of these national and international hubs, the Macau University of Science and Technology and the University of Macau's Institute of Chinese Medical Sciences each welcomed their first-ever Chinese state key laboratories in 2011 (Meneses 2022, 54; Lam 2017, 161), putting science rather than miracles at the forefront of Chinese medicine.

In comparison to the Macau-Portuguese government, the Macau SAR government has shown an unprecedented interest in TCM. What are the underlying motivations behind these national policies and investments? Why are the government and TCM practitioners so enthusiastic about developing, industrialising, and promoting the TCM sector in Macau? In the final section, I argue that Chinese medicine offers the Macau SAR government and local TCM practitioners an opportunity to express their patriotism by actively promoting a relatively unchallenged form of cultural nationalism.

Nationalism and Traditional Chinese Medicine

Sixty years after Mao Zedong endorsed Chinese medicine as 'a great treasure house' that 'should be diligently explored' (1958), Xi Jinping, current president of the People's Republic of China, gave a very similar speech during a visit to the Guangdong-Macau TCM Park (GMTCM Park) in 2018. President Xi said, 'TCM is a treasure of Chinese civilization. More efforts should be made to explore the essence of TCM and advance the industrialization, modernisation and globalisation of TCM'.

Long before the reunification of Macau and China in 1999, Macau's TCM practitioners had hoped to establish a closer relationship with the TCM sector in China. In Macau, the majority of TCM practitioners are patriots and nationalists who believe that TCM is a remarkable national heritage that has plenty to offer to the world. This kind of sentiment can be found in numerous speeches and publications produced by not only Macau's TCM communities but also their counterparts in neighbouring Hong Kong (Pang 2018). For example, in an article published in *The Journal of Chinese Medicine Doctors in Macau* in 1991, a TCM doctor wrote: 'Every Chinese medicine practitioner should be proud of our nation. We are responsible for exalting our nation's traditional medicine. To achieve this, we should make use of modern science and research new ways of improving our field'.

Even though Traditional Chinese Medicine is a communist project and an invented tradition for cultural nationalism in the 1950s (Croizier 1965; Farquhar 1996; Taylor 2004; Scheid 2007; Hsu 2008; Hsu 2021), this fact has not and will not dampen Macau doctors' enthusiasm for making Chinese medicine great again. Similar to other forms of cultural nationalism in China (Guo 2004), such as the promotion of Confucianism (Cheung 2012; Hubbert 2019) and the Han Clothing movement (Carrico 2017), cultural nationalism derived from TCM is 'marked by idealism and pride in China's ancient philosophy and cultural heritage' (Hsu 2008, 465). However, as political scientist Kelvin Cheung rightly points out, 'the sentiment born of "the century of national humiliation" is insufficient to explain the phenomenon of Chinese new nationalism' (Cheung 2012, 205). 'Instead of continuing to rely on the West as the benchmark against which it defines its success', Cheung argues, 'China is becoming more assertive in its own perspectives and values' (Cheung 2012, 206).

With respect to Traditional Chinese medicine, this new trend of nationalism can be discerned in its globalisation and the strategic integration of TCM with biomedicine. As Elisabeth Hsu notes, while 'Chineseness continues to be celebrated' and nationalistic sentiments remain strong (Hsu 2008, 466), the Chinese government's commitment to integrating traditional and modern medicine is 'remarkable if not unique' (Hsu 2008, 469), given that most governments in the world 'discourage the integration of biomedical and local medical theory and practice' (Hsu 2008, 469). In highlighting the innovativeness of such integration, where Chinese medicine is given equal footing with Western medicine instead of relying solely on Western medicine as the benchmark of good science, Chinese medicine is 'becoming more assertive about its own values and perspectives' (Cheung 2012, 206), thereby engendering new China imaginaries. Moreover, by emphasising the uniqueness of such a system, the notion of 'Chinese characteristics' (*Zhongguo tese* 中國特色) constitutes 'the new parameters within which China's future development derives its legitimacy' (Cheung 2012, 207). This is evident in the discourses of 'socialism with Chinese characteristics', 'development with Chinese characteristics' or 'higher education with Chinese characteristics' (Cheung 2012, 207).

To play their part in the internationalisation of TCM, the Macau SAR government and the TCM practitioners in Macau are expected not only to eulogise TCM's history and achievements – an imaginary practice exemplified in the quote from *The Journal of Chinese Medicine Doctors in Macau* – but also to help TCM gain a share in the lucrative global health market. The culture of demonstrating patriotism can be traced back to the Chinese Communist Party's (CCP) emphasis on absolute devotion and loyalty to the party. However, unlike in the early years, the CCP is no longer 'reliant on an ascriptive understanding of loyalty based on class labels' when the party needed to 'recruit beyond the so-called revolutionary classes of workers and peasants' (Doyon and Yang 2022, 388). Instead, the ascriptive approach to loyalty is now superseded by a behavioural approach, which expects local officials and anyone who have a close tie with the CCP to publicly display and declare their loyalty (Doyon and Yang 2022; Shih 2008). Since Macau's economy is highly dependent on China's patronage, it is important for Macau to actively declare its loyalty to China and contribute to its various development plans.

One of the crucial ways in which Macau has made itself useful to China is by facilitating communication and cooperation between China and Portuguese-speaking countries (Santos 2020). In 2003, Beijing decided to take advantage of Macau's unique historical and geopolitical position and designate it as a Sino-Lusophone interface between Macau, China, Portugal, and the former Portuguese colonies (Santos 2020, 36). Since then, Macau has hosted numerous events and initiatives aimed at promoting trade, investment, and cultural exchange between China and Lusophone countries. The establishment of the Forum for Economic and Trade Cooperation between China and Portuguese-speaking Countries (hereafter the Macau Forum) is widely regarded as a breakthrough in 'turning Macau into a hub of commercial arbitration between entrepreneurs' from China and many Lusophone countries (Santos 2020, 50).

In Macau, TCM is among the first sectors to leverage Macau's connection with Portuguese-speaking countries. Consequently, promoting TCM among Portuguese-speaking countries has become one of the top priorities of the Macau Forum (Meneses 2022, 60). Since 2017, Macau has established partnerships with medical authorities in Portugal, Mozambique, and Cape Verde, offering TCM training to doctors in these countries. In 2022, the Macau SAR government enacted Decree-Law No. 11/2021 to regulate pharmaceutical activities in the realm of TCM. The law allows the industry to create markets for TCM beyond Macau, opening up opportunities for its expansion. Prior to this legislation, Chinese medicines manufactured or registered in Macau were restricted from entering the market of Mainland China, let alone Portuguese-speaking countries (Meneses 2022, 49). With this law, the Macau SAR government hopes to facilitate the global distribution of Chinese medicine produced or registered in Macau and consolidate the city's role as a Sino-Portuguese platform for TCM.

The proactive development and industrialisation of TCM in Macau is a directive by the Central government to strengthen Macau's position in the global TCM market and boost China's exports. According to *The Paper News*, in 2021, China's export rate of TCM products and its international market share were very low. Only 20% of Chinese TCM products are exported overseas, with an international market share of less than 3%. In contrast, Japan holds a high international market share of 90% for traditional herbal medicine (Wang 2021). Naturally, with Macau's long-term connections with Lusophone countries and being the home of the first and only National Key Laboratory for Chinese Herbal Pharmacology, it is regarded as the ideal platform for the global expansion of TCM and Chinese Herbal Pharmacology (Wang 2021).

The industrialisation of TCM in Macau is also a response to Beijing's order to diversify its economy, which has been heavily dependent on revenues from the gambling industry since the Portuguese government legalised gambling in 1849 (Godinho 2014). Failure to respond to Beijing's demand would not only signify a lack of competence but also a lack of loyalty. Despite its unambiguous ambition, many of Macau's economic diversification projects end up like castles in the sky, including the Guangdong-Macau TCM Park. A recent report by the Commission of Audit questioned if the 14.7 billion Renminbi spent on the Park will ever break even (All About Macau 2021). Still, with the display of patriotism being a top priority, the Macau SAR government has to ride on this wave of cultural nationalism and reimagine itself as a bridge between the 'East' and the 'West', with or without fiscal benefits. This was evident in the Macau SAR government's incorporation of TCM in their anti-COVID policy. Although the overall effectiveness of TCM as a COVID treatment is inconclusive (Cyranoski 2020), the Chinese government insists on using TCM drugs to treat the disease. It is reported that 92% of the country's COVID-19 cases were treated with TCM to some extent (Jakhar 2020). Closely following the national policy, the Macau SAR government gave every resident of Macau a free pack of *Lianhua qingwen* 蓮花清瘟 – a TCM-formulated drug used for the treatment of influenza – in addition to the generic paracetamol during the peak of the pandemic. However, it is unclear what the take-up rate of *Lianhua qingwen* was.

The persistence of developing China's own COVID vaccines and using TCM to treat the pandemic is one of the most compelling examples of China's new nationalism, wherein new discourses of 'Chinese characteristics' are used to support an alternative medical model that is independent of Western prescriptive (Cheung 2012, 209). As the deputy head of the National Administration of Traditional Chinese Medicine elaborated, China is 'willing to share the Chinese experience and Chinese solution of treating COVID-19 with other countries, and let more countries learn about Chinese medicine, understand Chinese medicine, and use Chinese medicine' (Jakhar 2020).

Conclusion

This chapter examined the impact of colonial legacy and the transfer of sovereignty on the legitimacy of Traditional Chinese Medicine in Macau today. Contrary to the prevalent perception that TCM relies on miracle-making to establish its legitimacy, I argued that the legitimacy of TCM in Macau is established through three main strategies: first, by fostering empathy and building mutual medical references with TCM patients; second, by reimaging TCM in light of the discourses of modernity, science, and technology; and finally, by aligning TCM with a new form of cultural nationalism. Like the promotion of Confucianism, the internationalisation of TCM is China's latest endeavour to reinvent traditional Chinese culture as a source of soft power. Given its earlier success in curing malaria with Artemisia carvifolia (*qinghao* 青蒿) (Hsu 2006), TCM may indeed have a better chance than more contested forms of cultural nationalism, such as New Confucianism, to exert its influence on the global community. As to Macau, it has always taken pride in being the first Chinese city where 'Chinese' medicine met 'Western' medicine. With the influence of nationalism, it will spare no effort to extend this 16th-century legacy to the 21st century.

Bibliography

Afonso, José da Conceição. 2007. 'Macau: Contributos Para a História Do Abastecimento de Á Gua Potável à Cidade'. *Revista Da Administração Pública de Macau* 75, no. 1: 1269.

All About Macau Media. 2021. 'It Is Doubtful Whether the 14.7 Billion Chinese Medicine Industrial Park Can Break Even'. *All about Macau Media*, 19 January. https://shorturl.at/iuDW7.

Amaro, Ana Maria. 2008. 'Aomen yixue mingyi yaofang liuxingbing ji yiwu zhiliao 澳門醫學、名醫、藥房、流行病及醫務治療 [Macau Medicine: Famous Doctors, Pharmacies, Epidemiology and Medical Treatment]'. In *Nova História de Macau/ Aomenshi xinbian* 澳門史新編, vol. 3, edited by Guoping Jin and Haijian Tang, 993. Macau: Fundação Macau.

Barnes, Linda L. 2007. *Needles, Herbs, Gods, and Ghosts China, Healing, and the West to 1848*. Cambridge: Harvard University Press.

Bloch, Harry. 1988. 'Medicine and Science in the 19th and 20th Centuries'. *Journal of the National Medical Association* 80, no. 2: 229–32. https://www.ncbi.nlm.nih.gov/pmc/articles/PMC2625730/?page=1.

Buchillet, Dominique. 2010. 'The 1895 Epidemic Outbreak of Bubonic Plague in Macao: A Portuguese View on the Transmission and Spread of Plague'. *Review of Culture* 34: 77–91.

Carrico, Kevin. 2017. *The Great Han. Race, Nationalism, and Tradition in China Today.* Berkeley: University of California Press. https://doi.org/10.1525/california/9780520295490.001.0001.

Cheung, Kelvin Chi-Kin. 2012. 'Away from Socialism, towards Chinese Characteristics: Confucianism and the Futures of Chinese Nationalism'. *China Information* 26, no. 2: 205–18. https://doi.org/10.1177/0920203x12440548.

Croizier, Ralph C. 1965. 'Traditional Medicine in Communist China: Science, Communism and Cultural Nationalism'. *The China Quarterly*, no. 23: 1–27. https://doi.org/10.1017/s0305741000009863.

Cultural Affairs Bureau. 2023. 'AM019: Consulate General of Portugal in Macao and Hong Kong (Building of the Former St. Raphael Hospital and Garden)'. Cultural Heritage of Macao. 2023. https://www.culturalheritage.mo/(X(1)S(dqyunkof2vp2kxguj5c2xuqg))/en/detail/99972?AspxAutoDetectCookieSupport=1#:~:text=reconstruction%20in%201939.-.

Cyranoski, David. 2020. 'China Is Promoting Coronavirus Treatments Based on Unproven Traditional Medicines'. *Nature*, May. https://doi.org/10.1038/d41586-020-01284-x.

Doyon, Jérôme, and Long Yang. 2022. 'Shades of Red: Changing Understandings of Political Loyalty in the Chinese Communist Party, 1921–2021'. *Journal of Current Chinese Affairs* 51 no. 3. https://doi.org/10.1177/18681026221119220.

DSEC. 2021. 'Health Statistics 2021'. *Official Statistics*. Documentation and Information Centre of the Statistics and Census Service. https://www.dsec.gov.mo/getAttachment/1b795d1d-3dbb-40f0-be66-712e46d07ade/C_SAU_PUB_2021_Y.aspx.

Farquhar, Judith. 1994. *Knowing Practice: The Clinical Encounter of Chinese Medicine*. 1st ed. New York: Routledge. https://doi.org/10.4324/9780429499449.

Ferzacca, Steve. 2000. '"Actually, I Don't Feel That Bad": Managing Diabetes and the Clinical Encounter'. *Medical Anthropology Quarterly* 14, no. 1: 28–50. https://doi.org/10.1525/maq.2000.14.1.28.

France, Honoré, and Carmen Rodriguez. 2019. 'Traditional Chinese Medicine in Canada: An Indigenous Perspective'. *Chinese Medicine and Culture* 2, no. 1: 1. https://doi.org/10.4103/cmac.cmac_2_19.

Godinho, Jorge. 2014. 'Casino Gaming in Macau: Evolution, Regulation and Challenges'. *UNLV Gaming Law Journal* 5, no. 1. https://scholars.law.unlv.edu/glj/vol5/iss1/7.

Godinho, Jorge A.F. 2012. 'A History of Games of Chance in Macau: Part I — Introduction'. Papers.ssrn.com. Rochester, NY. 10 October. https://ssrn.com/abstract=2263185.

Good, Byron J. 1993. *Medicine, Rationality, and Experience: An Anthropological Perspective*. Cambridge: Cambridge University Press. https://doi.org/10.1017/cbo9780511811029.

Guo, Yingjie. 2004. *Cultural Nationalism in Contemporary China: The Search for National Identity under Reform*. London: Routledge.

Hsu, E. 2008. 'The History of Chinese Medicine in the People's Republic of China and Its Globalization'. *East Asian Science, Technology and Society* 2, no. 4: 465–84. https://doi.org/10.1215/s12280-009-9072-y.

Hsu, Elisabeth. 2002. '"The Medicine from China Has Rapid Effects": Chinese Medicine Patients in Tanzania'. *Anthropology & Medicine* 9, no. 3: 291–313. https://doi.org/10.1080/13648470216335.

Hsu, Elisabeth. 2006. 'Reflections on the "Discovery" of the Antimalarial Qinghao'. *British Journal of Clinical Pharmacology* 61, no. 6: 666–70. https://doi.org/10.1111/j.1365-2125.2006.02673.x.

Hsu, Elisabeth. 2021. 'Traditional Chinese Medicine History, Ethnography, and Practice'. In *The Routledge Handbook of Religion, Medicine and Health*, edited by Lüddeckens Dorothea, Philipp Hetmanczyk, Pamela E. Klassen, and Justin B. Stein. London: Routledge.

Huang, Yanhong. 2019. '1895 nian Aomen gongong weisheng de fazhan 1895年澳門公共衛生的發展' [The Plague of 1895 and the Development of Public Health in Macao]. *Revista da Universidade Politecnica de Macau* 3: 174–82. https://journal.ipm.edu.mo/images/journal_c/2019_3/201903-174-182.pdf.

Huang, Yanhong. 2021. 'Aomen gongong weisheng de fazhan yu jinbu Cong shuyi SARS dao xinguan feiyan 澳門公共衛生的發展與進步：從鼠疫、SARS到新冠肺炎' [The Development and Progress of Public Health in Macao: From Plague, SARS to New Coronary Pneumonia]. *Administração* 34, no. 131: 1–17. https://safp.gov.mo https://www.safp.gov.mo › WCM_075676.

Hubbert, Jennifer Ann. 2019. *China in the World: An Anthropology of Confucius Institutes, Soft Power, and Globalization*. Honolulu: University of Hawai'i Press.

Jakhar, Pratik. 2020. 'Covid-19: China Pushes Traditional Remedies amid Outbreak'. *BBC News*, 28 June, sec. Asia. https://www.bbc.co.uk/news/world-asia-53094603.

Kadetz, Paul, and Michael Stanley-Baker. 2022. 'About Face: How the People's Republic of China Harnessed Health to Leverage Soft Power on the World Stage'. *Frontiers in Human Dynamics* 3 (February). https://doi.org/10.3389/fhumd.2021.774765.

Kirby, William C. 1989. 'Technocratic Organization and Technological Development in China'. In *Science and Technology in Post-Mao China*, edited by Merle Goldman and Denis Fred Simon, 23–44. Cambridge, MA: Harvard University Asia Center. https://doi.org/10.2307/j.ctt1sq5t6m.6.

Lam, Nogueira Oi Ching Bernice. 2017. 'Traditional Chinese Medicine in Health Care in Macao'. *Revista de Enfermagem Referência* IV Série, no. 13: 157–64. https://doi.org/10.12707/riv17007.

Leung, Angela Ki Che. 2009. *Leprosy in China: A History*. New York: Columbia University Press. https://doi.org/10.7312/leun12300.

Lei, Sean Hsiang-lin. 2014. *Neither Donkey nor Horse: Medicine in the Struggle over China's Modernity*. Chicago: University of Chicago Press. https://doi.org/10.7208/chicago/9780226169910.001.0001.

Lieber, Marylène. 2012. 'Practitioners of Traditional Chinese Medicine in Switzerland: Competing Justifications for Cultural Legitimacy'. *Ethnic and Racial Studies* 35, no. 4: 757–75. https://doi.org/10.1080/01419870.2011.577227.

Lo, Vivienne, and Michael Stanley-Baker. 2012. 'Chinese Medicine'. In *The Oxford Handbook of the History of Medicine*, edited by Mark Jackson, 150–68. Oxford University Press. https://doi.org/10.1093/oxfordhb/9780199546497.013.0009.

Lou, Loretta. 2016. 'Beyond Miracles: How Traditional Chinese Medicine Establishes Professional Legitimacy in Post-Colonial Macau'. *Somatosphere*, 9 December. http://somatosphere.net/2016/beyond-miracles-how-traditional-chinese-medicine-establishes-professional-legitimacy-in-post-colonial-macau.html/.

Lou, Loretta. 2022. 'From Hygienic Modernity to Green Modernity: Two Modes of Modern Living in Hong Kong since the 1970s'. In *Design and Modernity in Asia: National Identity and Transnational Exchange 1945–1990*, edited by Yunah Lee and Megha Rajguru, 105–20. Bloomsbury Publishing. https://doi.org/10.5040/9781350091498.ch-6.

Macau Memory. 2019. 'Yiliao weisheng 醫療衛生' [Health Care]. Macau Memory. Fundação Macau. https://www.macaumemory.mo/category_55c328a7ed86f568b3751d9c.

Meneses, João Paulo. 2022. 'Special Report: Traditional Chinese Medicine Breathing a New Life'. *Macau Business*, January.

Pang, Ka Wei. 2018. 'The Making of Chinese Medicine in Hong Kong'. *Social Transformations in Chinese Societies* 14, no. 1: 17–28. https://doi.org/10.1108/stics-01-2018-0003.

Platt, Jerome J., Maurice E. Jones, and Arleen K. Platt. 1998. *Whitewash Brigade: Hong Kong Plague of 1894*. London: Dix Noonan Webb.

Santos, Jose Carlos Matias Dos. 2020. 'Macau and China-Portuguese Speaking Countries Relations: From Nation Branding to Soft Power'. In *Macau 20 Years after the Handover: Changes and Challenges under "One Country, Two Systems"*, edited by Meng U Ieong, 36–53. London: Routledge. https://doi.org/10.4324/9780429323157.

Scheid, Volker. 1999. 'The Globalisation of Chinese Medicine'. *The Lancet* 354 (SIV10). https://doi.org/10.1016/S0140-6736(99)90353-7.

Scheid, Volker. 2002. *Chinese Medicine in Contemporary China: Plurality and Synthesis*. Durham: Duke University Press. https://doi.org/10.1215/9780822383710.

Scheid, Volker. 2007. *Currents of Tradition in Chinese Medicine, 1626–2006*. Seattle: Eastland Press.

Sinn, Elizabeth. 2003. *Power and Charity: A Chinese Merchant Elite in Colonial Hong Kong*. Hong Kong: Hong Kong University Press.

Shih, Victor Chung-Hon. 2008. '"Nauseating" Displays of Loyalty: Monitoring the Factional Bargain through Ideological Campaigns in China'. *The Journal of Politics* 70, no. 4: 1177–92. https://doi.org/10.1017/s0022381608081139.

Tao, Fei Ya. 2010. 'Chuanjiaoshi zhongyiguan de bianqian 传教士中医观的变迁 [Changes in Missionaries' Views on Traditional Chinese Medicine]. *Lishi yanjiu* 5: 60–78. https://www.globethics.net/pdfs/CNKI/CPFD/ZSKS200908001005.pdf.

Taylor, Kim. 2004. *Chinese Medicine in Early Communist China, 1945–1963*. London: Routledge. https://doi.org/10.4324/9780203311271.

Wang, Ning. 2021. 'Why Is the Hengqin Guangdong-Macau In-Depth Cooperation Zone Focused on Traditional Chinese Medicine?'. *Paper News*. https://m.thepaper.cn/newsDetail_forward_14425859.

Wu, Zhiliang, Kaijian Tang, and Guoping Jin, eds. 2009. *Aomen biannianshi Disijuan* 澳門編年史：第四卷 [Chronicle of Macau, Vol. 4]. Guangdong: Guangdong renmin chubanshe.

Zhan, Mei. 2001. 'Does It Take a Miracle? Negotiating Knowledges, Identities, and Communities of Traditional Chinese Medicine'. *Cultural Anthropology* 16, no. 4: 453–80. https://doi.org/10.1525/can.2001.16.4.453.

Scheid, Volker. 2009. *Other-Worldly Making Chinese Medicine through Transnational Frames*. Durham: Duke University Press. https://doi.org/10.2307/j.ctv1198xrp.

Biography

Loretta I.T. Lou is assistant professor in Social Anthropology at Durham University. She has a DPhil in Anthropology from Oxford University and specialises in the study of environment, health, healing, and social movements in East Asia. She is currently the Degree Director for the MSc in Global & Planetary Health and Medical Anthropology at Durham University.

Index

For Product Safety Concerns and Information please contact our EU representative GPSR@taylorandfrancis.com Taylor & Francis Verlag GmbH, Kaufingerstraße 24, 80331 München, Germany

Batch number: 10725973

Printed by Printforce, the Netherlands